Antiinflammatory Agents

CHEMISTRY AND PHARMACOLOGY

VOLUME I

MEDICINAL CHEMISTRY

A Series of Monographs

EDITED BY

GEORGE deSTEVENS

CIBA Pharmaceutical Company, A Division of CIBA Corporation
Summit, New Jersey

Volume 1. GEORGE deSTEVENS. Diuretics: Chemistry and Pharmacology. 1963

Volume 2. RUDOLFO PAOLETTI (ED.). Lipid Pharmacology. 1964

Volume 3. E. J. ARIENS (ED.). Molecular Pharmacology: The Mode of Action of Biologically Active Compounds. (In two volumes.) 1964

Volume 4. MAXWELL GORDON (ED.). Psychopharmacological Agents. Volume I. 1964. Volume II. 1967. Volume III. 1974.

Volume 5. GEORGE deSTEVENS (ED.). Analgetics. 1965

Volume 6. ROLAND H. THORP AND LEONARD B. COBBIN. Cardiac Stimulant Substances. 1967

Volume 7. EMIL SCHLITTLER (ED.). Antihypertensive Agents. 1967

Volume 8. U. S. VON EULER AND RUNE ELIASSON. Prostaglandins. 1967

Volume 9. G. D. CAMPBELL (ED.). Oral Hypoglycaemic Agents: Pharmacology and Therapeutics. 1969

Volume 10. LEMONT B. KIER. Molecular Orbital Theory in Drug Research. 1971

Volume 11. E. J. ARIENS (ED.). Drug Design. Volumes I and II. 1971. Volume III. 1972. Volume IV. 1973

Volume 12. PAUL E. THOMPSON AND LESLIE M. WERBEL. Antimalarial Agents: Chemistry and Pharmacology. 1972

Volume 13. ROBERT A. SCHERRER AND MICHAEL W. WHITEHOUSE (Eds.). Antiinflammatory Agents: Chemistry and Pharmacology. (In two volumes.) 1974

ANTIINFLAMMATORY AGENTS

Chemistry and Pharmacology

VOLUME I

Edited by

ROBERT A. SCHERRER

RIKER LABORATORIES, INC.
3M CENTER
ST. PAUL, MINNESOTA

MICHAEL W. WHITEHOUSE

DEPARTMENT OF EXPERIMENTAL PATHOLOGY
THE JOHN CURTIN SCHOOL OF MEDICAL RESEARCH
THE AUSTRALIAN NATIONAL UNIVERSITY
CANBERRA A.C.T., AUSTRALIA

ACADEMIC PRESS   New York   San Francisco   London 1974

A Subsidiary of Harcourt Brace Jovanovich, Publishers

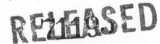

ACADEMIC PRESS, INC.
111 Fifth Avenue, New York, New York 10003

United Kingdom Edition published by
ACADEMIC PRESS, INC. (LONDON) LTD.
24/28 Oval Road, London NW1

Library of Congress Cataloging in Publication Data

Scherrer, Robert Allan, Date
        Antiinflammatory agents.

        (Medicinal chemistry; a series of monographs,   )
        Includes bibliographies.
        1.   Antiphlogistics.   I.   Whitehouse, Michael W.,
joint author.   II.   Title.   III.   Series.
[DNLM: 1.   Antiinflammatory agents.   WIME64/QV55
A629]
RM121.S37   615'.7   73-9447
ISBN 0−12−623901−0 (v.1)

PRINTED IN THE UNITED STATES OF AMERICA

To all those investigators who paved the way for our present under-standing of inflammation and its regulation, and to our wives, secre-taries, and others without whose loyal support these chapters would not have been written

Contents

Part I   Inflammatory Diseases

Chapter 1   Some Inflammatory Diseases in Man and Their Current Therapy

Harold E. Paulus

Part II   Preparation, Physical and Chemical Properties, and Structure–Activity Relationships

Chapter 2   Introduction to the Chemistry of Antiinflammatory and Antiarthritic Agents

Robert A. Scherrer

Chapter 3   **Aryl- and Heteroarylcarboxylic Acids**

Robert A. Scherrer

Chapter 4   **Aryl- and Heteroarylalkanoic Acids and
              Related Compounds**

Peter F. Juby

List of Contributors

Numbers in parentheses indicate the pages on which the authors' contributions begin.

MICHAEL J. DiMARTINO (209), Smith Kline & French Laboratories, Philadelphia, Pennsylvania

J. D. FISHER (363), Biochemistry Research Department, Armour Pharmaceutical Co., Kankakee, Illinois

THOMAS J. FITZGERALD* (295), Department of Pharmacology, University of Kansas Medical Center, Kansas City, Kansas

PETER F. JUBY (91), Bristol Laboratories, Division of Bristol-Myers Company, Syracuse, New York

JOSEPH G. LOMBARDINO (129), Pfizer Central Research, Pfizer, Inc., Groton, Connecticut

GEORGE G. I. MOORE (159), Riker Laboratories, Inc., 3M Center, St. Paul, Minnesota

HAROLD E. PAULUS (3), Department of Medicine, University of California School of Medicine, Los Angeles, California

THOMAS L. POPPER (245), Schering Corporation, Bloomfield, New Jersey

ROBERT A. SCHERRER (29, 45), Riker Laboratories, Inc., 3M Center, St. Paul, Minnesota

T. Y. SHEN (179), Merck Sharp & Dohme Research Laboratories, Rahway, New Jersey

*Present address: School of Pharmacy, Florida Agricultural and Mechanical University, Tallahassee, Florida.

BLAINE M. SUTTON (209), Smith Kline & French Laboratories, Philadelphia, Pennsylvania

DONALD T. WALZ (209), Smith Kline & French Laboratories, Philadelphia,
Pennsylvania

ARTHUR S. WATNICK (245), Schering Corporation, Bloomfield, New Jersey

Preface

Callimachus, the Alexandrian poet, once wrote: "A big book is a big evil." On the whole, we must agree with this view. This two-volume work is therefore a compromise between trying to lessen this evil while still doing justice, with an adequate review, to the tremendous outlay of effort and ingenuity expended by physicians, chemists, and experimental biologists through the years in seeking new drugs to treat arthritis and other severely debilitating chronic inflammatory diseases.

This treatise is a review of the current status of antiinflammatory research from the laboratory to the clinic. It is directed toward the student and investigator concerned with the design of new and better agents and with their critical evaluation in the laboratory and in man. Emphasis is given to factors which could lead to new and better agents.

One of the advantages of having a multiauthored volume is to introduce a variety of viewpoints. Authors have been encouraged to express their personal opinions. Inevitably there is a certain amount of duplication and even contradiction among some of the individual contributions. Some of the reviews are the first generally available in English. We hope they may provide a suitable foundation and appropriate stimulus for the preparation of more evenly balanced, second generation surveys at some time in the future. Certainly this present offering owes much to its antecedents, the reviews and literature surveys which have accumulated over the past twenty years. A list of some of the more recent reviews can be found following the Introduction for the benefit of those who wish to read the earlier literature not detailed in the succeeding chapters.

The work is divided into three parts, presented in two volumes. The first part, comprising one chapter only, discusses the medical background and describes the current therapy for the more prominent inflammatory diseases. The chemistry of diverse types of compounds with antiinflammatory activity is then surveyed in the remaining chapters of Volume I, comprising the second part. The last four of these chapters deal with gold compounds, corticosteroids, colchicine, allopurinol, and some natural antiinflammatory agents, including their special pharmacology as well as chemistry. The more general biological properties of antiinflammatory (and immunosuppressive) agents are then discussed in the third part which comprises the second volume. Two of the chapters are devoted to the clinical assessment of these agents in man and the concluding chapter to some aspects of metabolism related to the design and evaluation of antiinflammatory drugs.

Regrettably, it has not been feasible to include any systematic discussion of topical antiinflammatory agents other than the steroids. The inadequacy of current assays has necessarily obscured the possible utility of such agents as dimethyl sulfoxide or glycyrrhetic acid derivatives, to mention but two types of locally active agents, as "leads" in developing new drugs to treat rather localized inflammatory states. Several topics have inevitably received less attention than they deserve. To those investigators whose work has been undervalued or, worse still, ignored, we offer our regrets and apologies.

Whatever merits this treatise possesses lie with the contributing authors, each of whom found time amidst a full and active schedule to share his insights and enthusiasm with us and cheerfully accepted the thankless burden of authorship. For its shortcomings, only the editors are responsible.

We would like to acknowledge our gratitude to Riker Laboratories, Inc., for assisting us in many ways, to Rosemary Baatz for preparing the Subject Index, and to the staff of Academic Press for their patience, encouragement, and ready assistance in translating this book from a nebulous concept into concrete reality.

While this work was in preparation we were saddened to hear of the death of C. V. (Steve) Winder (1909–1972) who contributed greatly to our present understanding of the pharmacological control of inflammation. Through his life and his work he was an inspiration to many who knew him.

ROBERT A. SCHERRER
MICHAEL W. WHITEHOUSE

Contents of Volume 11

Introduction

It seems appropriate in noting the progress made in drug development to comment on a few points, not all of which are elaborated *in extenso* in the chapters comprising this two-volume work.

1. The need for antiarthritic drugs. This is not so much indicated by the current United States annual sales figures for this class of drugs of well over 200 million dollars (see tabulation below) as by the estimated (The Arthritis Foundation) current annual expenditure of 400 million dollars on quack remedies and the 1000 million dollars on medical care for arthritic patients in the United States alone. This represents only a fraction of the world need and cost.

Approximate Sales (Manufacturers Level)
of Antiarthritic Agents in the United States in 1970

Drug	Millions of dollars
Aspirin and salicylates	50[a]
Aspirin combinations	88[a]
Antiarthritics (nonsteroidal; not included below)	70
Corticoids, systemic	10[b]
Antigout agents	22
Gold compounds	0.4
Antimalarials	0.2[b]

[a] Estimated at one-half of total sales.

[b] Based on figures in *Chemical and Engineering News*, August 12, 1968, p. 46. The total sales of systemic corticoids was 73 million dollars in 1970, while that of quinoline antimalarials was about 0.8 million dollars.

2. The truly long history of the salicylates, dating back to the perception of early Greek physicians that certain plants were a good source of "medicine" to treat pain and inflammation.

3. The haphazard discovery of nearly all the other antiarthritic drugs

introduced into clinical use [before the advent of the fenamates (in 1962) and indomethacin and ibufenac (in 1963)] whose efficacy was noted first in man (often quite by accident) and which were only subsequently investigated in detail in laboratory animals. With both the fenamates and indomethacin, this order of discovery was notably reversed. The very slow increase in numbers of post-indomethacin drugs accepted into the armamentarium of the rheumatologist may underscore not only the difficulties in introducing any novel agent (proving safety, efficacy, etc.), but also perhaps the limitations in repeating the strategy of drug testing to find anything other than an indomethacin-like drug.

4. The stimulus given to the development of antiinflammatory drugs by the advances in drug testing in the late 1950's to the early 1960's. The carrageenan-induced rat paw edema assay of C. A. Winter, the UV erythema assay of G. Wilhelmi and C. V. Winder, and the adjuvant arthritis assay of C. M. Pearson and B. B. Newbould were certainly notable. These scientists in turn benefited from work and ideas of their respective colleagues and forerunners.

5. The pioneer chemists on whose work we build are rarely acknowledged. This is easily understood. Their contribution comes early in the sequence of events leading to the discovery of a drug and is usually associated with a single class of agents. One can associate the names of E. Fisher with indoleacetic acids, F. Ullman and A. W. Chapman with the fenamic acids, C. Friedel and J. Crafts and C. Willgerodt and K. Kindler with arylacetic acids, and, of course, H. Kolbe and R. Schmitt with the salicylic acids. The list could be lengthy. Let our debt to these pioneers be recognized, if not always specifically acknowledged.

6. The great diversity of synthetic chemical and natural products legitimately classified as either antiinflammatory or antiarthritic agents. They range from pure inorganic compounds (e.g., gold sodium thiosulfate) through basic or acidic, alicyclic or aromatic compounds of low molecular weight, to hormones and other naturally occurring biological regulators with molecular weights of up to several thousand daltons.

7. The volume of disclosures of "new antiinflammatory agents" in the patent literature, currently at the rate of about 120 patents yearly of compounds deemed worthy of patent protection outside their country of origin, e.g., Belgian patents noted in the Derwent Index during 1972.

8. The variety and complexity of the biological systems and animal models which have been suggested as being appropriate for the preclinical investigation of any compound to establish its value as a potential antiarthritic agent.

9. The alarmingly small ratio of progress (however measured) to effort invested in bringing new agents to clinical trial, emphasizing how much

either a real "breakthrough" or further effort is still needed in synthesizing new structures, devising new isolation procedures, or further developing appropriate assays.

10. The many difficulties in the clinical assessment of new agents against the background of placebo reactors, natural remissions, and free access to salicylates, further complicated by the variety of inflammatory conditions against which assessment can be made. This is illustrated by conflicting clinical reports concerning the utility of even some well-established drugs as well as several new drug candidates.

11. Ignorance of the mechanisms by which even one of the well-established antiinflammatory drugs, such as aspirin or cortisol, may act *in vivo* to regulate an inflammatory process.

12. The virtual impossibility of any one individual, no matter how determined or gifted, being able to keep track of all the appropriate literature concerning those advances in both chemistry and physiology which are germane to finding the superior antiarthritic agents of the future.

Whether we admit it or not, future developments in antiinflammatory pharmacology would seem to belong to the well-knit team of researchers, drawn from a diversity of backgrounds and disciplines but possessing a single-minded vision and determination, while retaining their multidisciplinary competence.

At the risk of emphasizing the obvious, we must allude to the problem of nomenclature. We have tried to adhere to the practice of calling those agents *antiarthritic drugs* which benefit human suffering in arthritic disorders, in a capacity beyond analgesia alone. The description *antiarthritic* is preferred to *antirheumatic* mainly because it may include more agents, and it is usually easier to distinguish the conditions affected as an "arthritis" rather than as "a rheumatic disorder." Where such drugs unequivocally depress a generally acceptable model of inflammation induced in man or laboratory animal, we designate such activity as *antiinflammatory* and prefer this to the alternative designation *antiphlogistic*. Many antiarthritic agents are certainly antiinflammatory but some are probably not, e.g., gold preparations, quinoline-based antimalarials; conversely, many drugs, which are antiinflammatory in animals have not proved to be more than analgesics (if that) in man and so fail to qualify as antiarthritic agents. It is important to distinguish, therefore, between these descriptions while realizing that the terms antiinflammatory and antiarthritic may be synonymous or superimposable within the context of describing one particular drug, but nonoverlapping or even at distant ends of the spectrum in describing other drug entities. Since certain types of chronic inflammation are initiated and sustained by a continuing immunogenic or allergic response and are adequately treated by drugs primarily undercutting the immune/allergic mechanisms, the pragmatic description of a drug as antiinflammatory should not exclude its possible pharmacological activity as an *immunosuppressant* or *antiallergic drug* (or even vice versa). Again, as pointed out above, the term antiinflammatory may be almost synonymous with (one or both of) these two latter descriptions in one context, but totally removed in another.

For the reader wishing more detailed coverage of earlier developments, a listing of selected reviews follows.

ROBERT A. SCHERRER
MICHAEL W. WHITEHOUSE

Selected Reviews Dealing with Anti-inflammatory Drugs

The early history of these drugs has been surveyed by G. P. Rodnan and T. G. Benedek, *Arthr. Rheum.* **13**, 145 (1970). The articles listed below deal with nonclinical properties (chemistry, pharmacology, etc.). References to clinical reviews are included in Chapter 1, Volume I.

H. K. von Rechenberg, "Phenylbutazone." Edward Arnold, Ltd., London, 1962.

J. S. Nicholson, *Rep. Progr. Appl. Chem.* **49**, 192 (1964).

M. W. Whitehouse, *Progr. Drug Res.* **8**, 321 (1965).

R. A. Scherrer, *Annu. Rep. Med. Chem.* **1965**, 224 (1966).

C. A. Winter, *Annu. Rev. Pharmacol.* **6**, 157 (1966); *Progr. Drug Res.* **10**, 139 (1966).

M. J. H. Smith and P. K. Smith, "The Salicylates, A Critical, Bibliographic Review." Wiley (Interscience), New York, 1966.

R. Domenjoz, *Advan. Pharmacol.* **4**, 143 (1966).

S. S. Adams and R. Cobb, *Progr. Med. Chem.* **5**, 59 (1967).

T. Y. Shen, *in* "Topics in Medicinal Chemistry" (J. L. Rabinowitz and R. M. Myerson, eds.), Vol. I, p. 29. Wiley (Interscience), New York, 1967.

I. F. Skidmore and K. Trnavský, *Acta Rheumatol. Balneol. Pistiniana* **3** (1967).

T. Y. Shen, *Annu. Rep. Med. Chem.* **1966**, 217 (1967); *Annu. Rep. Med. Chem.* **1967**, 215 (1968).

J. S. Nicholson, *Rep. Progr. Appl. Chem.* **53**, 208 (1968).

W. Kuzell, *Annu. Rev. Pharmacol.* **8**, 357 (1968).

W. Moll, *Progr. Drug Res.* **12**, 165 (1968).

K. J. Doebel, M. L. Graeme, N. Gruenfeld, L. J. Ignarro, S. J. Piliero, and J. W. F. Wasley, *Annu. Rep. Med. Chem.* **1968**, 207 (1969); *Annu. Rep. Med. Chem.* **1969**, 225 (1970).

M. L. Tainter and A. J. Ferris, "Aspirin in Modern Therapy, A Review." Bayer Co., New York, 1969.

H. O. J. Collier, *Advan. Pharmacol. Chemotherap.* **7**, 333 (1969).

K. J. Doebel, *Pure Appl. Chem.* **19**, 49 (1969).

R. W. Rundles, J. B. Wyngaarden, G. H. Hitchings, and G. B. Elion, *Annu. Rev. Pharmacol.* **9**, 345 (1969).

W. E. Coyne, *in* "Medicinal Chemistry" (A. Burger, ed.), p. 953. Wiley (Interscience), New York, 1970.

M. Weiner and S. J. Piliero, *Annu. Rev. Pharmacol.* **10**, 171 (1970).

P. F. Juby and T. W. Hudyma, *Annu. Rep. Med. Chem.* **1970**, 182 (1971); *Annu. Rep. Med. Chem.* **1971**, 208 (1972).

R. Domenjoz, *in* "Rheumatoid Arthritis" (W. Müller, H. G. Harwerth, and K. Fehr, eds.), pp. 513–550. Academic Press, London, 1971.

H. E. Paulus and M. W. Whitehouse, *in* "Search for New Drugs" (A. Rubin, ed.), pp. 1–114. Marcel Dekker, New York, 1972.

T. Y. Shen, *Angew. Chem. Int. Ed. Engl.* **11,** 460 (1972).

H. E. Paulus and M. W. Whitehouse, *Annu. Rev. Pharmacol.* **13,** 107 (1973).

M. E. Rosenthale, *Annu. Rep. Med. Chem.* **8,** 214 (1973).

S. H. Ferreira and J. R. Vane, *Annu. Rev. Pharmacol.* **14,** 57 (1974).

Antiinflammatory Agents

CHEMISTRY AND PHARMACOLOGY

VOLUME I

Part I

INFLAMMATORY DISEASES

Chapter 1

Some Inflammatory Diseases in Man and Their Current Therapy

HAROLD E. PAULUS

Department of Medicine
University of California School of Medicine
Los Angeles, California

I. INTRODUCTION

Inflammation is an essentially protective and normal response to any noxious stimulus that may threaten the well-being of the host, varying from an acute, transient, and highly localized response to the simplest mechanical injury, such as a pin prick, to a complex, sustained response involving the whole organism that may lead to the immunological rejection of (transplanted) foreign tissues. When tissue injury is caused by a single finite event, such as mechanical trauma, a thermal or chemical burn, or a single exposure to a nonreplicating antigen, the inflammatory and reparative process progresses smoothly from injury to healing. In these circumstances, the whole inflammatory process is truly beneficial and provides an example of a complex homeostatic mechanism restoring the affected tissue to its former normal, healthy state. By contrast, when the injurious agent is a self- replicating parasite (bacterium, virus, or neoplasm), the ensuing inflammatory response becomes much more complex because some form of tissue injury will continue for as long as the agent itself persists. With certain noxious agents that cannot be destroyed or readily eliminated, the inflammatory response attempts to isolate them from the rest of the organism by forming a granuloma, as seen in pulmonary tuberculosis and silicosis, or a gumma, as in syphilis.

There are many chronic disabling, inflammatory conditions of as yet unknown etiology that affect single or multiple organ systems of the body; examples include those affecting the skin (psoriasis, scleroderma), the gastrointestinal tract (ulcerative colitis), and the nervous system (multiple sclerosis) and many conditions affecting the connective tissues. These chronic inflammatory conditions of unknown etiology, with which I am chiefly concerned in this chapter, fluctuate rather unpredictably, with spontaneous remissions and exacerbations. The rapidity with which the disease progresses and its prognosis depend on the organ systems involved.

Although antiinflammatory drugs may be used to modify the inflammatory response in diseases of unknown etiology, such as rheumatoid arthritis, or to symptomatically relieve inflammation in conditions of known etiology, such as gout, they are unlikely to be curative in the sense of removing the underlying cause of the disease. Ideally, such a drug should not interfere with the normal inflammatory response to invading microorganisms, etc., or the patient will be unable to protect himself against his environment. Almost by definition, therefore, antiinflammatory agents are symptomatic therapy and cannot be expected to significantly alter the course of the underlying disease. Agents that relieve inflammation by specifically altering or removing a known causative factor are not considered to be antiinflammatory drugs.

There are at least four distinct target areas available for pharmacological attack. The methods of investigation, realistic goals, and inherent toxicity of therapy differ for each of these four areas. It seems reasonable to assume that for each individual with a chronic inflammatory disorder there is some etiological factor that in some way produces tissue injury. This tissue injury triggers the normal protective inflammatory response, which attempts to repair the injury and restore normal function to the injured tissue. In the case of chronic inflammation, however, restoration of function is prevented by continuing tissue injury or by some abnormality of the inflammatory response, impairing healing and often leading to progressive loss of function. The four potential targets for pharmacological attack are, therefore, as follows: (1) the etiological factor (prime cause); (2) mediators of the initial tissue injury released by, or produced in response to, the etiological factor; (3) the nonspecific, normal, protective inflammatory response evoked by this tissue injury; and (4) the process(es) attempting to restore normal function. A drug aimed at target (1), if effective, would have much more specificity than drugs aimed at targets (3) and (4).

No attempt is made in this chapter to discuss all inflammatory diseases. Such an effort would encompass much of medicine if a broad definition of inflammation were used. Nor are all rheumatological conditions and their appropriate therapies discussed. Instead, a few chronic inflammatory conditions have been selected to illustrate (1) the range of factors that may cause the inflammation, ranging from physical irritation in gout to immunological incompatabilities in renal transplantation, and (2) the interaction of some of these causative agents with those drugs found to be effective clinically. The clinical conditions discussed in Sections II–VI are arranged in the order of an increasing probability that they have an immunopathic etiology. An illustrative classification of some inflammatory conditions and presently available therapy is presented in Table I. Hollander's book (1972), those of Boyle and Buchanan (1971) and Copeman (1969), and the "Primer on the Rheumatic Diseases" (edited by Rodnan, 1973) are recommended as supplemental reading to this chapter.

Although I wish to stress that chronic inflammatory diseases rarely affect only the joints, it may be helpful to review briefly the anatomy and physiology of a joint before discussing specific diseases primarily involving the articular tissues (Fig. 1).

Most joints are designed to permit controlled movement between two articulating bones. The opposing surfaces of the bones are covered with cartilage, a smooth translucent material that minimizes friction during joint motion. Apposition of the two bones is maintained by the tough fibrous joint capsule as well as by muscles that span the joint. The space between the joint capsule and the articulating cartilages is occupied by the synovial

TABLE I

Classification of Some Inflammatory Conditions and Available Therapy

Disease	Prime cause	Mediator of initial tissue injury	Manifestations of disease	Drugs available to:[a]		
				Eradicate prime cause	Prevent initial tissue injury	Moderate the inflammatory response
A. Infection						
Tuberculosis	*Mycobacterium tuberculosis*	Direct injury; immune response?	Caseating granuloma	INH, PAS, streptomycin	?	Salicylates
Syphilis	*Treponema pallidum*	Direct bacterial injury; immune response?	Varied, gumma	Penicillin	?	?
Tetanus	*Clostridium tetanus*	Tetanus toxin	Neuromuscular spasm	Penicillin	Tetanus anti-toxin (active or passive immunization)	Muscle relaxant, curare
Infectious mononucleosis	Epstein-Barr virus	?	Varied	?	?	Corticosteroids
Whipple's disease	Bacilli?	Immune response?	Arthritis, enteritis, lymphadenopathy	Tetracycline	?	Corticosteroids
B. Physical or chemical						
Silicosis	Silica	Silicic acid	Granuloma	?	?	?
Wilson's disease	Abnormal gene	Copper	Cirrhosis of liver, encephalopathy	?	Penicillamine, BAL	Corticosteroids
Gout	Na-urate microcrystals	Polymorphonuclear leukocytes	Tophus	Probenecid, allopurinol	Colchicine	Indomethacin, phenylbutazone

C. Immunological

Disease	Antigen	Mechanism	Manifestations	Specific treatment	Immunosuppressive	Symptomatic treatment
Rheumatic fever	Streptococcal antigen	Antistreptococcal antibody (cross-reacting with myocardium)	Carditis, arthritis, rash, Aschoff body	Penicillin	? (Immunosuppressive)	Salicylates, corticosteroids
Glomerulonephritis	Streptococcal (or other antigen)	Soluble antigen–antibody complex	Nephritis, nephrotic syndrome	Penicillin?	Immunosuppressive	Corticosteroids
Serum sickness	Foreign antigen (drug or serum)	Antigen–antibody–complement complex	Arthritis, hives, nephritis	Discontinue antigen administration	Immunosuppressive	Corticosteroids, salicylates
Contact dermatitis	Exogenous antigen	Sensitized lymphocyte	Dermatitis	Avoid the antigen	?	Topical steroids
Renal homotransplantation	Homograft antigens	Antigen–antibody complex	Rejection		Immunosuppressive (azathioprine, ALG, etc.)	Corticosteroids

D. Unknown causes

Disease	Antigen	Mechanism	Manifestations	Specific treatment	Immunosuppressive	Symptomatic treatment
Osteoarthritis	?	?	Arthritis, osteophyte formation, Heberden's nodes	?	?	Salicylates, indomethacin, phenylbutazone
Rheumatoid arthritis	?	? (Globulin–antiglobulin–complement complex)	Synovitis, rheumatoid nodule, vasculitis	?	Immunosuppressive	Salicylates, indomethacin, gold, corticosteroids
Ankylosing spondylitis	?	?	Syndesmophyte, synovitis, iritis, aortitis	?	?	Indomethacin, phenylbutazone
Reiter's syndrome	Mycoplasma? Bedsonia?	? ?	Urethritis, arthritis, conjunctivitis, dermatitis	? Antibiotic	?	Phenylbutazone, indomethacin, salicylates, (methotrexate?)

TABLE I (*continued*)

Disease	Prime cause	Mediator of initial tissue injury	Manifestations of disease	Drugs available to:[a] Eradicate prime cause	Prevent initial tissue injury	Moderate the inflammatory response
Systemic lupus erythematosus	? Virus	Probable antigen–antibody complex and/or sensitized lymphocytes	Arthritis, pleuritis, pericarditis, nephritis, dermatitis, carditis, encephalitis, anemia, thrombocytopenia, leukopenia, etc.	?	Immunosuppressive	Corticosteroids, salicylates, antimalarial drug, indomethacin
Polyarteritis	?	?	Inflammation of small and medium-sized arteries	?	?	Corticosteroids
Wegener's granulomatosis	?	?	Arteritis, venulitis, granulomas	?	?	Corticosteroids, cyclophosphamide
Dermatomyositis	?	Sensitized lymphocytes?	Dermatitis, myositis	?	Methotrexate	Corticosteroids

Scleroderma	?	?	Dermopathy, arthritis, smooth muscle dysfunction (GI tract), pulmonary fibrosis, nephritis, carditis	?	?	?
Psoriasis	?	?	Dermoproliferation, arthritis	?	Methotrexate	Topical coal tar derivatives, etc.
Ulcerative colitis	Antibody?	?	Inflammation of the bowel	?	Immunosuppressive?	Azulfidine, corticosteroids—topical or systemic
Sarcoidosis	?	?	Granuloma	?	Immunosuppressive	Corticosteroids
Chronic active hepatitis	Sensitized lymphocytes? Antibody?	?	Piecemeal necrosis	?	Immunosuppressive	Corticosteroids
Multiple sclerosis	Sensitized lymphocytes?	?	Demyelination	?	?	Corticosteroids

[a]Note: No available agents to enhance tissue repair. INH, Isonicotinic acid hydrazide (Isoniazid); PAS, 4-aminosalicylic acid; Penicillamine, β,β-dimethylcysteine; BAL, 2,3-dimercaptopropanol; ALG, antilymphocyte globulin; Azulfidine, salicylazosulfapyridine.

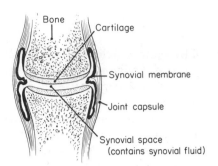

Fig. 1   A stylized representation of a joint.

membrane. The synovial membrane has a generous blood supply and secretes synovial fluid, which supplies nutrients to the avascular articular cartilage. Normal synovial fluid also contains hyaluronic acid–protein complexes, macromolecules that are intimately involved in lubrication and decreasing joint friction.

Inflammation of the vascular synovial membrane impairs joint function in a number of ways. The inflamed membrane is more permeable to plasma constituents, which exude into the joint space, producing a synovial effusion, often described as a "pathological" synovial fluid. Joint friction is increased because hyaluronic acid is not only diluted but is sometimes also chemically degraded by the effusion. Inflammatory cells migrate into the inflamed synovial membrane and into the effusion. When these cells die, they release lytic enzymes that decrease the resilience and slipperiness of cartilage by digesting some of its constituents. With chronic inflammation, the synovial membrane becomes packed with inflammatory cells, hypertrophies, and grows over the already damaged articular cartilage in a form of granulation tissue called "pannus." Wherever pannus grows, it digests and erodes away the cartilage and underlying bone, eventually destroying the joint. Locally, the critical pathological event is the transition from the reversible synovial inflammation (synovitis) to the irreversible pannus overgrowth and sub-pannus cartilage destruction.

II. GOUT

Gout is an excellent example of an inflammatory condition that can be well controlled with currently available drugs. Its etiology and patho-genesis are fairly well understood, and effective drugs are available to treat both the causative agent and the inflammatory response.

A. Pathology

Gout is characterized by acute and chronic inflammatory responses to the deposition of microcrystals of sodium urate (monohydrate) in the joints and tissues. Acute arthritis occurs when the crystals enter the synovial cavity; tophi form when they are deposited in other tissues. When gout is implicated as a cause of death, it is usually because of renal failure resulting from the chronic inflammation occurring secondary to urate crystal deposition in the renal parenchyma. Urate deposits in the tissues when its concentration exceeds its solubility in the extracellular fluid. The extracellular concentration of urate may rise if either its urinary excretion is decreased or the total metabolic production of urate is increased (Fig. 2). Many causes of

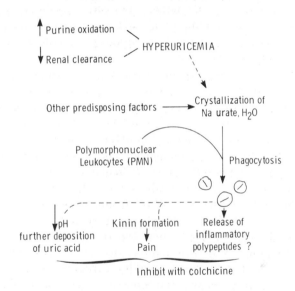

Fig. 2 Pathogenesis of gout.

underexcretion and overproduction of urate have been established clinically; they include uremia, acidosis, competition of diuretic drugs, excessive purine production in leukemia or psoriasis, and hereditary deficiency of the enzyme phosphoribosyltransferase. Cytostatic drugs, irradiation, and tumor chemotherapy may stimulate nucleic acid catabolism with a concomitant increase in urate production from the purine breakdown products. If the concentration of uric acid exceeds its solubility in the urine, uric acid may precipitate to form kidney stones.

B. Therapy

When a patient presents with acute arthritis caused by gout, treatment must be directed at two therapeutically independent aspects of his disease. First, the painful acute arthritis must be relieved; then the plasma urate concentration must be decreased so that it no longer deposits in the tissues and so that already formed tophi will be dissolved. At the present time it is not possible to accomplish both of these aims effectively with a single drug.

Acute inflammatory, gouty arthritis usually can be controlled with an antiinflammatory drug; colchicine, phenylbutazone, or indomethacin is commonly used for this purpose. Aspirin and other salicylate preparations are less effective for gouty arthritis. Colchicine is the preferred drug for the initial attack; because it is relatively ineffective in other types of arthritis, a dramatic clinical improvement with colchicine therapy usually confirms the diagnosis of gout. Colchicine is not an analgesic and has no effect on the metabolism, excretion, or solubility of urate but abolishes the pain of acute gout entirely by its antiinflammatory action. It may be given intravenously (1 or 2 mg in 15 ml of 5% glucose in water with a maximum of 5 mg in any 24-hour period) or orally (0.6 mg every hour until symptomatic relief is obtained or gastrointestinal toxicity occurs). Significant amounts of colchicine are excreted in the bile and reabsorbed from the intestine, which perhaps partly explains the prominence of intestinal symptoms with overdosage. Dramatic relief of the pain, swelling, and inflammation of acute gout usually occurs within 6–12 hours after intensive therapy is initiated; complete recovery of joint function occurs within 24–48 hours. A dose of 0.6 mg of colchicine 1 to 3 times daily is frequently given prophylactically to to prevent gouty attacks, even though the underlying hyperuricemia is not altered by this drug.

Because diarrhea is frequently caused by therapeutic doses of colchicine, other antiinflammatory agents are often used to treat acute gout. The most effective substitutes seem to be phenylbutazone (200 mg every 8 hours) or indomethacin (50 mg every 4–6 hours).

The underlying hyperuricemia responsible for gout may be pharmacologically controlled by agents that increase uric acid excretion or by agents that decrease uric acid production. Urate is filtered by the renal glomeruli, reabsorbed in the proximal tubule, and secreted by the distal tubule. Substances that decrease (distal tubular) urate secretion tend to produce hyperuricemia; examples are organic anions such as lactate or salicylate (at low doses), and most diuretics. Substances that decrease (proximal tubular) urate reabsorption increase the urate clearance by the kidney and lower serum uric acid levels. Salicylate, phenylbutazone, sulfinpyrazone, and probenecid are among the drugs that have been found to inhibit the renal tubular transport of urate. Small doses of these agents decrease urate clearance, presumably by inhibiting its secretion, but larger doses apparently also block reabsorption and, therefore, have a uricosuric effect. Probenecid (200–600 mg daily) and sulfinpyrazone (100 or 200 mg every 6 hours) are the two most effective uricosuric agents currently used to treat hyperuricemia.

The immediate metabolic precursor of uric acid is xanthine; it is formed from hypoxanthine and is also oxidized to uric acid by the same enzyme, xanthine oxidase, which is present in the liver. A structural isomer of hypoxanthine, allopurinol (4-hydroxypyrazolo[3,4-*d*]pyrimidine), decreases uric acid production by inhibiting xanthine oxidase (Fig. 3). This raises the levels of xanthine and hypoxanthine in the urine. Perhaps because these two oxypurines are somewhat more soluble than uric acid and are rapidly cleared by the kidneys, xanthine crystal deposition is not a problem in patients treated with allopurinol. Hyperuricemia can usually be controlled by 200–600 mg/day of the drug.

Neither the uricosuric agents nor allopurinol have any antiinflammatory or analgesic effects so they are not useful for treating the inflammation of gouty arthritis. Thus, in gout there is a complete separation of the therapy for inflammation from the therapy for the underlying cause. One can effectively treat the acute inflammatory attack without influencing the underly-

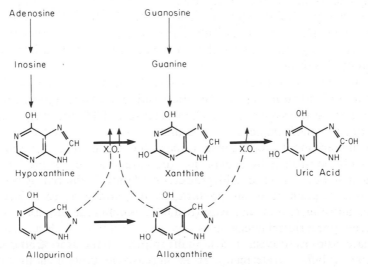

Fig. 3 Inhibition of uric acid synthesis by allopurinol (X.O. = xanthine oxidase).

ing hyperuricemia and, conversely, effectively lower the blood urate level without altering the course of an acute attack of gouty arthritis.

The causes of the conditions discussed hereafter in this chapter are not nearly so well understood as that of gout, but the lesson taught by an analysis of gout is equally applicable to them; i.e., successful treatment of the symptoms of inflammation may have no effect on the underlying etiology or the course of the basic disease.

III. THE RHEUMATOID VARIANTS

The so-called rheumatoid variants are a group of rheumatic disorders characterized by the absence of detectable antiglobulin (rheumatoid factor) and antinuclear antibodies in the serum. Examples include ankylosing spondylitis, Reiter's syndrome, psoriatic arthritis, and the arthritis as-associated with regional enteritis and ulcerative colitis. These conditions do not occur predominantly in females, in contrast to the higher incidence of both rheumatoid arthritis and systemic lupus erythematosus in females. Certain clinical characteristics or complications, such as inflammation of the sacroiliac joints and spine, the iris of the eye (iritis), or the media of the root of the aorta, and dermatological manifestations tend to be shared by some or all of this group of variants. Arthritis of the joints in the extremities tends to be episodic and asymmetrical, with an acute onset and relatively less joint destruction than occurs in rheumatoid arthritis. Arthritis of the sacroiliac joints and spine may progress insidiously to produce complete fusion of the vertebrae of the entire spine.

Therapy

The inflammation of these variants responds somewhat better to phenyl-butazone (or oxyphenbutazone) and indomethacin than it does to salicylate, in contrast to rheumatoid arthritis, which responds more satisfactorily to salicylates. Effective doses are somewhat lower than those used in acute gout: 200–400 mg daily of phenylbutazone and 50–150 mg daily of indo-methacin. Because it may depress the activity of the bone marrow, prolonged therapy with phenylbutazone is usually avoided unless other less toxic drugs are ineffective. When it is used, the number of blood leukocytes should be monitored regularly.

Symptoms of psoriatic arthritis usually improve if the psoriatic dermatitis improves either spontaneously or during treatment with methotrexate, azauridine triacetate, or other antimetabolites. Similarly, the articular inflammation of the arthritis associated with regional enteritis or ulcerative colitis usually parallels that of the bowel disease and remits if the inflamed colon is surgically removed.

IV. RHEUMATOID ARTHRITIS

It must be admitted that a claim for a role of autoimmunity in the pathogenesis of rheumatoid arthritis receives its strongest support from the absence of any stronger claimant. Nevertheless, despite the circumstantial nature of the evidence, extremely strong support can be adduced for the autoimmune hypothesis. Some of the evidence has been marshalled by Ziff (1973) and Zvaifler (1972).

A. Pathology

Interest in the immunological aberrations of the rheumatic diseases was greatly stimulated by the finding of rheumatoid factor (an antiglobulin antibody) in patients with rheumatoid arthritis by Rose and associates in 1948. Further intensive study has conclusively demonstrated that, depending on the methods used, rheumatoid factor occurs in 70–80% of adults with rheumatoid arthritis but has failed to clearly elucidate its role in the pathogenesis of the disease. The demonstration that rheumatoid synovium can produce rheumatoid factor and that leukocytes in the synovial fluid ingest immune complexes (containing rheumatoid factor, globulin, and complement) suggest that these immunological abnormalities may be involved in the mediation of inflammation in rheumatoid arthritis, but the overall picture remains puzzling. One popular viewpoint assumes that the phagocytic leukocytes, in the course of ingesting immune complexes, release into the joint cavity lysosomal hydrolases that attack the joint cartilage and other supportive structures.

This apparent localization of an immunological event in the joint tempts one to conclude that rheumatoid arthritis is a localized disease and then, accordingly, to restrict therapeutic efforts to the joint. Such reasoning is almost certainly fallacious. It is more likely that the many manifestations of rheumatoid arthritis are expressions of a generalized systemic disease, and the joints are merely the most obvious target organ. Monoarticular juvenile rheumatoid arthritis is the most benign form of rheumatoid arthritis, involving only one joint, and the sedimentation rate of the erythrocytes in freshly drawn blood is frequently normal. This juvenile disease would certainly seem to be an ideal candidate for curative intraarticular or localized therapy. Yet, patients with monoarticular juvenile rheumatoid arthritis have a high incidence of inflammation of the iris of the eye, which may cause blindness if not adequately suppressed. Interestingly, the iritis may occasionally precede the first symptom of arthritis by months or years, or it may occur during complete remission of the joint inflammation, in addition to the more usual concurrence of the two clinical findings. This suggests that both the iritis and the arthritis are rather independent dysfunctions of two target organs, resulting from a more generalized pathological process.

Rheumatoid arthritis, therefore, continues to be an enigmatic clinical condition characterized by symmetrical polyarthritis that occurs more frequently in females and usually has a chronic course with cyclic exacerbations and remissions of symptoms. Systemic manifestations vary but are usually present to some degree. One of the commonest extraarticular symptoms is vasculitis (inflammatory degeneration of the small blood vessels), which may manifest itself in various ways, the most typical example being the rheumatoid nodule. The arthritis may progress rapidly to crippling disability, it may "smolder" for years with little apparent deterioration, or it may spontaneously remit at any time. The very variability of the disease and the frequency of these spontaneous remissions makes objective evaluation of drug therapy rather difficult. The symptoms and inflammation of rheumatoid arthritis can be suppressed readily in all patients by corticosteroid therapy and in some patients by intramuscular injection of gold derivatives. Long-term controlled studies have shown repeatedly that joint damage may progress continuously despite an almost complete suppression of symptoms with corticosteroids, and exacerbation tends to occur whenever suppressive therapy is discontinued. These observations clearly indicate that suppression of inflammation does not truly affect the underlying etiology to significantly alter the normal course of the disease (Berntsen and Freyberg, 1961).

B. Therapy

Intensive salicylate therapy (3–10 gm of aspirin daily), combined with rest and physical therapy, continues to offer the best balance of beneficial antiinflammatory effect and minimal toxicity for the long-term management of rheumatoid arthritis (Fig. 4). Indomethacin and phenylbutazone seem to add little to salicylate therapy, and the need to use these drugs usually indicates that the patient is not getting sufficient rest. Gold therapy has a delayed effect but seems to be associated with remissions somewhat more frequently than would be anticipated from the natural history of the disease. The use of corticosteroids is discouraged because of the well-known compli-

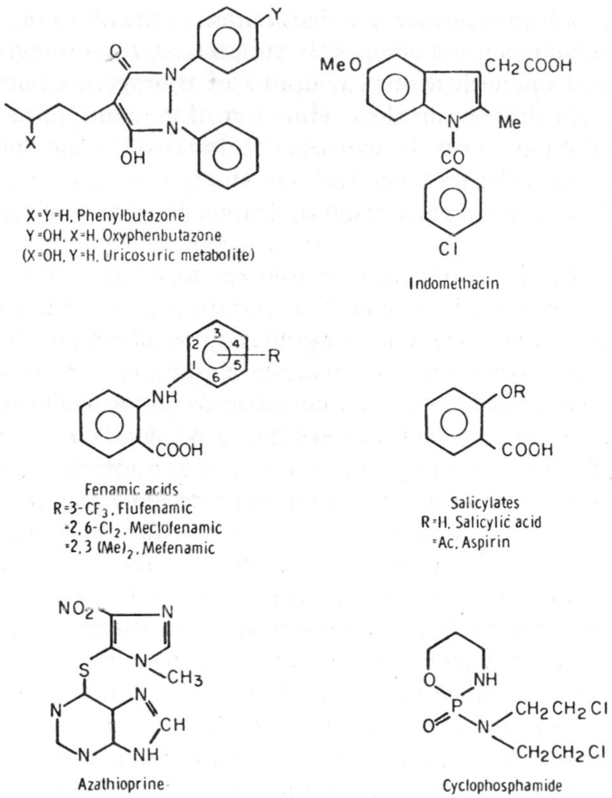

X=Y=H, Phenylbutazone
Y=OH, X=H, Oxyphenbutazone
(X=OH, Y=H, Uricosuric metabolite)

Indomethacin

Fenamic acids
R=3-CF₃, Flufenamic
=2,6-Cl₂, Meclofenamic
=2,3 (Me)₂, Mefenamic

Salicylates
R=H, Salicylic acid
=Ac, Aspirin

Azathioprine

Cyclophosphamide

Fig. 4 Some drugs used to treat rheumatic diseases.

cations of administering them over a long term. Antimalarial drugs related to chloroquine are no longer used extensively because they may cause damage to the retina with prolonged use, and they seem to lack any clear advantage over more conservative therapy. In countries where they are available, the fenamates (*N*-arylanthranilates) and certain phenylacetic acid derivatives, e.g., Ibuprofen, are also used to treat rheumatoid arthritis (Adams *et al.*, 1969; Davies and Avery, 1971).

Immunosuppressive (cytostatic) agents, such as azathioprine (Imuran) and cyclophosphamide (Cytoxan, Fig. 4), are currently undergoing clinical trials. Many patients who are resistant to other drugs benefit from them and complete remissions may be seen in some patients after 6–18 months of therapy (Fosdick *et al.*, 1969). One controlled study reports that new erosions of articular cartilage do not develop during treatment with cyclophosphamide (Cooperating Clinics Committee of the American Rheumatism

Association, 1970). Even if they reliably induce remissions of the disease, the toxicity of the presently available cytostatic agents will probably prove to be too great to allow them to be used very widely and over a long term for treating rheumatoid arthritis. However, they clearly point toward a pharmacological approach to treating the disease at a more fundamental level than just treating the inflammatory symptoms.

Several blind studies, especially the Empire Rheumatism Council Subcommittee cooperative study in Britain (reported in 1961), demonstrate significantly greater improvement of gold-treated patients when compared to patients receiving only placebo. The occasional occurrence of a complete clinical remission during gold therapy is particularly noteworthy. The usual weekly dose contains about 25 mg of gold. The time sequence of the clinical response to gold therapy parallels the metabolism and excretion of gold preparations. When soluble gold compounds are injected intramuscularly, the circulating gold is bound to α_1-globulin and albumin as a gold–protein complex. Plasma levels rise rapidly and are maintained over at least the next 24 hours but urinary excretion is greatest during the first 2 hours and decreases markedly thereafter. With constant weekly dosage, much of the injected gold is retained in the body (Freyberg, et al. 1972). It presumably accumulates in the various tissues. It has been found that gold may be continuously excreted in the urine for up to 15 months beyond the last weekly injection. The half-life of body retention of [^{195}Au] aurothiomalate tracer is about 30 days (Gerber et al., 1972). The onset of clinical improvement is very subtle and is usually seen 2–3 months after beginning the weekly therapy. If remission occurs, it may persist for 12–18 months after injections are discontinued, suggesting that the therapeutic response is related to the quantity of gold retained in the tissues. In the Empire Rheumatism Council study, the average clinical condition of the gold-treated group of patients was better than that of the placebo-treated group for 13 months following termination of the 5-month course of weekly injections but by the twenty-fifth month this advantage had all but disappeared. It is still not known whether patients who fail to respond to gold derivatives fail to accumulate sufficient gold in the target tissues or whether they are simply resistant to its effects in vivo. Extensive clinical use of gold derivatives is limited by the relatively high incidence of toxicity (hematological, renal, and mucocutaneous), the rather discouraging delay before any therapeutic benefit is apparent, and the fairly large proportion of patients who fail to respond at all.

Depletion of the circulating lymphocytes in rats by thoracic duct drainage has been found to ameliorate certain experimental immunopathic diseases, including the lymphocyte-mediated arthritis that can be induced with Freund's adjuvant (Whitehouse et al., 1969, 1972). Depletion of thoracic duct lymphocytes has also been found to temporarily relieve the inflammation of patients with rheumatoid arthritis, even though they had been withdrawn from all antiinflammatory drug therapy (Paulus *et al.*, 1973). These studies indicate that lymphocytes play a crucial role in at least some chronic inflammatory conditions.

V. SYSTEMIC LUPUS ERYTHEMATOSUS

Systemic lupus erythematosus is characterized by its many immunological abnormalities. During the course of the disease, a single patient may develop antibodies to many of his own tissue components; one or more of a number of antibodies, i.e., antinuclear, anticytoplasmic, antithyroid, antierythrocyte, or antithrombocyte (platelet), may be demonstrable at various times. The patient may have immunologically mediated disease of the kidneys, skin, joints, heart, formed blood elements, and blood vessels. However, despite its rich serology and extensive immunological investigation, its etiology remains unknown. The finding of viruslike particles in electronmicrographs of glomerular endothelium from lupus nephritis patients (Norton, 1969; Györky *et al.*, 1969) and some evidence that diseases in Aleutian minks and NZB mice, which rather closely resemble systemic lupus erythematosus in man, may be transmitted by a viruslike particle (Williams, 1968) have intensified interest in the possibility that this disease has a viral origin.

Clinically, the disease runs an undulating course, involving many tissues simultaneously or independently. The prognosis for the disease varies with the nature of the organs primarily involved. For example, if it is limited to the skin and joints, life expectancy is not decreased, whereas if the kidneys or heart are significantly involved, the prognosis is indeed grave.

Therapy

The potency of the therapeutic measures required to treat the ongoing disease varies according to the importance of the organs involved. Because no available therapy is curative, the preferred treatment is to use the least toxic agents that will relieve the symptoms without otherwise debilitating the patient. Salicylates (3–6 gm/day) or antimalarial drugs, such as chloroquine (250 mg/day) or hydroxychloroquine (200–400 mg/day), may be the only treatment needed if only arthritis and dermatitis are present. However, if there is any life-threatening involvement of the heart or central nervous system, large doses of corticosteroid drugs (> 100 mg/day of prednisone) may be needed to prevent death. It should be noted that even when steroids have this dramatic effect, they are not really much more effective than salicylates in the sense that they, too, are incapable of curing the disease and, like the salicylates, treat only the symptoms.

Cytostatic immunosuppressive agents, such as azathioprine, are being studied in systemic lupus erythematosus because of their ability to interfere with the immunological mediators of the disease. Preliminary reports suggest that the combination of prednisone and an immunosuppressive drug may delay the progress of early renal lesions, but the ultimate role of such therapy in the general management of this disease remains to be determined. The number of deaths caused by involvement of the central nervous system has dramatically decreased with aggressive steroid therapy (Dubois, 1966), and similar reductions in mortality caused by pericarditis, fever, and hemolytic anemia have also occurred. Combination therapy with steroids and azathioprine seems to improve the prognosis of patients with mild nephritis (Drinkard et al., 1970). Unfortunately, however, many patients continue to die of lupus nephritis, complications of therapy, and uncontrollable progression of disease.

VI. RENAL TRANSPLANTATION

Although it is really not a natural disease, renal homotransplantation is mentioned here because it is a well-studied unnatural condition in which the causative factor, immunological incompatibility, is fairly well understood, and the time of onset of the inflammatory state can be precisely determined. Clearly, rejection of the transplanted organ is initiated by normally protective immunological reactions (meant to be defensive but actually manifest as aggression) but mediated by the familiar sequelae to an inflammatory stimulus leading to the cardinal signs of inflammation and, above all, loss of function.

Therapy

Prevention of a rejection crisis requires potent immunosuppressive therapy, commonly with azathioprine (1–3 mg/kg body weight daily) combined with potent antiinflammatory therapy, nearly always with corticosteroids (20 to > 100 mg/day). The frequent occurrence of serious infections during such drastic immunosuppressive and antiinflammatory therapy emphasizes the hazards of interfering too efficiently with the natural protective mechanisms of the host. Nevertheless, with appropriate caution, such combination therapy is sufficiently effective for it to be acceptable clinically as a necessary adjunct to renal transplantation.

It should be noted that even in the fairly well-understood context of organ transplantation the attainment of specific immunological tolerance remains an elusive goal, except for transplants between identical twins. In addition, even with the maximum degree of chronic immunosuppressive and antiinflammatory therapy that can be tolerated, it probably does not prevent persistent or episodic low-grade inflammation in the transplanted organ, so that its physiological function and life-expectancy may still be rather limited. Some patients have in fact already required second organ grafts, which clearly demonstrates that any inflammation may be too much.

More specific depression of lymphocyte-mediated immunity has been attempted by two methods: (1) administration of heterologous anti-human-lymphocyte globulin and (2) removal or destruction of circulating (thoracic duct) lymphocytes by other means.

The administration of heterologous anti-human-lymphocyte globulin (ALG), although not universally practiced, is used extensively enough to be considered a common, adjunctive, immunosuppressive measure. To prepare ALG an animal, usually a horse, is immunized with human lymphocytes (collected from human spleen, thymus, or cultured lymphoblasts). The immune serum is collected; partially fractionated; absorbed with appropriate human red cells, platelets, and plasma to remove unwanted antibodies; and administered intramuscularly to homotransplant recipients. Therapy with ALG usually is begun 3–5 days before transplantation and is continued, in gradually decreasing doses, for about 4 months. Mortality and homograft loss may be decreased with ALG, renal function improved, and the quantities of azathioprine and prednisone needed to achieve these results considerably reduced when ALG is used in conjunction with these two drugs.

Because a number of problems are associated with it, ALG is not universally used as an immunosuppressive agent. Injection of foreign proteins may result in serum sickness or anaphylactic reactions, even in patients receiving immunosuppressive therapy. Failure to absorb all hemagglutinins and antiplatelet antibodies may cause anemia and thrombocytopenia. Pain and swelling at the injection site commonly occur. The risk of ALG enhancing a malignancy (by its immunosuppressive action) is emphasized in a number of reports (Deodhar et al., 1969; Zipp and Kountz, 1971; McKhann, 1969). Indeed, ALG has been described, not too inaccurately, as an oncogenic agent.

Fish and his associates (1969) cannulated the thoracic duct of potential renal transplant recipients: the collected lymph was dialyzed against tap water to destroy the lymphocytes or centrifuged to remove them and then reinfused in the patients to prevent protein depletion. Over 70 patients were treated in this manner for at least 4–6 weeks prior to transplanting cadaver kidneys and for up to 68 days after the transplant. Following transplantation, no immunosuppressive drugs or prednisone were given until the patients recovered from the surgical procedure, when azathioprine and prednisone therapy were begun. Despite the lack of drug therapy, rejection rarely occurred during thoracic duct drainage. Immunoglobulin levels in blood and lymph remained normal during the period that the circulating lymphocytes were depleted, whereas skin tests for delayed hypersensitivity diminished in intensity but were not completely abolished.

VII. OSTEOARTHRITIS (DEGENERATIVE JOINT DISEASE)

"Osteoarthritis is a non-inflammatory disorder of movable joints characterized by deterioration and abrasion of articular cartilage, and also by formation of new bone at the joint surfaces" [Leon Sokoloff (1966)]. Although this definition implies a single disease with a well-defined pathophysiology, clinical experience suggests that the one diagnosis, osteoarthritis, includes several distinct constellations of symptoms. One is seen in weight-bearing joints as the residue of a lifetime of physical labor or because of injury to a particular joint and appears to be caused by mechanical wearing out of the joints. Active inflammation is rarely present, and abortive attempts to repair the damaged joint result in the characteristic pathologic findings of eburnation (formation of a dense, polished, bony articular surface to replace the lost cartilage) and osteophyte formation. However, only a small proportion of patients with the characteristic X-ray findings and pathological lesions of degenerative joint disease have notable symptoms and, with a few exceptions, disability is minimal. When symptoms occur, therapy with analgesic doses of salicylates (1–3 gm/day) and physical rest usually suffice.

A contrasting clinical picture is seen in some women at the onset of menopause. Their syndrome, described by Kellgren (1954) and emphasized by Peter et al. (1966), consists of rather conspicuous inflammation of the distal joints of the fingers that persists for 1 or 2 years and resolves with the formation of painless Heberden's nodes. These are hard knobs on the sides of the distal finger joints produced by bony overgrowth. Biopsy of the acute lesion shows an infiltration of inflammatory cells into the synovium, sometimes indistinguishable from that seen in rheumatoid arthritis. The other non-weight-bearing and weight-bearing joints are often extensively involved. A prominent familial predisposition also characterizes the syndrome. Severe impairment of joint function is rare. Therapy of the acute stages usually requires antiinflammatory doses of salicylates, phenylbutazone, or indomethacin.

Still another picture is seen with osteoarthritis of the hip joint (*malum coxae senilis*). It may occur as part of generalized osteoarthritis, as a result of a predisposing mechanical derangement (coxae plana, dysplasia of the acetabulum, congenital subluxation, etc.), following avascular necrosis of the femoral head, or spontaneously as an isolated occurrence with no apparent predisposing cause. Regardless of the onset, the end result is degeneration of cartilage, sclerosis of subchondral bone, and marginal osteophyte formation, producing severe pain and marked disability. Treatment is primarily by surgical correction or replacement of the damaged joint, but symptomatic therapy with phenylbutazone, indomethacin, and sometimes mild narcotics aids in controlling pain.

These few examples should make it clear that osteoarthritis, which is the most frequently encountered joint disease, really represents a collection of somewhat diverse clinical syndromes that share only a common pathological outcome. Although they are not usually severely disabling or fatal, in aggregate they cause a great deal of discomfort.

VIII. PSORIASIS

Psoriasis is a benign skin disease characterized by patches of thick white scales on a base of erythematous skin that occurs in 1–2% of white-skinned individuals. It is thought to be genetically determined, being dominantly inherited, with incomplete penetrance. In most patients, for most of the time, the inflammatory component is minimal but episodes of acute severe inflammation (called "pustular psoriasis") or of generalized redness (called "erythrodermic psoriasis") may occur. Psoriatic epidermis has been demonstrated to renew itself every 48 hours, which is excessively rapid compared to the turnover time of normal epidermis (usually 12–14 days). Treatment with the folic acid antagonist, amethopterin (methotrexate), selectively inhibits multiplication of the abnormally replicating basal cells and increases the turnover time toward normal (Weinstein and Frost, 1969).

Because of its essentially irreversible inhibition of dihydrofolate reductase and its rapid clearance by the kidneys, the toxicity and optimal dose of methotrexate depend not so much on the size of the dose as on the duration of cellular exposure to the drug. Thus, 2.5 mg daily by mouth may not be tolerated for more than 5–7 days, whereas 50 mg intravenously once weekly may cause no toxicity because of the ample recovery period allowed by the dosage schedule. Folinic acid (citrovorum factor) terminates the effects of methotrexate by bypassing the need for folate reductase and has been used to rescue patients following large doses of methotrexate. Triacetylazauridine and other antimetabolites have also been used to treat psoriasis.

Psoriasis also illustrates the propensity of the chronic inflammatory diseases for involving more than one organ system; in the case of psoriasis, a characteristic type of peripheral joint arthritis that exacerbates or remits when the skin lesions do so sometimes occurs.

IX. OTHER SKIN DISEASES

Most dermatological conditions consist of acute, subacute, or chronic inflammatory reactions to various known and unknown prime causes. They differ from other inflammatory diseases in that the extent and severity of the inflammation (as it involves the skin) is readily assessed visually and also because, by shedding, the skin is sometimes able to rid itself of the actual cause of inflammation. Such skin diseases as pemphigus, pemphigoid, and discoid lupus apparently involve circulating antibodies and respond to immunosuppressive therapy (Ebringer and Mackay, 1969). Contact dermatitis, in contrast, is a manifestation of delayed hypersensitivity. There are dermatological manifestations of many bacterial and viral infections, and rashes are often a part of some generalized chronic inflammatory diseases (e.g., rheumatic fever, juvenile rheumatoid arthritis, ulcerative colitis). Inflammation of the small blood vessels (vasculitis) and inflammatory cell infiltrates are a prominent part of many skin diseases, just as they are in many systemic inflammatory states.

Therapy

Except for the use of baths, compresses, and mild irritants (such as coal tar ointments) to stimulate shedding and self-renewal of the skin and ointments to protect it from external irritation, the drug therapy of skin diseases is rather similar to that used for other inflammatory conditions. Corticosteroids or immunosuppressives may be administered systemically. In addition, if properly formulated and administered, topically applied corticosteroids are absorbed sufficiently well to relieve local symptoms while sparing the host much of their systemic toxic effects. Their efficacy is not entirely limited to the skin, however, and the chronic application of steroid-containing creams to large areas of skin may result in adrenal suppression, especially if absorption is enhanced by the use of occlusive dressings. In small animals, topically applied steroids will dramatically reduce the mass of the thymus within a very few days, clearly demonstrating that even a topically applied steroid may carry considerable systemic toxicity (DiPasquale *et al.*, 1970). The nonsteroidal acidic antiinflammatory drugs are not used very often for skin diseases, probably because it is so readily apparent that they are not very effective for this purpose.

X. CONJUNCTIVITIS, EPISCLERITIS, AND UVEITIS

The specialized epithelial structures of the eye are subject to a number of inflammatory conditions that usually are readily apparent to the observer. These may be caused by bacterial or viral infections, physical or chemical trauma, exposure to antigens, or other unknown factors. Usually the inflammation is readily relieved with topical corticosteroid preparations. However, if steroids are inadvertently used to treat a viral infection, such as that caused by the herpesvirus, the persistent infection may cause progressive ulceration and scarring of the cornea and may result in blindness, illustrating once again the potential hazards of potent symptomatic antiinflammatory therapy.

REFERENCES

Adams, S. S., Bough, R. G., Cliffe, E. E., Lessel, B., and Mills, R. F. N. (1969). *Toxicol. Appl. Pharmacol.* **15**, 310.

Berntsen, C. A., and Freyberg, R. H. (1961). *Ann. Intern. Med.* **54**, 938.

Boyle, J. A., and Buchanan, W. W. (1971). "Clinical Rheumatology." Davis, Philadelphia, Pennsylvania.

Cooperating Clinics of the American Rheumatism Association (1970). *N. Engl. J. Med.* **283**, 883.

Copeman, W. S. C., ed. (1969). "Textbook of the Rheumatic Diseases," 4th ed. Livingstone, Edinburgh.

Davies, E. F., and Avery, G. S. (1971). *Drugs* **2**, 416.

Deodhar, S. D., Kuklinca, A. G., Vidt, D. G., Robertson, A. L., and Hazard, J. B. (1969). *N. Engl. J. Med.* **280**, 1104.

DiPasquale, G., Rassaert, C. L., and McDougall, E. (1970). *J. Pharm. Sci.* **59**, 267.

Drinkard, J. P., Stanley, T. M., Dornfeld, L., Austin, R. C., Barnett, E. V., Pearson, C. M., Vernier, R. L., Adams, D. A., Latta, H., and Gonick, H. (1970). *Medicine (Baltimore)* **49**, 411.

Dubois, E. L. (1966). "Lupus Erythematosus." McGraw-Hill, New York.
Ebringer, A., and Mackay, I. R. (1969). *Ann. Intern. Med.* **71**, 125.
Empire Rheumatism Council Subcommittee (1961). *Ann. Rheum. Dis.* **20**, 315.
Fish, J. C., Sarles, H. E., Remmers, H. R., Tyson, K. R. T., Canales, C. C., Beathard, G. A., Fukushima, M., Ritzmann, S. E., and Levin, W. C. (1969). *Surg., Gynecol. Obstet.* **128**, 777.
Fosdick, W. M., Parsons, J. L., and Hill, D. F. (1969). *Arthritis Rheum.* **12**, 663.
Freyberg, R. H., Ziff, M., and Baum, J. (1972). *In* "Arthritis and Allied Conditions" (J. L. Hollander and D. J. McCarty, Jr., ed.), 8th ed., 455–482. Lea & Febiger, Philadelphia, Pennsylvania.
Gerber, R. C., Paulus, H. E., and Bluestone, R. (1972). *Abstr. Int. Congr. Pharmacol., 5th, 1972* p. 80.
Györky, F., Min, K-W., and Györky, p. (1969). *Arthritis Rheum.* **12**, 300.
Hollander, J. L., and McCarty, D. J., Jr., ed. (1972). "Arthritis and Allied Conditions" 8th ed. Lea & Febiger, Philadelphia, Pennsylvania.
Kellgren, J. H. (1954). *Bull. Rheum. Dis.* **4**, 46.
McKhann, C. F. (1969). *Transplantation* **8**, 209.
Norton, W. L. (1969). *Arthritis Rheum.* **12**, 320.
Paulus, H. E., Machleder, H., Bangert, R., Stratton, J. A., Goldberg, L., Whitehouse, M. W., Yu, D., and Pearson, C. M. (1973). *Clin. Immunol. Immunopathol.* **1**, 173.
Peter, J. B., Pearson, C. M., and Marmor, L. (1966). *Arthritis Rheum.* **9**, 365.
Rodnan, G. P., (1973). "Primer on the Rheumatic Diseases." Arthritis Found., New York; also *J. Amer. Med. Ass.* **224**, No. 5 (1973) (Supplement)
Rose, H. M., Ragan, C., Pearce, E., and Lipman, M. O. (1948). *Proc. Soc. Exp. Biol. Med.* **68**, 1.
Sokoloff, L. (1972). *In* "Arthritis and Allied Conditions" (J. L. Hollander and D. J. McCarty, Jr., ed.), 8th ed., p. 1009. Lea & Febiger, Philadelphia, Pennsylvania.
Weinstein, G. D., and Frost, P. (1969). *Nat. Cancer. Inst., Monogr.* **30**, 255.
Whitehouse, D. J., Whitehouse, M. W., and Pearson, C. M. (1969). *Nature (London)* **224**, 1322.
Whitehouse, M. W., Pearson, C. M., and Paulus, H. E. (1972). *Proc. Carlo Erba Symp., Rheumatoid Arthritis, 1971* (in press).
Williams, R. C. (1968). *Arthritis Rheum.* **11**, 593.
Ziff, M. (1973). *Fed. Proc., Fed. Amer. Soc. Exp. Biol.* **32**, 131.
Zipp, P., and Kountz, S. L. (1971). *Amer. J. Surg.* **122**, 204.
Zvaifler, N. J. (1972). *In* "Inflammation Mechanisms and Control," (I. Lepow and P. Ward, eds.), pp. 223–237. Academic Press, New York.

Part II

PREPARATION, PHYSICAL AND CHEMICAL PROPERTIES, AND STRUCTURE–ACTIVITY RELATIONSHIPS

Chapter 2

Introduction to the Chemistry of Anti-inflammatory and Antiarthritic Agents

ROBERT A. SCHERRER

Riker Laboratories, Inc.
3M Center
St. Paul, Minnesota

I. SCOPE OF THESE CHAPTERS*

Few aspects of the antiinflammatory field are free of controversy. Debate ranges from the proposed mechanisms of action of antiinflammatory agents, through the selection of areas in which chemists should be concentrating

*It may be helpful to define a few abbreviations that are used throughout this volume. Routes of administration of a compound are indicated by i.p. (intraperitoneal), i.m. (intramuscular), p.o. (oral), s.c. (subcutaneous), and i.v. (intravenous). ED_{50} and LD_{50} are, respectively, 50% effective and 50% lethal dose levels. MED stands for minimum effective dose.

their efforts, to methods for evaluating compounds in the laboratory. It even extends to the proper clinical evaluation of these agents. The authors of these chemically oriented chapters cannot avoid bringing in the controversy in other disciplines as each chemist (or research team) must evaluate to his (its) own satisfaction the biological and clinical reports concerning efficacy on which plans for future work are based.

Synthetic routes to the various classes of compounds covered in this volume are not discussed extensively. General routes, where it is felt they are of interest, are included. Two topics receive a little greater chemical emphasis. Because Chapter 10, by Fitzgerald, is the first extensive review of colchicine in the context of inflammation, more detail on the chemistry of this class of alkaloids is included. Improved routes for synthesizing fenamic acids are scattered throughout the patent literature so this subject is also given special attention.

Although many of the nonsteroidal antiinflammatory agents are antipyretic and peripheral analgesics, these properties, in general, are not considered in discussing structure–activity relationships. I find it difficult to accept as meaningful, attempts to quantitatively assess analgesic (antinociceptive) activity in animal models that have inflammatory components (Wilhelmi et al., 1968; Winter and Flataker, 1965) or are subject to nonspecific effects, e.g., in various writhing tests (Hendershot and Forsaith, 1959). As an example of interpretative complications, bradykinin-induced writhing is now felt to be mediated by a prostaglandin (Moncada et al., 1972) so the property being tested in this assay may be inhibition of prostaglandin synthesis, the same as in many antiinflammatory assays.

II. CHEMICAL AND PHARMACOLOGICAL CLASSES; INTERACTION POTENTIAL

The chapters in this volume cover the variety of antiarthritic agents under study today. They are broadly categorized by chemical class. This has the disadvantage of artificially separating some compounds that seem to fall within the same pharmacological class. However, this division accords with the special experience of the authors, and serves to categorize the agents for ready location. The division by chemical class does separate out those compounds having distinctly different pharmacological profiles and probably acting by different mechanisms and at different sites. It is worthwhile to keep in mind the theoretical therapeutic advantages to be gained by using a combination of agents acting by different mechanisms. It is a mathematical necessity (Black, 1963) that agents effective independently at different points in the same pathway (e.g., initiation ——>inflammation ——>tissue damage) be synergistic. (Synergism, loosely defined here as an effect greater than expected from the summation of the separate effects, is more fully discussed by Black.) Compounds acting on different pathways to produce the same end may be synergistic or additive in their effects. Compounds of the same mechanistic class acting at the same site may have either additive or partially antagonistic activities (Ariëns et al., 1964). Willoughby's "cocktail" for the treatment of rheumatoid arthritis (Shen, 1972) would include different pharmacological classes of agents.

III. ASSESSMENT OF PHARMACOLOGICAL DATA IN THE EVALUATION OF LITERATURE REPORTS

Much of the material covered in the chemistry section (Chapters 3–11) is from the patent literature. Patents are one of the most valuable sources of early information on developments in medicinal chemistry. Test methods, synthetic procedures, and often activity and toxicity data may appear in these sources and nowhere else. Certainly they often appear many years earlier in patents, even if they do eventually reach other scientific publications. The difficulty in using this source is in sorting out potentially important new clinical candidates from the borderline and the incidentally claimed compounds. This sorting is often done on the basis of limited data and is influenced by personal experience, bias, and reputation of the originating laboratory. It may be helpful to discuss some of the criteria one might use in selecting compounds as being of particular interest. In the main it involves trying to assess the meaningfulness of reported results. Chapter 2 by Swingle in Volume II should be especially valuable to the reader in this regard.

One problem encountered in reading the literature in this area is trying to attach significance to a specific activity level for a compound (particularly in the carrageenan edema assay). The problem arises because the same reference compounds tested in two laboratories in the same assay can be quoted as having activities varying by more than tenfold. Phenylbutazone ED_{50} values against carrageenan rat paw edema have been reported as anywhere from 25 mg/kg to 380 mg/kg. Many laboratories agree in reporting this particular ED_{50} as being in the range of 80–100 mg/kg. Would a compound that is equal to phenylbutazone at 250 mg/kg in an insensitive assay also be equally active at 25 mg/kg in a very sensitive assay? I doubt that it necessarily would. The source of this variation should be examined. Activity figures reported without comparative data for a reference drug are difficult to evaluate.

An important feature of carrageenan-induced paw edema is the biphasic course of its development (Vinegar et al., 1969; Swingle, Fig. 2, Chapter 2, Volume II). During the first hour the inflammation (30% or more) is mediated by histamine and serotonin, and only the later phase is sensitive to true antiinflammatory agents. Some points that may have influenced reported test results and should be considered in interpreting them are the following:

1. The influence of nonantiinflammatory agents on the first phase of the edema (e.g., antihistamines, antiserotonins).

2. Temporal factors in relation to the degree of development of the second phase. At least one laboratory that obtained high ED_{50} values for phenylbutazone measured inhibition after only 2 hours instead of 3 or 4.

3. The edemagenic property of the particular carrageenan preparation used (with reference to both the vascular and cellular phases of the inflammation); the influence thereof on the maximum percent inhibition obtainable with a true antiinflammatory agent.

4. The possible variation with strain of rat in the phase profile of carrageenan-induced edema.

Other aspects of the evaluation of carrageenan test results are documented by Swingle (Chapter 2, Volume II), but some are worth emphasizing here. Nonspecific activity is found for toxic doses of many compounds (mercuric chloride and carbon tetrachloride are two examples), as well as for irritating materials (e.g., carrageenan or powdered glass, i.p.). Niemegeers et al. (1964) reported that 38 of 49 miscellaneous drugs (without established antiarthritic value) had ED_{50} values of 160 mg/kg or less (where the ED_{50} of phenylbutazone was 25 mg/kg) and only eight compounds were without some antiedema activity at the highest dose. These authors suggested that greater reliability would be attained by discarding those compounds obviously exhibiting other biological properties at the effective dose level. For this reason claims of antiinflammatory activity for compounds having other recognized drug effects (other than antipyretic or analgesic activity) must be evaluated with caution.

With precautions the carrageenan assay can be very useful, as exemplified by Wiseman (Chapter 6, Volume II). The behavior of a variety of drug classes on some paw edema assays (formalin, yeast, egg white) shows such poor correlation with known clinical antiinflammatory and antiarthritic activities that it is surprising these assays are still used (see, e.g., Winter, 1965). Unfortunately, many claims for antiinflammatory activity in the patent literature are still based on these rather unpredictive assays.

IV. CLASSICAL NONSTEROIDAL ANTIINFLAMMATORY AGENTS

We propose to define as "classical" any nonsteroidal antiinflammatory agent that is active in the carrageenan and adjuvant arthritis assays, is anti-pyretic, and is active in the UV-erythema assay. The last two criteria eliminate steroids, chloroquine, gold compounds, colchicine, immunosup-pressants, hydroxyphenylbutazone, and basic compounds such as benzy-damine. The adjuvant arthritis assay (therapeutic, rats) and the UV-erythema assay (guinea pigs) in each of which, for example, phenylbutazone is active in the 5–10 mg/kg range are highly sensitive to these classical agents. It is appropriate from a historical viewpoint that the "classical" designation include the salicylates and those compounds classed as "aspirin-like." The neutral compounds indoxole and bimetopyrol (see Shen, Chapter 7 in this volume) are of the classical type by this definition. A common property reported for many of these classical agents is the ability to inhibit prostaglandin synthetase *in vitro*. Some of the consequences of this categorization are discussed below.

If all classical compounds act by the same mechanism(s) and at the same receptor site(s), there is a basis for considering that a biochemical or pharmacological property of one member, if not held by the others, is not important for their primary mechanism of action. On the biochemical level one may expect unique properties for the nonclassical agents, but common biochemical properties between the latter and classical agents cannot be expected to provide reassurance of clinical utility when the assessment has already been made that the classes are different. Are common properties of different classes more likely, in fact, to be irrelevant to the basic mechanism of antiinflammatory action of any of the classes? For example, Carrano and Malbica (1972) recently reported that all antiinflammatory agents tested enhanced $N,N,N'N'$-tetramethylazoformamide-induced lysosomal labil-ization at $10^{-4} M$. These included indomethacin, flufenamic acid, aspirin, hydrocortisone, and chloroquine, representing three classes of agents. I suggest that this is sufficient reason to question whether this assay really represents a fundamental property of any class of antiinflammatory agent.

A consequence of categorization of agents is that new classes of com-pounds can be evaluated more objectively. On the one hand, they have the highly desirable potential for acting by a new mechanism: otherwise re-fractory patients may be benefited; possibilities for synergistic or additive effects may be present. On the other hand, the high predictability from animal model to man is no longer applicable. Clinically useful agents out-side of the classical group deserve to have attention focused on their unique properties. An example would be the specific antiinflammatory activity of colchicine in gout.

V. RECEPTOR SITE FOR CLASSICAL ANTIINFLAMMATORY AGENTS

A number of years ago a hypothetical receptor outline was proposed (Fig. 1) (Scherrer et al., 1964). It was based on structure–activity relationships in a number of chemical series and on the assumption that these agents (Fig. 2) and others not shown acted at the same site. Two primary features where a cationic site and a trough to accept a twisted ring. Shen (1965) proposed a similar receptor based on a careful analysis of structure activity relationships and the preferred configuration in the indomethacin series indicated by spectral and physical data. This was further defined by the activity of a benzylideneindene (Shen, 1967; Shen et al., 1966) (Fig. 3).

Within the last 2 years the very high activity and specificity of many nonsteroidal antiinflammatory agents for the inhibition of prostaglandin synthetase has led to proposals (e.g., Flower et al., 1972) that this property may explain the mode of action of these agents in vivo. This is discussed in detail by Hichens (Chapter 8 Volume II). At the Alza Conference on Prostaglandins, Ham et al. (1972) reported that kinetic studies indicated the conversion of arachidonic acids to PGE_2 (below) is competitively inhibited

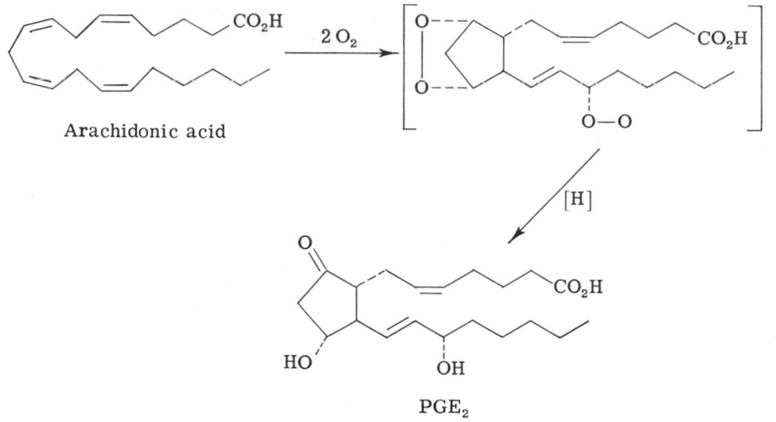

Arachidonic acid

PGE_2

by indomethacin. This means (Ariëns, 1971) that a "relationship in chemical structure may be expected" between the natural substrate–product and the antiinflammatory agent. (Details of the biosyntheses of the prostaglandins have been recently reviewed by Oesterling et al., 1972.)

Prostaglandin E_2 closely resembles classical nonsteroidal antiinflammatory agents in the conformation indicated in Fig. 4. If the role of the receptor is to hold the unsaturated fatty acid in the proper orientation, it may be hypothesized that the trough is the site where the oxygenation–cyclization occurs. The receptor seems to naturally require that the benzoyl-

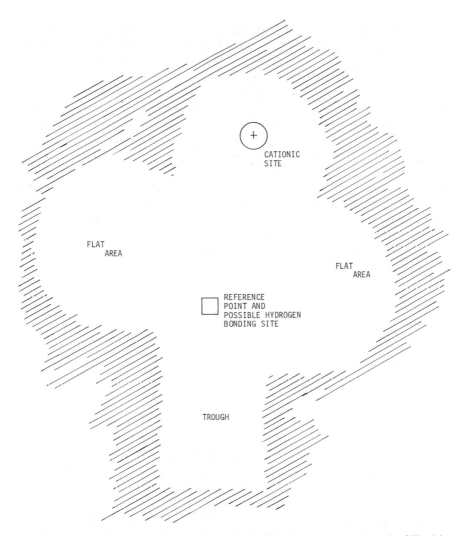

Fig. 1 A hypothetical receptor site derived by superimposing the compounds of Fig. 2 in the orientations indicated (Scherrer *et al.*, 1964). The same receptor design is a model for prostaglandin synthetase. The classical antiinflammatory agents now seem better accomodated on the same receptor in the orientations indicated in Figs. 4 and 5. The reference point underlies the N and carbonyl carbon, respectively, of the fenamic acids and indomethacin. It is about 4.5 Å from the cationic site.

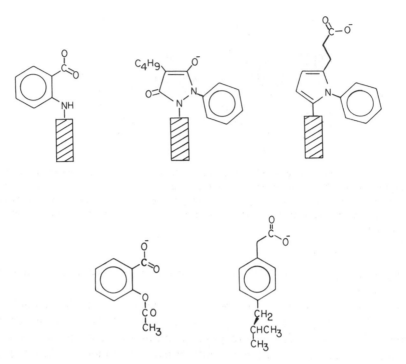

Fig. 2 Relative orientations of some antiinflammatory agents originally used in defining the features of the receptor of Fig. 1. Compounds represented are a fenamic acid, phenyl-butazone, a 1,3-diarylpyrrole-2-propionic acid, aspirin, and ibufenac.

group of indomethacin be situated below the benzo ring as originally proposed by Shen (1965). Reorienting antiinflammatory agents on the receptor of Fig. 1 as indicated in Fig. 5 gives a better fit and the correct absolute configuration for active α-methylarylacetic acids. Comparison of Figs. 3 and 4 will show that these are not merely mirror image changes.

Hoyland and Kier (1972) calculate that PGE_1 should have a preferred conformation in solution that is nearly planar, with both chains extended in parallel arms. This may be the form for some biological activities. However, just as histamine and acetylcholine have multiple receptors, we propose that wherever the classical antiinflammatory agents are potent inhibitors of the action of a *preformed* prostaglandin, this action more likely occurs at a receptor at which the prostaglandin has a conformation similar to that in Fig. 4. An example may be the inhibition of $PGF_{2\alpha}$-induced contraction of human bronchial muscle by meclofenamic acid at 0.1 μg/ml. As meclofenamic acid does not inhibit $PGF_{2\alpha}$-induced bronchoconstriction in the guinea

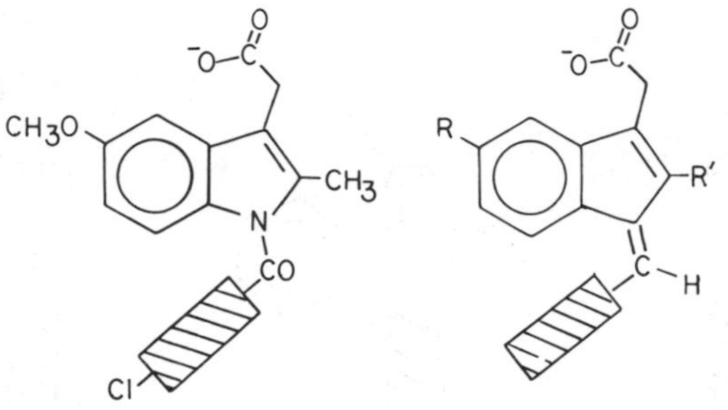

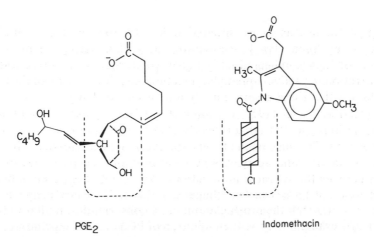

Fig. 3 The configuration of indomethacin as proposed to fit a hypothetical antiinflammatory receptor (Shen, 1965). This receptor has the main features indicated in Fig. 1, but with a different orientation for the trough. The finding of higher antiinflammatory activity in the *cis*-indene compared with the *trans*-indene isostere supports the Shen receptor proposal (Shen, 1967).

pig (Collier, 1971), the $PGF_{2\alpha}$ may be acting in a different conformation in this species.

The UV-erythema assay may be one of the best *in vivo* models available for the inhibition of prostaglandin synthetase. There are very few false positives from this assay. With rare exception, compounds active in this assay are antiedemic (versus carrageenan) and antipyretic (Winder *et al.*, 1967). The reverse correlation from anticarrageenan activity is not nearly as good. Because the UV-erythema assay is more specific, it appears likely that its

PGE₂   Indomethacin

Fig. 4 A possible conformation of PGE_2 at the prostaglandin synthetase antiinflamatory receptor (absolute configuration) compared with indomethacin, a potent inhibitor.

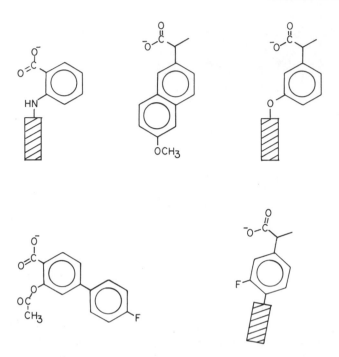

Fig. 5 Some antiinflammatory compounds as they are currently envisioned fitting the receptor of Fig. 1. The location of the cationic site is determined by the requirement to satisfy these diverse agents. Compounds represented are a fenamic acid, *S*-naproxen, *S*-fenoprofen, flufenisal, and *S*-flurbiprofen.

pathology is less complex than the edema models. Winder *et al.* (1958) called UV-erythema an "antipreinflammatory model." It is tempting to propose that the delayed erythema of this model is primarily caused by a prostaglandin. A prostaglandinlike lipid has been detected after UV irradiation of skin (Søndergaard and Greaves, 1970). The carrageenan edema is more complex, although the later phase is mediated by prostaglandin (DiRosa and Willoughby, 1971). Some years ago, H. O. J. Collier tested a large number of compounds in several chemical series (deliberately selected to cover a wide range of UV-erythema potencies) for their ability to inhibit the bronchoconstrictor action of bradykinin and SRS-A in guinea pigs. The rank order correlation of the activity of these dozens of compounds on the latter assays with the UV-erythema potency is highly significant in each series (reported by Winder *et al.*, 1967). There is evidence suggesting SRS-A causes the release (synthesis) of prostaglandin in the guinea pig lung (Piper and Vane, 1969). (Surprisingly the bronchoconstriction induced by bradykinin and SRS-A is almost identically inhibited by a wide variety of antiinflammatory agents—Collier, 1967; Berry and Collier, 1964.)

A very recent development is the disclosure that a variety of antioxidants including phenols and naphthols are inhibitors of prostaglandin synthetase *in vitro*. (Lands *et al.*, 1973; Takeguchi and Sih, 1972). These seem to act reversibly while some of the classical antiinflammatory agents do not. Further study in this area in terms of the receptor and the mode of action and utility of these kinds of agents *in vivo* will be interesting.

VI. LATENT ANTIINFLAMMATORY AGENTS

In the process of categorizing antiinflammatory agents, a decision must be made on the handling of a large group of compounds that may be loosely classified as potential metabolic precursors, or latent drugs. These are compounds envisioned as being susceptible by known hydrolytic or biological pathways to conversion *in vivo* to carboxylic acids. A conservative estimate is that 20% of the current patent literature falls in this category. For the most part, those which are included are described only incidentally in relation to the corresponding acids. Examples of the wide range of compounds that fall into this category are various esters, amides, reduced forms (alcohols, aldehydes), and two-carbon homologs.

In some instances the presence of the active acid metabolite has been demonstrated (e.g., Juby *et al.*, 1972). In others, the identity of structure–activity relationships in the two classes is presumptive evidence that the parent acid is the active form. It might be that some of these compounds have inherent antiinflammatory activity. Activity *in vitro* in inhibiting prostaglandin synthetase would be especially interesting. Whitehouse and Famaey (1973) recently compared a large number of carboxylic antiinflammatory agents with the corresponding alcohols in *in vitro* assays that precluded conversion to the acids. With only one exception, the alcohols were more active than the corresponding acids in inhibiting the incorporation of $[6\text{-}^{3}\text{H}]$ thymidine into thymocytes and in other *in vitro* assays.

There are two classes of acidic agents related to carboxylic acids that are of interest. These are tetrazoles (**1**) and acylsulfonamides (**2**). In this volume they will be found with the related carboxylic acids in Chapters 3 and 4.

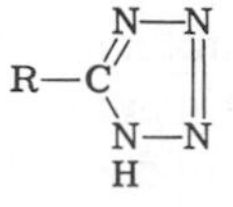

1 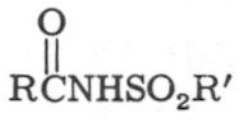   2

VII. TWO NONCLASSICAL ANTIINFLAMMATORY SERIES

A. Chloroquine and Hydroxychloroquine

Consideration was given to allotting a separate chapter to the chloroquine class of antimalarials (represented by **3** and **4**). This became unnecessary

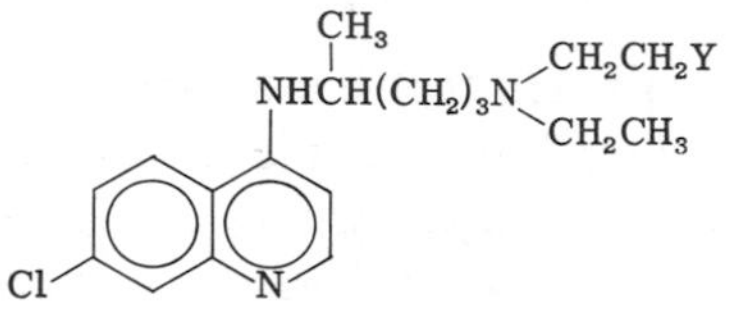

3 Y = H   Chloroquine
4 Y = OH Hydroxy-
            chloroquine

with the publication of "Antimalarial Agents", (a companion volume in this series by Thompson and Werbel, 1972). The problems are rather formidable. There is no biological assay agreed on as predictive of clinical utility for this class, even though Swingle, in Volume II, lists 33 noninfectious systems for the demonstration of various activities for chloroquine. The delay in man of up to 6 months before beneficial effects are prominent makes association with laboratory assays difficult and magnifies the problems in clinical evaluation. Finally, irreversible retinopathy is a serious problem with this class of agents. A recent report indicates some progress in the latter area, with an apparent means for detecting this toxicity while it is still reversible (Young *et al.*, 1972).

The mechanism of action of this class of agents as antiarthritics is certainly of interest because there are no other compounds like them. This topic was recently discussed by Bäumer (1971). Clinical aspects have most recently been reviewed by Lockie (1972). According to the latter author, hydroxychloroquine is the preferred of the two agents.

B. Benzydamine

Benzydamine (**5**) is not discussed elsewhere in this volume. Its inclusion at this point serves to emphasize some of the problems in the evaluation of new agents. Benzydamine is available in some countries outside the United States as an antiinflammatory analgesic. It is not a classical nonsteroidal agent (as defined in Section IV of this chapter), nor is it steroidlike, chloroquinelike, or goldlike. It is not antiarthritic in man. A substantial number of clinical reports indicate benzydamine provides some benefit against inflammation of a "primary" or "normal" type, such as a postoperative or posttraumatic inflammation (Silvestrini, 1968).

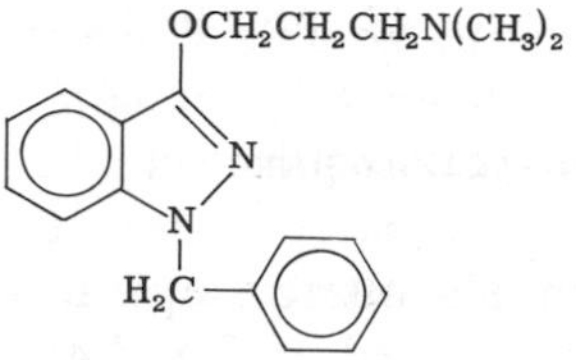

$OCH_2CH_2CH_2N(CH_3)_2$

5

The investigational approach that led to benzydamine was described by Silvestrini (1965,1968). Emphasis was placed on models of inflammatory pain. The pharmacology of benzydamine was outlined by Silvestrini (1965) and later detailed by Silvestrini *et al.* (1966). An interesting report appeared more recently (Boissier *et al.*, 1970) comparing **5** with five classical agents in ten common assays, with dose–response curves plotted. Briefly, benzydamine was active in inhibiting edema induced by a variety of agents, including carrageenan and kaolin. It was inactive in delaying UV-erythema (at 200 mg/kg) and had a weak effect on adjuvant-induced arthritis at 200 mg/kg. There is disagreement as to whether or not **5** is antipyretic and active in the Randall-Selitto yeast hyperesthesia assay for analgesic activity.

Silvestrini (1968) postulates that protection of albumin against denaturation as indicated by the Mizushima assay may have some bearing on the mechanism of action of benzydamine. This assay is increasingly being regarded as too nonspecific to be useful (discussed by Hichens, Chapter 8 in Volume II).

Drug absorption and metabolism studies have been reported (Catanese *et al.*, 1966). Numerous clinical studies are reviewed by De Gregorio (1965, 1968). Topical activity of a moderate degree has been demonstrated in a double-blind trial (Fantato and De Gregorio, 1971).

We are now beginning to see compounds in the patent literature referred to or implied as being "benzydaminelike" based on their pharmacological profiles. The reader is reminded that this kind of classification makes it easy to justify the false positives that would have been discarded in the past. Only careful clinical evaluation can establish whether any of these are truly useful.

VIII. GOALS OF FUTURE RESEARCH

Each author points out, within his own areas of coverage, future goals that might be sought. Gold research (see Chapter 8 by Walz, DiMartino, and Sutton) and steroid research (see Chapter 9 by Popper and Watnick) each deservedly receive new emphasis. The reader will, I feel, find especially interesting Chapter 7 by Shen, in which he discusses the search for new kinds of agents.

The introductory chapter to Volume II is especially thought provoking for anyone looking for new avenues to explore. Chapter 6 by Wiseman in Volume II can be rewardingly read following the chapter by Lombardino in this volume. One goal we can certainly hope to achieve is better predictability from animal to man. The approach outlined by Wiseman is worthy of further study.

REFERENCES

Ariëns, E. J. (1971). *In* "Drug Design" (E. J. Ariëns, ed.), Vol. 1. pp. 162–193. Academic Press, New York.

Ariëns, E. J., Simonis, A. M., and Van Rossum, J. M. (1964). *In* "Molecular Pharmacology" (E. J. Ariëns, ed.), Vol. 1, p. 287. Academic Press, New York.

Bäumer, A. (1971). *In* "Rheumatoid Arthritis" (W. Müller, H.-G. Harwerth, and F. Fehr, eds.), pp. 609–618. Academic Press, New York.

Berry, P. A., and Collier, H. O. J. (1964). *Brit. J. Pharmacol. Chemother.* **23**, 201.

Black, M. L. (1963). *J. Med. Chem.* **6**, 145.

Boissier, J. R., Lwolf, J. M., and Hertz, F. (1970). *Therapie* **25**, 43.

Carrano, R. A., and Malbica, J. O. (1972). *J. Pharm. Sci.* **61**, 1450.

Catanese, B., Grasso, A., and Silvestrini, B. (1966). *Arzneim.-Forsch.* **16**, 1355.

Collier, H. O. J. (1967). *Ann. Phys. Med., Suppl.* pp. 50–54.

Collier, H. O. J. (1971). *Nature (London)* **232**, 17.

De Gregorio, M. (1965). *Int. Symp. Non-Steroidal Anti-Inflammatory Drugs, Proc., 1964.* pp. 422–429.

De Gregorio, M. (1968). *Inflammation, Proc. Int. Symp. 1967.* pp. 175–183.

DiRosa, M., and Willoughby, D. A. (1971). *J. Pharm. Pharmacol.* **23**, 297.

Fantato, S., and De Gregorio, M. (1971). *Arzneim.-Forsch.* **21**, 1530.

Flower, R., Gryglewski, R., Herbaczyńska-Cedro, K., and Vane, J. R. (1972). *Nature (London), New Biol.* **238**, 104.

Ham, E. A., Cirillo, V. J., Zanetti, M., Shen, T. Y., and Kuehl, F. A., Jr. (1972). *In* "Prostaglandins in Cellular Biology" (P. W. Ramwell and B. B. Pharriss, eds.), pp. 345–352. Plenum, New York.

Hendershot, L. C., and Forsaith, J. (1959). *J. Pharmacol. Exp. Ther.* **125**, 237.

Hoyland, J. R., and Kier, L. B. (1972). *J. Med. Chem.* **15**, 84.

Juby, P. F., Hudyma, T. W., and Partyka, R. A. (1972). U. S. Patent 3,663,627 (to Bristol-Myers).

Lands, W. E. M., Letellier, P. R., Rome, L. H., and Vanderhoek, J. Y. (1973). *Adv. Biosciences* **9**, 15.

Lockie, L. M. (1972). *In* "Arthritis and Allied Conditions" (J. L. Hollander and D. J. McCarty, eds.), 8th ed., pp. 483–494. Lea & Febiger, Philadelphia, Pennsylvania.

Moncada, S., Ferreira, S. H., and Vane, J. R. (1972). *Int. Congr. Pharmacol. 5th, 1972* Abstract No. 959.

Niemegeers, C. J. E., Verbruggen, F. J., and Janssen, P. A. J. (1964). *J. Pharm. Pharmacol.* **16**, 810.

Oesterling, T. O., Morozowich, W., and Roseman, T. J. (1972). *J. Pharm. Sci.* **61**, 1861.

Piper, P. J., and Vane, J. R. (1969). *Nature (London)* **223**, 29.

Scherrer, R. A., Winder, C. V., and Short, F. W. (1964). *Nat. Med. Symp. Amer. Chem. Soc., Div. Med. Chem., 1964* Abstract, pp. 11a–11i.

Shen, T. Y. (1965). *Int. Symp. Non-Steroidal Anti-Inflammatory Drugs, Proc., 1964* pp. 13–20.

Shen, T. Y. (1967). *Top. Med. Chem.* **1**, 29–78.

Shen, T. Y. (1972). *Angew. Chem., Int. Ed. Engl.* **11**, 460.

Shen, T. Y., Ellis, R. L., Witzel, B. E., and Matzuk, A. R. (1966). *152nd Meet. Amer. Chem. Soc., 1966* Abstr., 3P.

Silvestrini, B. (1965). *Int. Symp. Non-Steroidal Anti-Inflammatory Drugs, Proc., 1964* pp. 180–189.

Silvestrini, B. (1968). *Inflammation, Proc. Int. Symp. 1967* pp. 26–36.

Silvestrini, B., Gocrau, A., Pozzatti, C., and Cioli, U. (1966). *Arzneim.-Forsch.* **16**, 59.

Søndergaard, J., and Greaves, M. W. (1970). *J. Pathol. Bacteriol.* **101**, 93.

Takeguchi, C., and Sih, C. J. (1972). *Prostaglandins* **2**, 169.

Thompson, P. E., and Werbel, L. M. (1972). "Antimalarial Agents: Chemistry and Pharmacology," pp. 150–196. Academic Press, New York.

Vinegar, R., Schreiber, W., and Hugo, R. (1969). *J. Pharmacol. Exp. Ther.* **166**, 96.

Whitehouse, M. W., and Famaey, J. P. (1973). *Agent. Actio.* **3**, 217.

Wilhelmi, G., Gdynia, K., and Ziel, R. (1968). *In* "Pain" (A. Soulairac, F. J. Cahn, and J. Charpentier, eds.), pp. 373–391. Academic Press, New York.

Winder, C. V., Wax, J., Beer, M., and Rosiere, C. (1958). *Arch. int. Pharmacodyn, Ther.* **116**, 261.

Winder, C. V., Kaump, D. H., Glazko, A. J., and Holmes, E. L. (1967). *Ann. Phys. Med., Suppl.* pp. 7–49.

Winter, C. A. (1965). *Int. Symp. Non-Steroidal Anti-Inflammatory Drugs, Proc., 1964* pp. 190–206.

Winter, C. A., and Flataker, L. (1965). *J. Pharmacol. Exp. Ther.* **150**, 165.

Young, P., Rardin, T., Lankford, B., Young, A., White, G., and Fry, J. (1972). *Arthritis Rheum.* **15**, 464.

Chapter 3

Aryl- and Heteroarylcarboxylic Acids

ROBERT A. SCHERRER

Riker Laboratories, Inc.
3M Center
St. Paul, Minnesota

I. N-ARYLANTHRANILIC ACIDS

A. Introduction

N-Arylanthranilic acids and related compounds are discussed here in more detail than space allows for other classes of agents covered in this volume. Primarily this is to illustrate, with specific examples, some of the problems in interpreting the literature and to give the reader an insight into the extent of work being done today to find new and better antiinflammatory agents of all types.

The *N*-arylanthranilic acids used in man have been given the generic name "fenamic acids." The specific clinically used anthranilic acids, structures (1)–(3), are discussed individually in Section I,C. This is one of

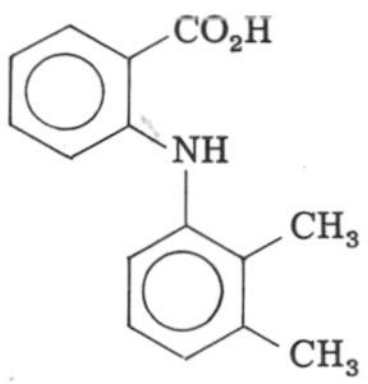

Mefenamic acid   Flufenamic acid   Meclofenamic acid
1   2   3

the earlier deliberately developed classes of agents, following the accidental discovery of the activity of phenylbutazone in man, to exhibit high clinical antiinflammatory activity.

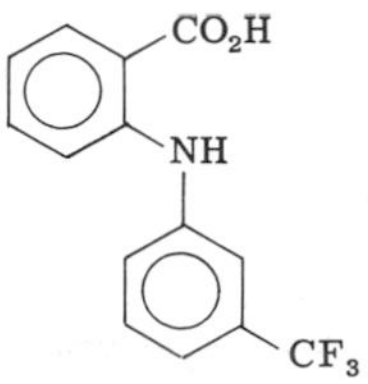

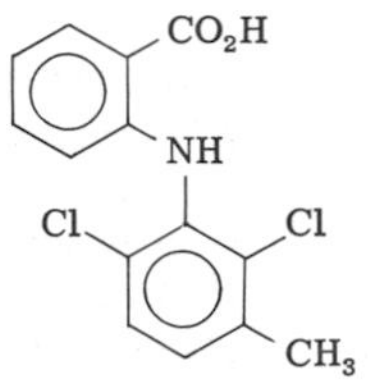

Since the first publication by Parke–Davis (Winder *et al.*, 1962), considerable attention has been given to the biological and biochemical properties of these compounds, their possible modes of action, and their activity in prospective assay procedures. Over 450 references have been compiled for mefenamic acid and over 300 for flufenamic acid through 1971.*

*Bibliographies compiled by the staff of Clinical Development, Parke, Davis and Company.

B. Structure–Activity Relationships

There are no detailed publications from Parke–Davis on structure–activity relationships for the N-arylanthranilic acids, but sufficient information is now available from combined sources to allow some conclusions and structure–activity correlations to be made. Some of these are discussed in the categories of (1) substitution effects, (2) replacement of the nitrogen atom, and (3) the acid function.

To anyone studying structure–activity relationships in this series, the conflicting claims from various laboratories are confusing. The conflict is basically between results from two different assay procedures: the delay of UV-erythema in guinea pigs and the inhibition of carrageenan-induced paw edema in rats. Even aside from interlaboratory variations, smooth relationships that allow some degree of predictability in the former assay are absent in the latter. Some comments on these test methods have been made in the preceding chapter. They are discussed in detail by Swingle (Chapter 2, Volume II).

It is interesting that inhibition of bronchoconstriction induced in the guinea pig by bradykinin, SRS-A, and anaphylaxis shows a high rank order correlation with UV-erythema activity for dozens of anthranilic acids (Winder *et al.*, 1967; Collier, 1967). The N-arylanthranilic acids are exceptional among nonsteroidal antiinflammatory agents in the lack of correlation between anticarrageenan activity and inhibition of prostaglandin synthetase (Ham *et al.*, 1972). The latter may correlate with UV-erythema activity.

Physical and pharmacokinetic factors, such as degree of absorption, half-life, and species variations, are difficult to evaluate. They remain as potential sources for explanations of unexpected or exceptional results.

1. SUBSTITUTION EFFECTS

It is convenient to designate the carboxyl-bearing ring as A and the N-aryl ring as B. The fenamic acids and some heterocyclic analogs seem to be exceptions among nonsteroidal antiinflammatory agents in the marked degree to which substitution can affect activity. Some structure–activity relationships were reported in a symposium on antiinflammatory agents (Scherrer *et al.*, 1964). In general, substitution on the A-ring reduces activity. Two examples are listed in Table I. Of B-ring-monosubstituted derivatives, the order of activity on the UV-erythema assay is generally $3 > 2 > > 4$. The 3-CF_3 derivative is exceptional in its degree of activity compared with other monosubstituted derivatives. This was also found for nicotinic acid analogs of the fenamates (Section II).

TABLE I

Antiinflammatory Activity of *N*-Arylanthranilic Acids

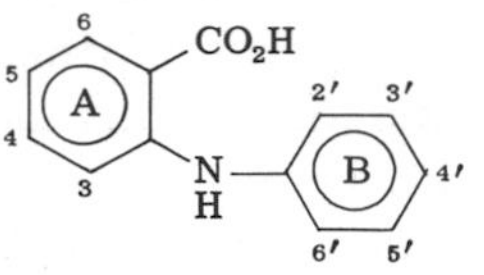

Substitution[a]	Anti-UV-erythema activity, ED_{50} (mg/kg)	Anticarrageenan activity, rat paw: % Inhibition/mg/kg	Anticarrageenan activity, rat paw: $ED_{40,50}$ (mg/kg)
Mefenamic acid	12[b], 16[c], 26[d], 50[e]	30/10[m]45/300[i] 27/40[j], 65/400[k]	50[g], 63[o], 20[e], 75[p,q] 9[r]
Flufenamic acid	4[b], 3.5[e], 11[c], 1.9[d]	39/128[l], 30/3[m], 63/30[n], 37/30[i] 52/40[j]	10[r], 300[i], 25[q]
Meclofenamic acid	0.5[b]	44/50[j]	128[l], 15[o]
Phenylbutazone	6[b], 3.5[d], 20[e], 16[f]	30/22[m], 52/30[n], 38/30[i], 53/100[j], 55/200[k]	100[o], 50[e], 25[r], 100[i], 60[q]
Indomethacin	2[b], 1.4[d]	57/10[j]	6.5[o], 2.2[r], 5[i], 2.4[q]
Aspirin	60[b]	—	150[o], 72[r], 60[m], 75[q]
Unsubstituted		8/150[l]	100[g], 50[e], >> 125[p]
$2\text{-}CH_3$	> 100[g]	10/30[n], 57/100[e]	
$3\text{-}CH_3$		16/30[n]	100[e], ≧ 100[p]
$4\text{-}CH_3$	25[e,h]	10/30[n]	100[e], ≧ 400[p]
2-Cl	—	25/150[l]	—
3-Cl	—	8/150[l]	—
4-Cl	—	0/150[l]	—
4-F	64[c]	—	—
$3\text{-}CF_3$, *see* Flufenamic acid			
5[A],$3\text{-}CH_3O,CF_3$	35[e]	—	—
$2,3\text{-}Cl_2$	3[f]	29/150[l]	—
$2,4\text{-}Cl_2$	200[f]	14/150[l]	—
$2,6\text{-}Cl_2$	—	29/150[l]	—
$2,5\text{-}F_2$	16[c]	—	—
$2,6\text{-}(CH_3)_2$	—	5/150[l]	250[p]
$2,3\text{-}(CH_3)_2$, *see* Mefenamic acid			
$2,3,6\text{-}(CH_3)_3$	6[g]	—	—
3[A],$2,3\text{-}(CH_3)_3$	> 100[g]	24/50[g]	—
$2,3,6\text{-}F_3$	6[c]	—	—
$2,3,5\text{-}F_3$	8[c]	—	—
$2,4,6\text{-}Cl_3$	—	4/150[l]	—
$2,6,3\text{-}Cl_2, CH_3$, *see* Meclofenamic acid			

TABLE I (*continued*)

Substitution[a]	Anti-UV-erythema activity, ED_{50} (mg/kg)	Anticarrageenan activity, rat paw: % Inhibition/ mg/kg	Anticarrageenan activity, rat paw: $ED_{40,50}$ (mg/kg)
2,3,4,6-F_4	50[c]	—	—
2,3,5,6-F_4	0.5[c]	—	—
2,3,5,6-Cl_4	5[c]	—	—
2,3,4,5,6-F_5	12[c]	—	—

[a] B-ring substitution unless otherwise specified.
[b] Winder *et al.* (1967).
[c] Gittos and James (1970).
[d] Alpermann (1970).
[e] Sota *et al.* (1969).
[f] K. F. Swingle (unpublished).
[g] Westby and Barfknecht (1973).
[h] Too low compared with reference agents.
[i] Carrano and Malbica (1972).
[j] Mörsdorf and Wolf (1972).
[k] De Marchi *et al.* (1968).
[l] Juby *et al.* (1968).
[m] Gryglewski *et al.* (1969).
[n] Fujihira *et al.* (1971).
[o] Flower *et al.* (1972).
[p] Izard-Verchere *et al.* (1971).
[q] Ham *et al.* (1972).
[r] Niemegeers *et al.* (1964).

In contrast to the UV results, Sota *et al.* (1969) found that in the carrageenan assay there was little difference in activity between isomeric nitro, methyl, or methoxy derivatives. They felt that the type of substitution was more important than the position of substitution. An example of an extreme in test differences is 6′-carboxyflufenamic acid (**4**), which is more active than

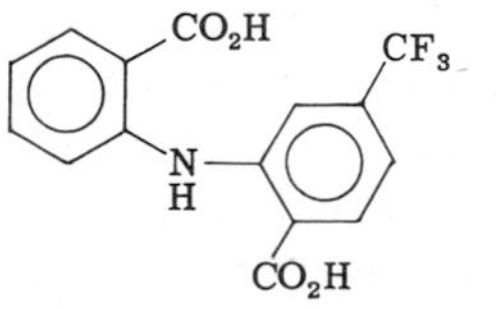

4

phenylbutazone in the carrageenan assay but is inactive against UV erythema. The simple 2′-, 3′-, and 4′-carboxyphenylanthranilic acids are inactive in both assays.

It has been reported that 4′-carbobutoxy (**5**) and related derivatives are more active than mefenamic acid in the formalin edema test (Picciola *et al.*, 1968). Because Winter (1965) has found flufenamic acid to be inactive in

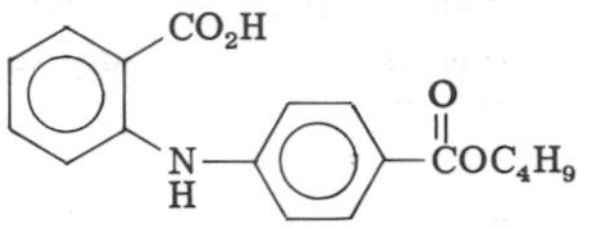

5

this test (at nontoxic doses) my tendency is to disregard all anthranilic acid results from this assay.

Juby *et al.* (1968) have found the 2'-chloro much more active than the 3'-chloro derivative and the latter about the same as the unsubstituted phenyl compound in the carrageenan assay (Table I). This contrasts with UV results, which place 3' > 2'.

2',3'-Disubstituted derivatives are usually the most active compounds with a given pair of substituents (Scherrer *et al.*, 1964). The marked effect of substitution pattern on activity is seen with the 2',3'- and 2',4'-dichloro isomers (**6**) and (**7**) (Table I). These isomers should have about the same

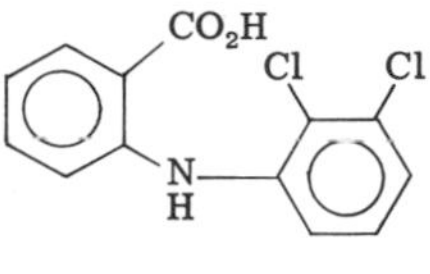

6 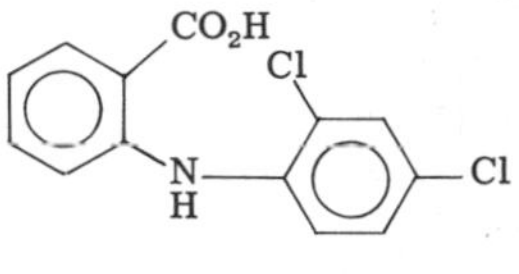   **7**

pK_a, the same partition coefficient, and the same degree of steric hindrance to coplanarity. They would provide a good test pair, along with active and inactive optical isomers, e.g., *S* and *R* isomers of naproxen, to challenge the specificity of *in vitro* and *in vivo* systems for the predictability of classical activity (as defined in the preceding chapter).

2',6'-Dichloro- (Egyesult Gyogyszer es Tapszergyar, 1968) and 3',5'-bistrifluoromethyl-substituted phenylanthranilic acid (Sallmann and Pfister, 1971c) are additional specifically claimed compounds. The latter is active in the range of 10–25 mg/kg in several assays (adjuvant, carrageenan, and UV).

2',3',6'-Trisubstituted compounds are generally the most active with three substituents. Other favorable multisubstituent B-ring patterns (2,3,5-; 2,3,4,6-; and 2,3,5,6-) are indicated in early patents (e.g., Scherrer and Short, 1965). The magnitude of some substitution effects can be seen in Table I (UV-erythema column).

A large number of 2',3'- and 2',3',6'-substituted *N*-arylanthranilic acids having high antiinflammatory activity have been disclosed from the Parke–Davis laboratories. These include nitro (Scherrer, 1963); halogen, alkyl, and alkoxy (Scherrer and Short, 1967); thio, sulfinyl, sulfonyl, and sulfamyl

(Scherrer, 1968a). trifluoromethyl (Scherrer, 1968b); amino (Scherrer, 1968d); and acyl and hydroxyalkyl derivatives (Scherrer, 1968c). (Invaluable support was given to this effort by F. W. Short, J. S. Kaltenbronn, and W. R. N. Williamson of Parke-Davis.)

Among more recent disclosures, the 2',3',5',6'-tetrafluorophenyl derivative of Aspro Nicholas (**8**) (Table I) (Gittos and James, 1970) has an

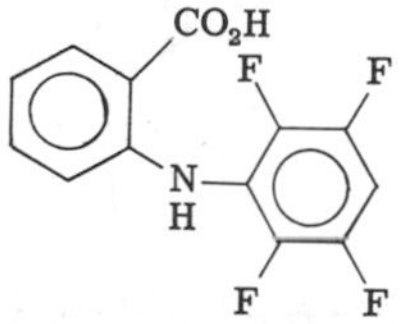

8

especially favorable acute therapeutic index. A report on the fibrinolytic activity of 2,6-dichloro-3-benzylthiophenylanthranilic acid, ASD-30 (Sandoz), has appeared (Van Riezen and Bettink, 1968).

A Russian patent (Yagupolskii *et al.*, 1972) discloses a variety of novelly substituted anthranilic acid derivatives in which the *N*-aryl substituents include $OCHF_2$, SF_3, SO_2CF_3, $SCHF_2$, OCF_3, and SO_2CHF_2 groups. The same laboratory has described adamantyl derivatives, including a 5-(1-adamantyl)mefenamic acid (**9**) (Stepanov *et al.*, 1971) and *N*-[*p*-(CH₂)ₙ-(1-

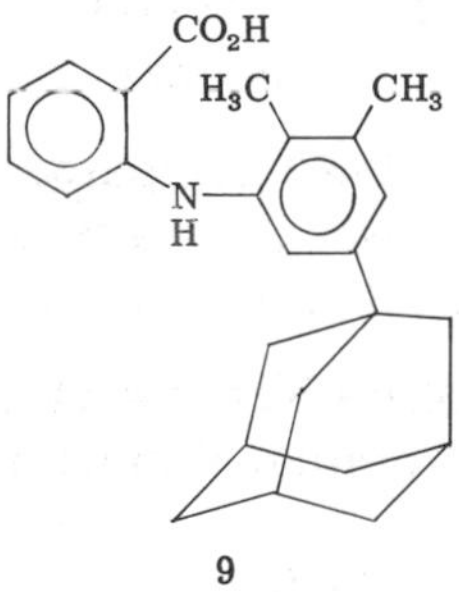

9

adamantyl)phenyl] anthranilic acids (Stepanov *et al.*, 1970, 1971). The latter ($n = 0$) is said to have significant antiinflammatory activity, although it does not fit the usual pattern for good antierythemic activity.

2. REPLACEMENT OF NITROGEN WITH OTHER GROUPS

a. MISCELLANEOUS.   Early reports disclosed that there was a high specificity for —NH— in retaining good antierythemic activity (Scherrer *et al.*, 1964). Single and double atom changes of —O—, —CH₂—, —CO—, —N(COC₆H₅)—, —N(COCH₃)—, —S—, —SO₂—, and —NHCO— were not fruitful in the systems examined.

b. N-NITROSO. A recent paper (Zoni *et al.*, 1971) examines *N*-nitroso-flufenamic acid (**10**, ITF-611) in a wide variety of pharmacological assays.

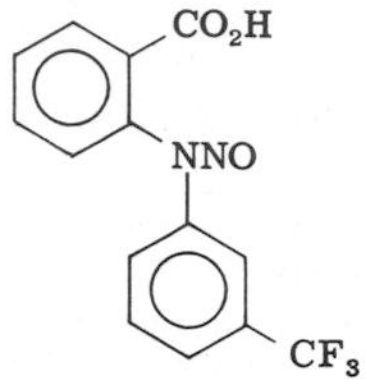

ITF-611

10

It is twice as active as flufenamic acid in antiinflammatory and analgesic assays, including carrageenan edema, cotton pellet granuloma, and yeast hyperesthesia models. On an acute basis, ITF-611 is half as toxic as flufenamic acid, and subacutely seems well tolerated at 20 times the proposed human dose (Zoni and Molinari, 1971). In view of the fact that these compounds readily hydrolyze under mild conditions to the corresponding *N*-arylan-thranilic acid and nitrous acid (Scherrer and Richter, 1965) this compound is not likely to be acceptable clinically. [The *Chemical Abstracts* citation of the latter reference contains an error. It should read a solution of *N*-(2,3-dimethylphenyl)-*N*-nitrosoanthranilic acid in ethanol containing 1% concentrated hydrochloric acid was heated 30 minutes not 30 hours. In a similar experiment hydrolysis was essentially complete by 5 minutes and in the absence of hydrochloric acid by 5 hours.]

c. N-METHYL. Sota *et al.* (1969) compared flufenamic acid and the *N*-methyl derivative. The latter was about a tenth as active as flufenamic acid on the UV assay and about a fourth as active against carrageenan edema.

d. OTHER. Some urea derivatives, e.g. (**11**) (O'Mant and Smith, 1972), are potential antiarthritics by virtue of immunosuppressant activity.

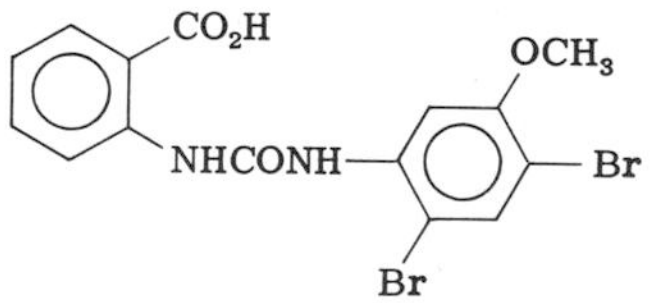

11

N-Alkyl- and *N*-acylanthranilic acids are generally inactive in the UV-erythema screen. Some recently described anthranilic acid derivatives of this type are listed in Table II. The likelihood that these have antiinflammatory activity of the classical type (as defined in the preceding chapter) seems low.

TABLE II

Miscellanous Anthranilic Acid Derivatives

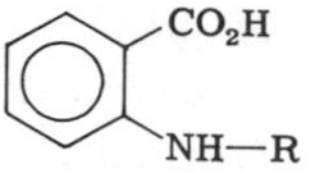

CO$_2$H ... NH—R (anthranilic acid structure)

R	Comments	Reference
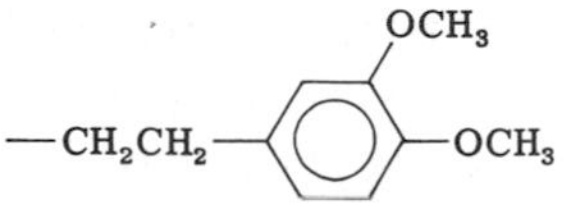 —CH$_2$CH$_2$— (2,4-dimethoxyphenyl)	ED$_{50}$ ca. 100 mg/kg, i.p. (carrageenan edema), but CNS activity at this dose	Gupta et al. (1970).
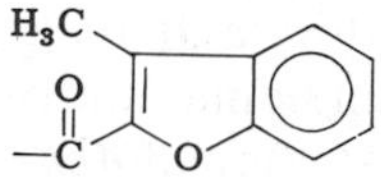 (methylbenzofuran carbonyl)	About equal to ASA; tested at 400 mg/kg	Saksena et al. (1971)
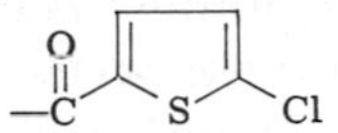 (chlorothiophene carbonyl)	ED$_{50}$ 230 mg/kg (carrageenan edema)	Queval and Falconnet (1972)
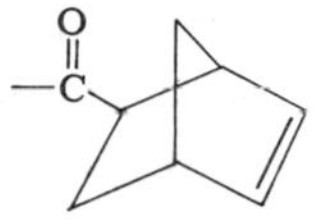 (norbornene carbonyl)	Antiinflammatory, but not primary claim	Yonan (1972)

3. THE CARBOXYLIC ACID FUNCTION

a. ACIDITY; ORTHO REQUIREMENT FOR ACTIVITY. The anthranilic acids are fairly acidic with pK_a's (extrapolated to water) of 4.2 for mefenamic acid, 3.9 for flufenamic acid, and 4 for meclofenamic acid (Winder et al., 1967). These pK_a's are difficult to determine directly with accuracy because of the low solubility of these compounds. The above values have been determined by a variety of methods, including calculation of the degree of ionization in methanol–water mixtures from the UV spectrum, and extrapolation to water (J. M. Vandenbelt, 1964, unpublished). A fair approximation is a pK_a 2.0–2.2 units below the titration value found in 67% dimethylformamide (Scherrer et al., 1964). The pK_a values determined for a series of anthranilic acids by titration in 5–10% acetone (Terada and Muraoka, 1972) appear to be in error from the absolute values and relative values.

The position of the carboxyl is critical for antiinflammatory activity. The m- and p-carboxydiarylamines are inactive (Scherrer et al., 1964). Some homologous acids having good activity are described in Section III,A.

Whitehouse (1967) has explored structure-activity relationships of anthranilic acids and related compounds in uncoupling oxidative phosphorylation. Some of the conclusions of requirements for optimal activity in this class (secondary amine, *o*-carboxyl, aromatic character) correspond with the requirements for antiinflammatory activity. The fenamic acids (1), (2), and (3) uncouple oxidative phosphorylation at 10^{-4} M. However, a number of compounds inactive in antiinflammatory assays also uncouple oxidative phosphorylation, including *N*-(2,4-dinitrophenyl)-anthranilic acid, 3,5-dibromoanthranilic acid, and *N*-benzoylanthranilic acid. It might be of interest to further challenge the correlation of uncoupling activity and antiinflammatory activity with isomeric pairs of active and inactive compounds, such as 2',3'- and 2',4'-dichlorophenylanthranilic acids. It does not seem likely this system will have the receptor specificity of a prostaglandin synthetase. The implications of uncoupling activity in antiinflammatory drugs are unknown.

b. TETRAZOLES. Tetrazoles are metabolically stable acidic functions that have been shown to substitute for carboxyl groups with retention of biological activity. Juby *et al.* (1968) describe a series of tetrazoles, such as (12), related to *N*-arylanthranilic acids, and report comparative anti-

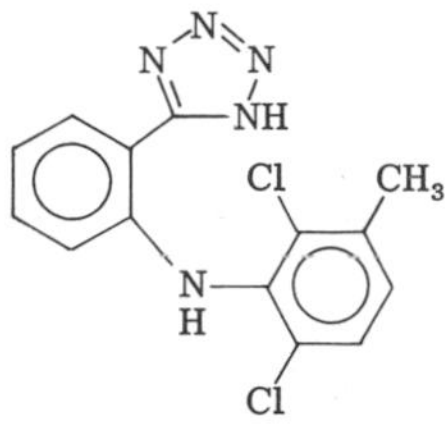

12

edemic activities for the two classes. Activities are generally similar with occasional large differences in both directions (but high dose levels were required for significant activity in this screen).

c. SULFONYLCARBOXAMIDES. Sulfonylcarboxamides (acylsulfonamides) approximate the acidity of carboxylic acids (Basu *et al.*, 1946; Hinman and Hoogenboom, 1961). These derivatives of fenamic acids are of the same order of antiinflammatory activity as the acids (Scherrer, 1969b). An example is *N*-mefenamylmethanesulfonamide (13).

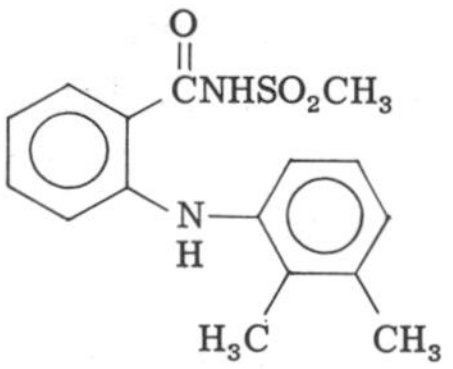

13

C. Fenamic Acids

The N-arylanthranilic acids are first described as antiinflammatory agents in a series of reports from Parke–Davis by Winder and associates on mefenamic acid (1) (1962), flufenamic acid (2) (1963), and meclofenamic acid (3) (1965). The pharmacology, toxicology, metabolism, and clinical tolerance in man, along with a historical background, are contained in the report of a symposium, *Fenamates in Medicine* (Winder et al., 1967). Other papers from the same symposium describe detailed clinical studies. The fenamic acids are discussed individually in Section I, C,1–3. Table III lists the activity levels found for these compounds in a variety of screens. Updated bibliographies on each compound are available from the Parke–Davis Clinical Investigation Department.

1. MEFENAMIC ACID

Mefenamic acid (1) is marketed in the United States as an analgesic with a strict 7-day limitation of its use. It is available overseas as an antiinflammatory analgesic. Considerable detail on its pharmacology, toxicology, and clinical properties is available in "Official Literature on New Drugs" (1968). Its efficacy as an analgesic has been supported in a recent large-scale multiagent trial at the 250-mg dose level (Moertel et al., 1972). However, its continued use has also been criticized (Anonymous, 1972). Apparently the liability of a possible allergic diarrhea (Winder et al., 1967) is a factor in limiting the period of administration. The initial trials of mefenamic acid as an analgesic were encouraged by the presumption that it had central analgesic activity like aminopyrine (Winder et al., 1962, 1967). This was determined by a procedure modified to minimize inflammation (pressure on the rat tail with a smooth bar). Mefenamic acid is the only member of the series to have this property at near the same level as its UV-erythema potency. The possibility of a counterirritant effect being responsible for the analgesic activity (Winter and Flataker, 1965a) is reduced by the subsequent finding of activity after p.o. as well as i.p. administration (Winder et al., 1967). The question whether antiinflammatory agents have independent analgesic activity or act by virtue of reducing inflammation is discussed in the preceding chapter. Collier (1967) believes that writhing data (see Table III) support the projection of clinical analgesic activity for all three fenamic acids. The yeast hyperesthesia results of Winter (Table III) are also felt to predict this. At any rate, many antiinflammatory agents, including flufenamic acid, do relieve pain in man (Van Coller, 1970; Kater, 1968).

Details of metabolism studies in man are disclosed by Glazko (Winder et al., 1967). Mefenamic acid is metabolized to a dicarboxylic acid, (15),

TABLE III

Selected Biological Properties of Fenamic Acids

	Mefen-amic acid, **1**	Flufen-amic acid, **2**	Meclo-fenamic acid, **3**	Phenyl-butazone	Indo-meth-acin	Aspirin
Dose level[a]						
Antiinflammatory dose in man						
gm/day	1.5–2.0	0.6	0.1	0.4[b]	0.07–0.1	2.5
mg/kg/day	21–28	8.5	1.4	5.7	1.0–1.4	36
UV-erythema, ED_{50}, guinea pig[c]	12	4	0.5	6	2	75
Carrageenan rat-paw edema, ED_{50}[e]	75	25	15[d]	60,100[d]	2.4	75
Prostaglandin synthetase, $\mu g/ml$[e]	0.50	0.70	0.03[d]	3.8,2.2[d]	0.16	15
Bradykinin-induced bronchoconstriction; MED, i.v., guinea pig[f]	—	—	0.06	—	2	2
Antianaphylactic, mepyramine pre-treated, MED, guinea pig[f]	32	4	1	—	—	64
Acetyl choline-induced writhing, mouse, ED_{50}[g]	77	33	11	62	0.5	54
Relative potencies						
Adjuvant arthritis, rats[h]						
18 days prophylactic	0.5	2.6	6.7[i]	1.0	—	0.06[i]
6 weeks, therapeutic	0.4	4.6[j]	—	1.0	—	—
Antipyretic, rat[c]	ca 1	> 1	> 20[k]	1.0	33–67	—
Yeast hyperesthesia[l]	2.0	10.3	—	—	27.7	1.0
Antigranulation, cotton pellet, rat, 7 days[c]	0.6	3.6	14[m]	1.0	32	
Toxicity						
Acute LD_{50}, rat[c]	1420	430	126	—	—	—
Subacute LD_{50}, rat						
14 days, 7-day dose[c]	415	107	38	702	6.7	—
Subacute LD_{50}, guinea pig, 14 days, 5-day dose (sodium salts)[f]	249	294	127	—	—	—

[a] Dose levels are mg/kg, p.o., unless otherwise stated. MED, minimum effective dose.
[b] The long half-life of phenylbutazone in man, 72 hours, must be considered in comparing animal and clinical potencies. See Wiseman, Chapter 6, Volume II.

[c] Winder et al. (1967).   [g] Collier et al. (1968a).   [k] −1.5°C at 5 mg/kg.
[d] Flower et al. (1972).   [h] Winder et al. (1969).   [l] Winter and Flataker
[e] Ham et al. (1972).   [i] Schardein et al. (1969).   (1965b).
[f] Collier et al. (1968b).   [j] At 0.4–3.6 mg/kg.   [m] At 0.7–7 mg/kg.

having a longer half-life in man (ca. 15 hours) than the parent molecule (2–4 hours). The intermediate (**14**) has moderate activity; (**15**) is inactive in

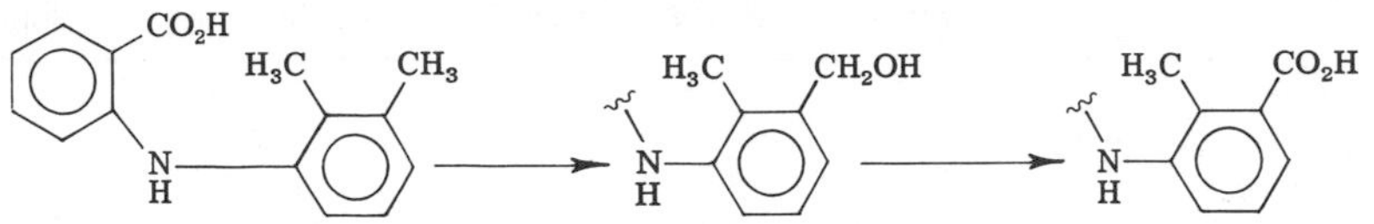

antiinflammatory screens. Interesting species differences in the metabolism are discussed by Ober (Chapter 10, Volume II).

A Russian paper on the pharmacology of mefenamic acid has appeared (Mokhort and Korkhova, 1968), as have studies of the activity and toxicity of a combination of mefenamic and salicylic acids (Kirichek, 1971; Kirichek and Trinus, 1971).

2. FLUFENAMIC ACID

Flufenamic acid (**2**) is widely available outside of the United States. It is also being marketed as the aluminum salt (by the Taisho Co.). The pharmacology is reviewed by Winder *et al.* (1963, 1967). The pharmacology of aluminum flufenamate is essentially the same as the acid, with some delay in peak effects in some acute models (Maruyama *et al.*, 1969).

Clinical studies on flufenamic acid are no longer being carried out in the United States (by Parke–Davis). Reports of about a dozen clinical trials are contained in the symposium proceedings *Fenamates in Medicine* (1967). Another series of clinical studies has appeared in *Profile of an Antirheumatic Compound* (1969). The clinically recommended dose is in the 600-mg/day range. Potential new applications may arise from the finding by Panse *et al.* (1971) that flufenamic acid is absorbed topically from an ointment through the intact skin of rabbits (blood levels) and the backs of rats (antiedema activity versus carrageenan).

The metabolism of flufenamic acid has been extensively studied. A fairly detailed review by Glazko is available (Winder *et al.*, 1967). As with mefenamic acid, there are considerable species differences in metabolism. The main course of metabolism in man is ring hydroxylation in the 4 and 4′ positions. Metabolite II, the 4′-hydroxy derivative, is formed to the extent of 42%. Flufenamic acid has a half-life of 2–4 hours in man but only reaches maximum blood levels at 6 hours (in one study). Enterohepatic circulation of drug and metabolites is evident in man and demonstrated in animals. A consequence of enterohepatic circulation in rats is that an intramuscular dose is 0.95 as ulcerogenic as one given p.o. (Wax *et al.*, 1970). Further details are given by Ober (Chapter 10, Volume II).

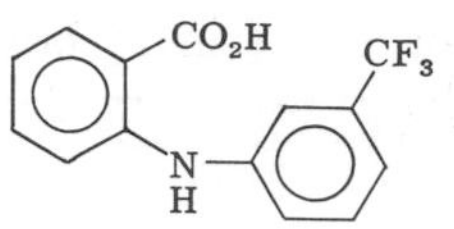

2

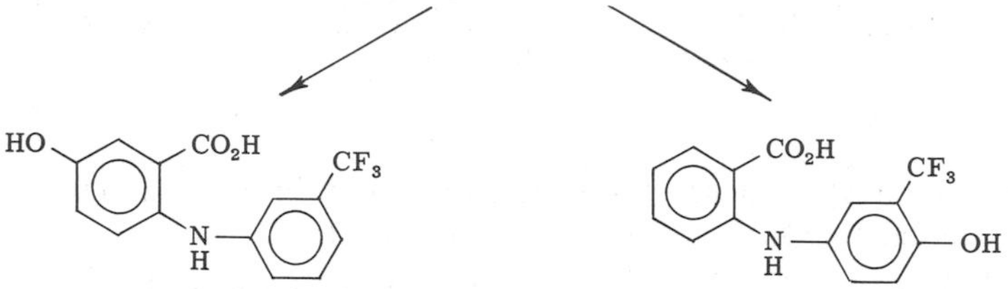

Metabolite I   Metabolite II

3. MECLOFENAMIC ACID

Meclofenamic acid (**3**, CI-583) is currently under clinical investigation by Parke–Davis. It is the most potent of the three in a variety of animal models and many *in vitro* assays (Table III) (Winder *et al.*, 1965). It is particularly active in inhibiting prostaglandin synthetase *in vitro* (Flower *et al.*, 1972), in which it had an ED_{50} value of 0.03 μg/ml. There is one report of a double-blind clinical study that indicated efficacy at 100 mg/day in rheumatoid arthritic patients (de Salcedo *et al.*, 1970). Neither meclofenamic, nor flufenamic, nor mefenamic acid is uricosuric (Robinson and Radcliff, 1972). Reproduction studies in rabbits and rats are reported by Schardein *et al.* (1969).

4. NEUTRAL AND BASIC POTENTIAL PRECURSORS

Some of the variety of carboxyl modifications that have the potential to act as metabolic precursors to a carboxyl group are listed in Chapter 2, Section VI. Many compounds of this type related to fenamic acids share in common a biologically similar activity and a patentably distinct structure. As mentioned earlier, the practical potential advantages are not usually determinable from the available literature. The listing in Table IV will serve to give the reader a feeling for this aspect of medicinal research. As one may expect, where metabolic activation is required, there is likely to be some degree of activity variation with species. Many of these, for example, are not active in the guinea pig (UV-erythema assay) but are active in the rat and could be active in man. Lower acute toxicities and lower ulceration potential in certain animal models are generally claimed as properties of this group. As noted in Section I,C,2, however, a recent study (Wax *et al.*, 1970) found that in rats, flufenamic acid is 95% as ulcerogenic given intramuscularly as

TABLE IV

Nonacidic Carboxyl Variations of the Fenamic Acids[a]

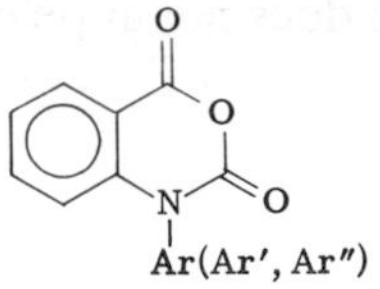

Scherrer (1966) 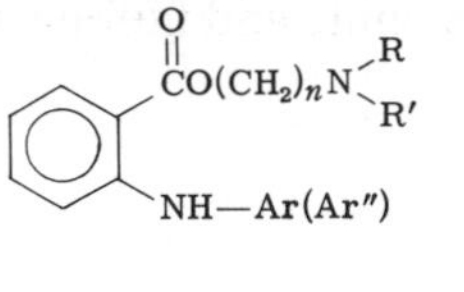   Scherrer and Short (1969) 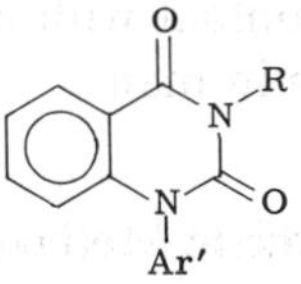   Yaburchi *et al.* (1971)

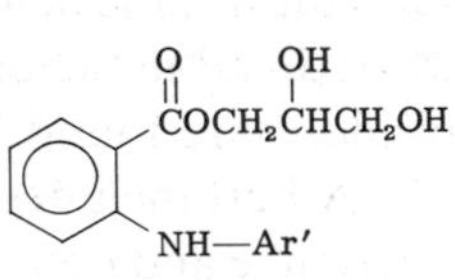

Sherlock (1972b) 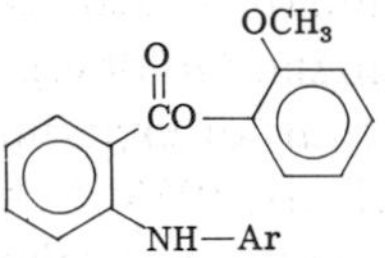   De Marchi *et al.* (1968)

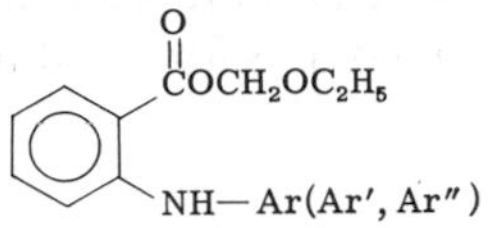

Manghisi (1972) 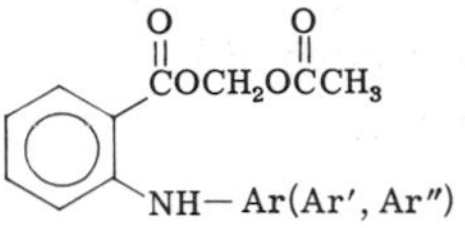   Manghisi (1972)

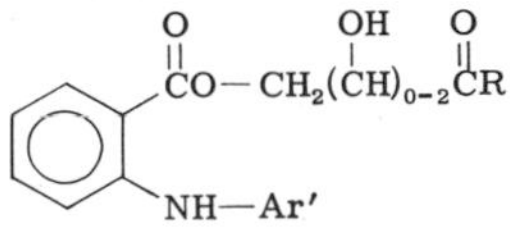

Boltze *et al.* (1971a) 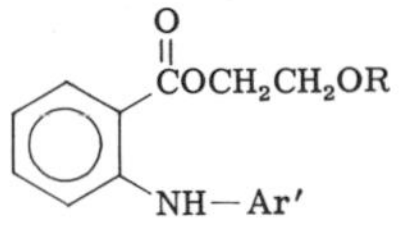   Boltze *et al.* (1971b)

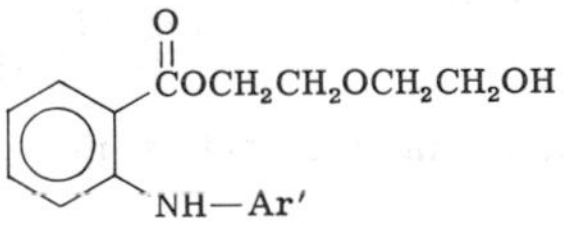

Boltze and Lorenz (1970) 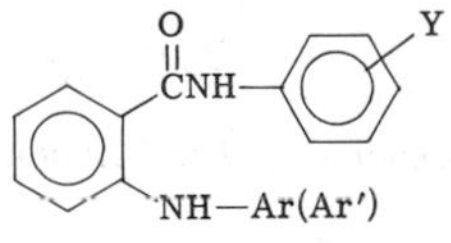   Spano and Marri (1968) Linari and Spano (1971)

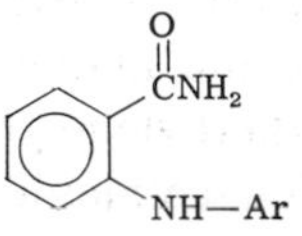

Nakanishi *et al.* (1967) 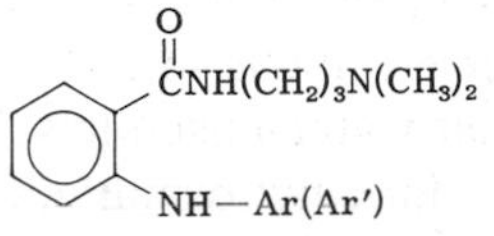   Alkede and Neuhold (1969) 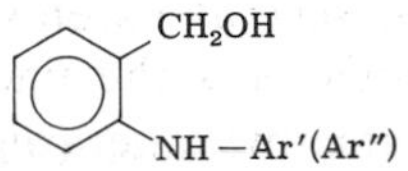   Ross and Zirkle (1970)

[a] Ar = 2,3-xylyl; Ar′ = α,α,α,-trifluoro-3-tolyl; Ar″ = 2,6-dichloro-3-tolyl.

orally because of an enterohepatic circulation of the free and conjugated drug. A real advantage for any latent drug of this class would seem to require the absence of enterohepatic circulation in man. Stomach ulceration from initial contact with mefenamic and flufenamic acid does not appear to be a problem in man.

D. Synthetic Methods

1. ULLMANN-GOLDBERG CONDENSATIONS

The most commonly used routes to N-arylanthranilic acids are the type I and type II Ullmann-Goldberg reactions* outlined in Scheme I. Extensive reviews with details of experimental procedure are found in two volumes on acridines (Albert, 1966; Acheson, 1956). Albert includes many personal observations from his own laboratory experience and detailed procedures. Both include extensive tabulations of N-arylanthranilic acids, with routes, yields, and melting points. Acheson lists several hundred compounds. These compounds have been of interest as intermediates for acridine antimalarials and phenothiazines.

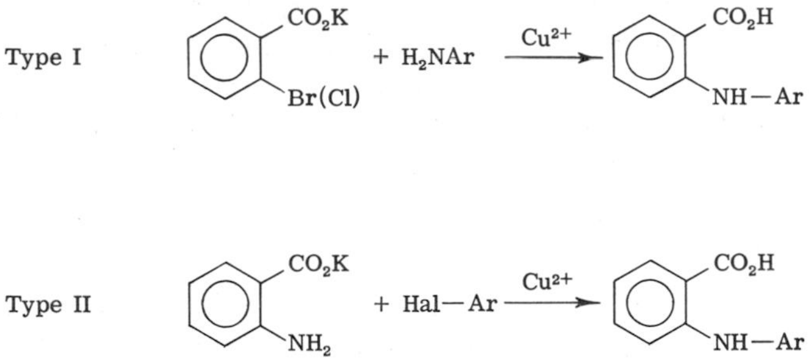

Type I

$$\text{(ring)} \begin{array}{c} CO_2K \\ Br(Cl) \end{array} + H_2NAr \xrightarrow{Cu^{2+}} \text{(ring)} \begin{array}{c} CO_2H \\ NH-Ar \end{array}$$

Type II

$$\text{(ring)} \begin{array}{c} CO_2K \\ NH_2 \end{array} + Hal-Ar \xrightarrow{Cu^{2+}} \text{(ring)} \begin{array}{c} CO_2H \\ NH-Ar \end{array}$$

Scheme I. The Ullmann N-arylanthranilic acid syntheses.

The condensation reactions (Scheme I) six decades after Ullmann's discovery, still maintain an aura of art rather than science about them. Modifications developed in the Parke–Davis laboratories are illustrated in several patents (Scherrer, 1968a–d). Of interest since the above two reviews is the finding that water-miscible solvents, e.g., diethylene glycol dimethyl ether (diglyme), dimethylformamide, and dimethylacetamide, are much more convenient to use than isoamyl alcohol. Special preparations

---

*This is often shortened to "the Ullmann reaction," even though the Ullmann diaryl coupling reaction is given the same name.

for metalic copper catalysts are described in the literature, but it appears that copper ion (cupric is assumed) is the actual catalyst. One will find that when preformed potassium o-bromobenzoate and copper metal are used with potassium carbonate as a base, there is an induction period when no CO_2 evolution (i.e., no reaction) occurs until the blue color of cupric ion appears. Cupric acetate is a satisfactory catalyst. The course of the reaction can be followed by CO_2 evolution.

In recent Russian work (Yagupolskii et al., 1972), the preferred route to these compounds was to use 2-chloro-5-nitrobenzoic acid for the Ullmann condensation and then to remove the nitro group by reduction and diazotization. A detailed example of this kind of process is described by Scherrer (1965a).

The type I Ullmann reaction with weakly basic hindered anilines (e.g., 2,6-dichloro-3-toluidine), a characteristic of precursors of many highly active anthranilic acids, leaves much to be desired. Anhydrous conditions are desirable because water (as well as any alcohol solvent) competes with the aniline to produce salicylic acid (or derivatives). The use of preformed potassium o-halobenzoate with or without small to equimolar amounts of N-ethylmorpholine is convenient. There must be some degree of Ar–X bond breaking in the transition state of the usual Ullmann reactions because the relative reactivity of the halogens in both type I and type II reactions is Br > Cl > F. o-Iodobenzoic acid under the usual conditions offers no advantages, possibly because of steric hindrance to formation of an intermediate copper chelate. Selective type II reactions with bromine over chlorine in mixed halogen-containing aromatic derivatives are practical.

2. CHAPMAN REARRANGEMENTS

a. TYPE I. The Chapman reaction now also has type I and type II counterparts. The first modification of the Chapman synthesis of diarylamines for N-arylanthranilic acids (type I) is described by Jamison and Turner (1937) and outlined in Scheme II. It has recently been reviewed by Schulenberg and Archer (1965). The modification is advantageous when a particular substituted salicylic acid is available. R of the N-arylimidate (16) may be phenyl, t-butyl, CCl=N—Ar, or a variety of other non-α-hydrogen-bearing functions (Scherrer, 1965b; cf. Scherrer, 1968a). The rearrangement takes place at a lower temperature when R = t-butyl instead of the usual phenyl.

b. TYPE II. A modification, outlined in Scheme II, was devised to allow phenols to be used as precursors to the B ring of N-arylanthranilic acids (Scherrer and Short, 1967; Westby and Barfknecht, 1973). It happens,

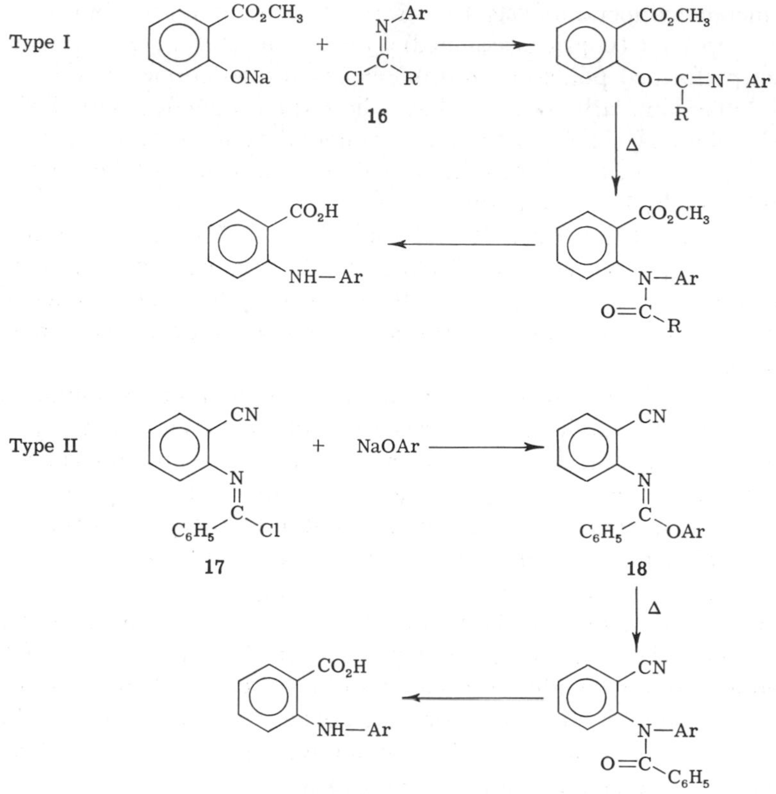

Scheme II. Chapman N-arylanthranilic acid syntheses.

conveniently, that steric hindrance and o-electron-withdrawing groups in the phenol (B-ring precursor Ar of **18**), factors that in $ArNH_2$ impede the type I Ullmann reaction, favor the type II Chapman. The required benz-imidoyl chloride (**17**) is conveniently prepared in one step from benzoylan-thranilamide, thionyl chloride, and collidine (Scherrer and Short, 1967). Simple benzoylanthranilic acid esters, under the usual conditions for imidoyl chloride formation, cyclize to the benzoxazinone (**19**).

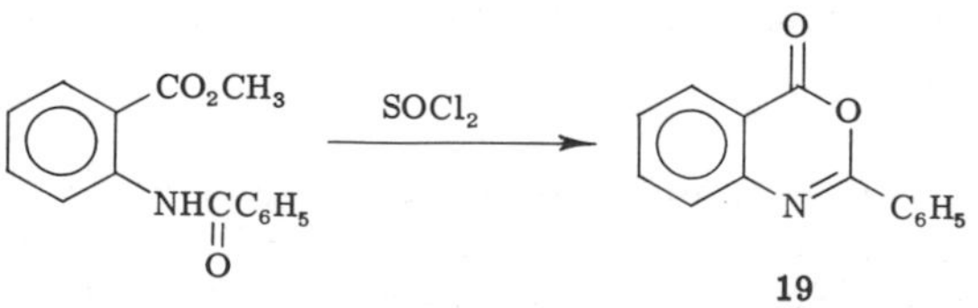

3. CHICHIBABIN REARRANGEMENTS

An alternative route to *N*-arylanthranilic acids, with a phenol as the B-ring precursor, is a Chapman equivalent in which the nitrogen is part of a heterocycle. The procedure outlined in Scheme III, makes use of a double rearrangement of 2,4–diaryloxyquinazolines (Scherrer, 1965c; Juby *et al.*, 1968). Further details of the rearrangement (Chichibabin rearrangement) have recently appeared (Scherrer and Beatty, 1972).

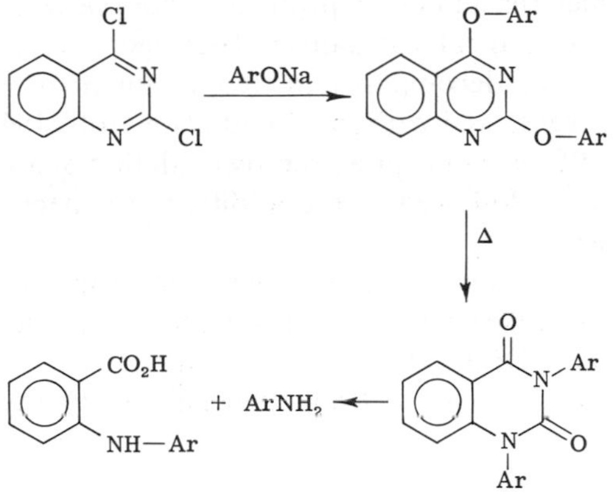

Scheme III

4. DIPHENYLIODONIO-2-CARBOXYLATE CONDENSATIONS

There is a new route to *N*-arylanthranilic acids, Scheme IV, the description of which has only appeared in the patent literature (Scherrer, 1965d). It has been found that diphenyliodonio-2-carboxylate (DPIC) undergoes cupric

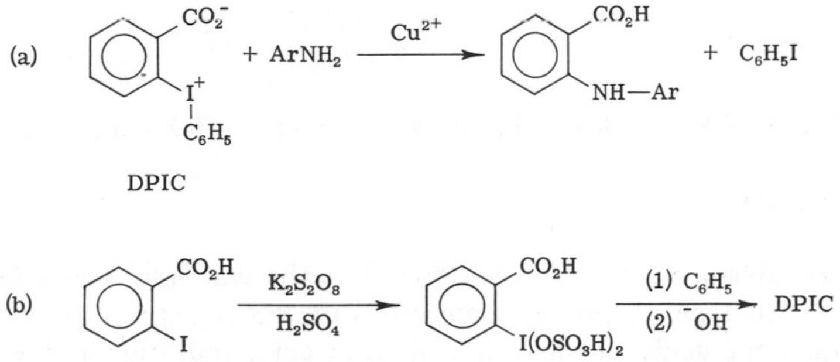

Scheme IV. Diaryliodonio-2-carboxylate (DPIC) route to *N*-arylanthranilic acids.

ion-catalyzed nucleophilic displacement reactions. This reaction corresponds to the type I Ullmann reaction in that it is a one-step reaction using an aniline as the B-ring precursor. This route is especially useful for weakly basic and/or hindered anilines. Condensations occur at 80°C or lower in such diverse solvents as isopropanol, 1,2-dichloroethane, and acetone. The reaction is cupric ion-catalyzed and is highly specific toward displacement of iodobenzene as opposed to *o*-iodobenzoic acid.

This selectivity and cupric ion catalysis contrasts with simple diaryliodonium salts, which react under cuprous ion catalysis with little selectivity, probably by a free-radical mechanism (Beringer and Falk, 1964). The iodonio-2-carboxylate decomposes at temperatures of about 160°C to benzyne, iodobenzene, and carbon dioxide (Le Goff, 1962; Beringer and Huang, 1964). DPIC is readily prepared by oxidation of *o*-iodobenzoic acid with persulfuric acid, followed by the addition of benzene to the reaction mixture (Scheme IV).

DPIC has a particular advantage over potassium *o*-halobenzoate in cupric-catalyzed displacement reactions with anionic nucleophiles. The transition state with DPIC involves a partial neutralization of charges in contrast to the requirement to bring two anions together in the second situation.

5. N-ARYLHYDROXYLAMINE CONDENSATIONS

A synthesis of *N*-arylanthranilic acids, remarkable for its high reported yields if not for the ready availability of starting materials, is the reaction of *o*-iodobenzoic acid with *N*-arylhydroxylamines in isopropanol or benzene to give flufenamic acid (90.5%) and meclofenamic acid (91.5%) (Moriyama *et al.*, 1971). The type II equivalent, with *N*-hydroxyanthranilic acid and an iodobenzene, also occurs in high yields.

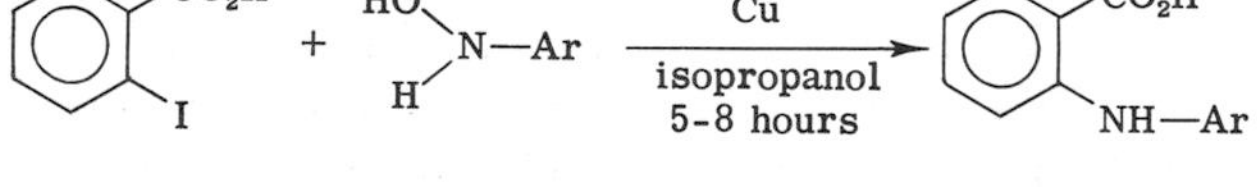

II. HETEROCYCLIC ISOSTERES OF N-ARYLANTHRANILIC ACIDS

A. Introduction

Considerable synthetic effort has gone into the search for active heterocycles of this type. Resulting compounds of special interest include the anilinonicotinic acids, clonixin and niflumic acid, and some highly active anilinothiophenecarboxylic acids. The B-ring structure–activity patterns seem to parallel those for the anthranilic acids (Sherlock and Sperber, 1967).

Synthetic procedures, in general, also parallel those for the anthranilic acids; exceptions are noted in the appropriate sections.

B. Anilinonicotinic Acids

1. CLONIXIN

The pharmacology of clonixin (**20**) has been described in detail (Watnick *et al*., 1971). Its activity is of the order of flufenamic acid and phenylbutazone in most assays. Beyond this the important factors to be considered are safety and freedom from side effects. Clonixin appears to be less ulcerogenic than flufenamic acid in rats. It is especially active as an analgesic in animal models, including the monkey (Ciofalo *et al*., 1972). In two double-blind trials against surgical and postpartum pain, 600 mg of clonixin have been found about equivalent to 10 mg of morphine, i.p. (Finch and De Kornfeld, 1971). Numerous related compounds are described by Sherlock and Sperber (1967). The glyceryl ester of clonixin, clonixeril, is apparently of special interest. A newer member of the series is flunixin which has a trifluoromethyl group in place of the chloro.

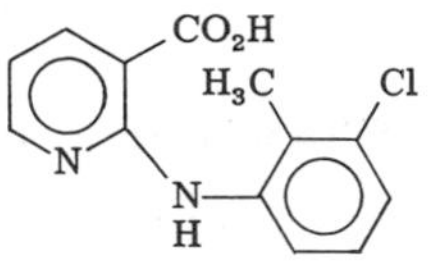

Clonixin

20

2. NIFLUMIC ACID

Another A-ring heterocycle studied in man is niflumic acid (**21**). The pharmacology of (**21**) has been directly compared with five other agents (Boissier *et al*., 1970). This interesting paper gives plots of dose–response curves for flufenamic acid, indomethacin, phenylbutazone, aspirin, and benzydamine in a variety of animal assays. The metabolism (Boissier *et al*., 1971) and clinical trials (Camus, 1968) have been described. The nicotinic acid isomer triflocin (**22**), interestingly, is diuretic as well as antiinflammatory (Littell *et al*., 1969; Cummings *et al*., 1968). It appears that 2-anilinonicotinic acids are generally, about as active in antiinflammatory assays as the corresponding fenamic acids (within a factor of two), depending on the particular test system.

Evans *et al*. (1967) compared flufenamic acid and three aza analogs in two assays. The 4-aza isomer (**23**) was essentially inactive (Table V).

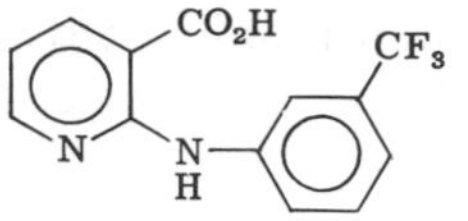

Niflumic acid	Triflocin	
21	**22**	**23**

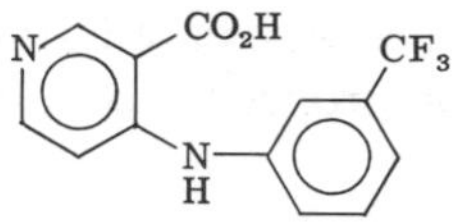

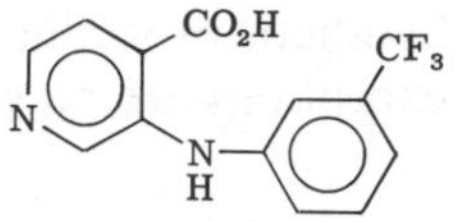

Tetrazole analogs are described for several 2-anilinonicotinic acids, e.g., (**24**), by Chausse (1971).

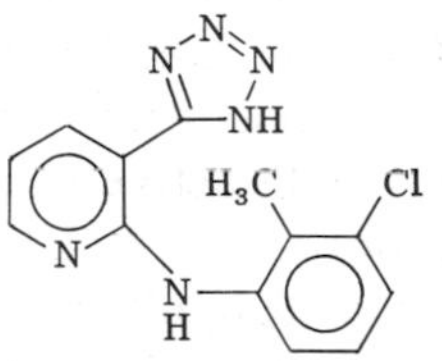

24

3. OTHER NICOTINIC ACID DERIVATIVES

a. 2-AMINO DERIVATIVES. Spano and Linari (1971) report high anticarrageenan edema activity for a series of N-substituted 2-aminonicotinic acids. Some of these activities are surprising in view of the general correspondence of the nicotinic and anthranilic acid series. It would be unexpected if, for example, the N-cyclohexyl and N-benzyl derivatives are active in the UV-erythema screen. A variety of anilinonicotinic acids and related derivatives have been prepared for antiinflammatory testing (Nantka-Namirski, 1967).

b. 2-ARYLOXY AND 2-ARYLTHIO DERIVATIVES. Two third-generation series are 2-aryloxy- and 2-arylthionicotinic acids (Blum, 1970, 1971). These are different from the arylamino derivatives in their structure–activity relationships. Unsubstituted phenyl derivatives are equal to, or more active than, derivatives substituted as the fenamic acids are (carrageenan assays). Some results are presented in Table VI. One must use reservation in interpreting results from compounds administered intraperitoneally.

TABLE V

Aza Derivatives of Flufenamic Acid

Compound	Inhibition of carrageenan-induced edema at 200 mg/kg (%)	Inhibition of UV erythema at 100 mg/kg (%)
2	70	78 (at 25 mg/kg)
21	69	94
22	40	88
23	30	0

TABLE VI

Nicotinic Acid Derivatives

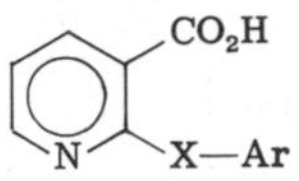

Ar	X	Inhibition of carra-geenan edema at 100 mg/kg (p.o.?) $(\%)^a$	Inhibition at 1/25 acute LD_{50}, i.p. $[\%/(mg/kg)]^b$
C_6H_5	O	43	71/48
C_6H_5	S	61	—
$3\text{-}CF_3C_6H_4$	S	60	—
$3\text{-}CF_3C_6H_4$	O	—	33/30
$2,4\text{-}Cl_2C_6H_3$	O	—	40/56
$3\text{-}CF_3C_6H_4$ (niflumic acid)	N	55	65^c

[a] Blum (1971).
[b] Blum (1970).
[c] At 100 mg/kg.

C. Other A-Ring Heterocycles

1. ANILINOTHIOPHENECARBOXYLIC ACIDS

Some 4-anilino-3-thiophenecarboxylic acids are highly active, equal to or more active than the corresponding anthranilic acids (Table VII; Alper-

TABLE VII

Anilinothiophenecarboxylic Acids

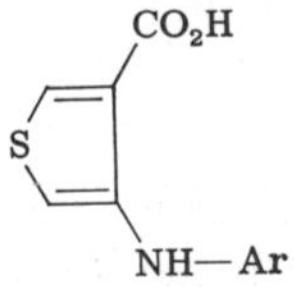

Ar	UV-erythema, ED_{50} $(mg/kg)^a$
$2,3\text{-}CH_3ClC_6H_3$	0.8
$2,6\text{-}Cl_2C_6H_3$	1.7
$2,3\text{-}(CH_3)_2C_6H_3$	$[3.5]^b$
Mefenamic	26^c
Flufenamic	1.9
Phenylbutazone	3.5

[a] Alpermann (1970).
[b] "Equal to phenylbutazone," Ruschig et al. (1969).
[c] Too high relative to reference values.

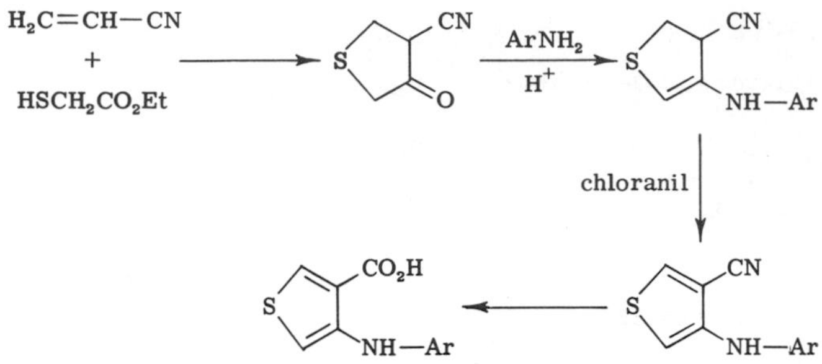

Scheme V

mann, 1970). Some are potent inhibitors of platelet aggregation (Von Kaulla and Thilo, 1970). A novel route to these compounds is outlined in Scheme V (Ruschig *et al.*, 1969).

2. PYRIMIDINECARBOXYLIC ACIDS

Juby (1967) found (25) to show activity on the order of phenylbutazone in the carrageenan assay. The pyrimidine is deactivating as is shown by the lack of significant activity in unsubstituted and monosubstituted derivatives. Other anilinopyrimidinecarboxylic acid derivatives have been patented (Jutz and Mueller, 1970).

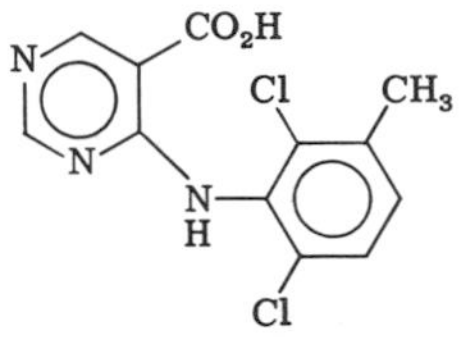

25

3. QUINOXALINECARBOXYLIC ACIDS

A variety of quinoxaline-2-carboxylic acid derivatives (26) were prepared by Lombardino (1966) but produced no usefully active compounds (carrageenan assay).

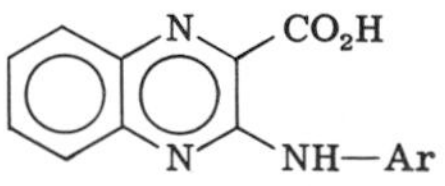

26

4. PYRROLECARBOXYLIC ACIDS

4-Anilino-1-phenyl-3-pyrrolecarboxylic acid derivatives (27) do not have significant anticarrageenan activity (Bauer and Safir, 1972). This is in marked contrast to the anilinothiophenes of Section II, C, 1.

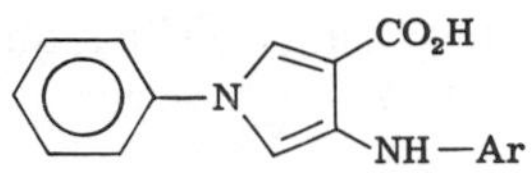

27

D. B-Ring Heterocycles

1. GLAPHENINE

Probably the most extensively studied of the B-ring heterocycles is glaphenine (**28**). It is marketed outside the United States primarily as an analgesic.

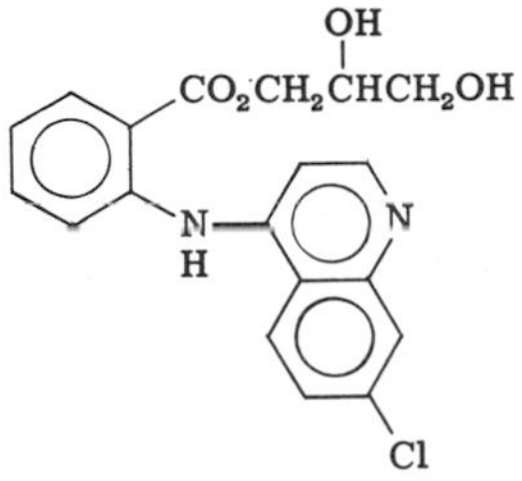

28

The greater activity of the ester over the acid (about sixfold in some assays) is attributed to better absorption than the acid. Boissier and Fichelle-Pagny (1967) feel the ester is a requisite part of the active compound. Glaphenine has been compared structurally with chloroquine (Ruedy and Bentley, 1969) but they share no important pharmacological properties (Boissier and Fichelle-Pagny, 1967; Peterfalvi *et al.*, 1966). Ruedy and Bentley (1969) describe a double-blind trial against dental pain in which 400 mg of glaphenine was preferred to 30 mg of codeine. Glaphenine has weak antiinflammatory activity by the UV-erythema assay (twice aspirin, one tenth of phenylbutazone; Allais and Meier, 1966).

Synthetic procedures and structure-activity relationships are detailed extensively by Allais *et al.* (1966) in terms of inhibition of acetic acid writhing and the inhibition of edema produced by naphthoylheparamine. In the latter little used assay glaphenine has an ED_{40} of 10 mg/kg and aspirin one of 100 mg/kg. This series is unusual in that simple esters, hydroxyalkyl esters, and aminoalkyl esters are up to 6 times more active than the corresponding acid against naphthoylheparamine-induced edema (Allais *et al.*, 1966). More recently the secondary glyceryl ester (Allais and Girault, 1970) and an 8-

trifluoromethyl analog of glaphenine (Allais and Meier, 1972) have been disclosed.

2. PYRIMIDINE DERIVATIVES

In general, B-ring heterocycles having nitrogen conjugated with the arylamine function are not highly active. Falch *et al*. (1968) prepared series of 2- and 4-pyrimidyl derivatives (29) and (30). The most active of these was (30) (R_2 = Cl, R_3 = CH_3), which at 300 mg/kg in the kaolin rat paw edema assay (57% inhibition) was about as active as 100 mg/kg of mefenamic acid or 50 mg/kg of phenylbutazone. A series of 4-pyrimidyl derivatives was examined for antiformalin edema and for analgesic and antipyretic activity (Mokhort, 1970).

Compounds of type (30), e.g., in which R_2 = R_3 = Cl, are claimed to have useful analgesic and antiinflammatory activity (Matter and Staehelin, 1968).

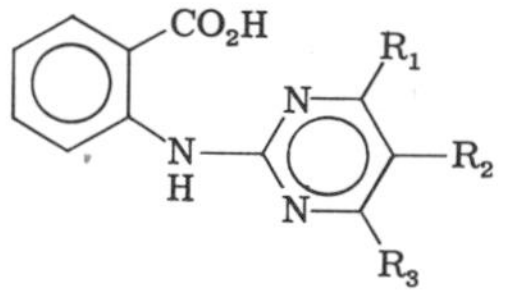

29 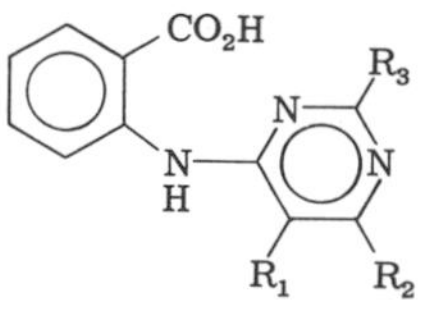   30

3. OTHERS

Compound (31), R = H, a hybrid of antipyrine and a fenamic acid, is reported to lack analgesic activity and to be antiinflammatory only at toxic levels (Galvez and Balasch, 1971). However, both the *o*- and *p*-carboxylic acid isomers (R = H or alkyl) are described as "especially useful as antiinflammatory drugs" (Kinoshita *et al*., 1971; assay not reported).

Compounds of types (32) (Scherrer, 1969a) and (33) (Scherrer, 1970) have activity on the order of mefenamic acid or greater by the UV-erythema assay.

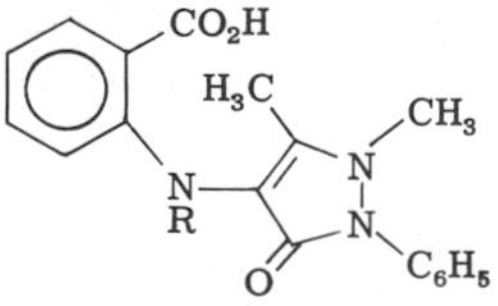

31 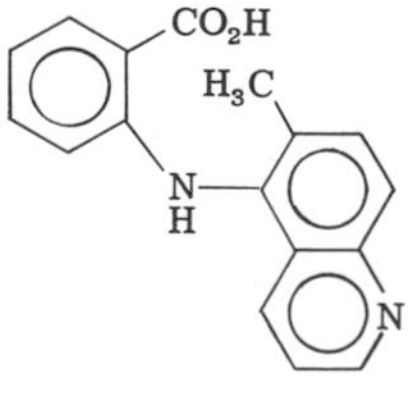   32 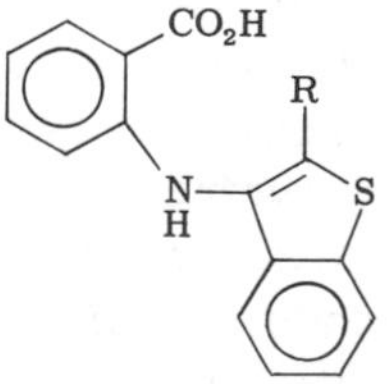   33

III. HOMOLOGS OF *N*-ARYLANTHRANILIC ACIDS AND HETEROCYCLIC ISOSTERES

A. Acetic Acids

1. DICLOFENAC SODIUM (GP 45840)

The most interesting compound in this group is GP 45840 (Ciba-Geigy), *o*-(2,6-dichloroanilino)phenylacetic acid sodium salt (Krupp *et al*., 1972). This compound appears highly active in a variety of assays. It is equal to indomethacin in the carrageenan edema assay and has about the same relative activity in the adjuvant arthritis model. It has the expected spectrum of properties and, based on an acute LD_{50}, a very favorable therapeutic index. Diclofenac sodium is the recently adopted generic name for this compound.

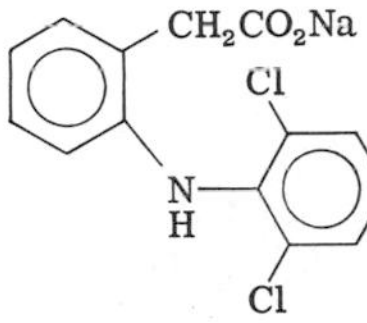

GP 45840

34

Of special interest for receptor and mechanism considerations is the unusually high activity of (**34**) in shorter duration *in vivo* and *in vitro* tests. In antibradykinin activity (guinea pig bronchoconstriction, intravenous dosing), it is 3 times indomethacin and 25 times phenylbutazone. It is 20 times indomethacin and 200 times phenylbutazone in inhibiting arachidonic acid peroxide-induced contraction of the guinea pig ileum *in vitro* (without inhibiting acetylcholine- or histamine-induced contraction). The higher relative activities in the shorter-term test systems may reflect a tendency for GP 45840 to be inactivated by cyclization to the inactive oxindole. If this is the case, 2,6 substitution should be an advantage because it decreases the tendency toward cyclization. Preparation from a diarylamine is outlined on page 72 (Sallmann and Pfister, 1971c).

Additional anilinophenylacetic acids of interest have the substitutions 3'-trifluoromethyl, 3',5'-bistrifluoromethyl, and 2',6'-dichloro-3'-methyl, corresponding to the substitutions in active fenamic acids (Sallmann and Pfister, 1971a,c).

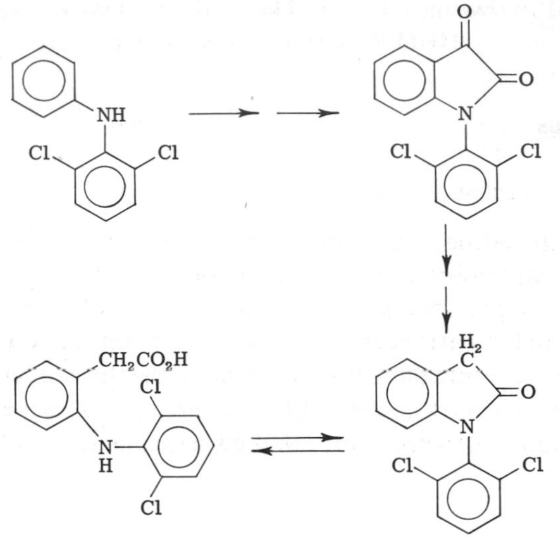

2. META AND PARA ISOMERS

The isomeric *m*-anilinophenylacetic acid (Marshall, 1972) and *p*-anilino-phenylacetic acid (Rhone-Poulenc, 1966) are also antiinflammatory, in contrast to the corresponding anilinobenzoic acids. Another distinction from fenamic acids and *o*-acetic acid homologs is that there is no indication of preference for substitution in the anilino portion of the *m*- and *p*-acetic acids. The meta-isomer is isosteric with Lilly's fenoprofen, α-methyl-3-phenoxyphenylacetic acid, also unsubstituted in the phenoxy ring (see Chapter 4 by Juby).

3. HOMOLOGS OF GLAPHENINE

The acetic and propionic homologs of glaphenine are described as anti-malarial (because they inhibit imidazole-*N*-methyltransferase) and as antiinflammatory (Wasley and Gruenfeld, 1972). The closest homolog

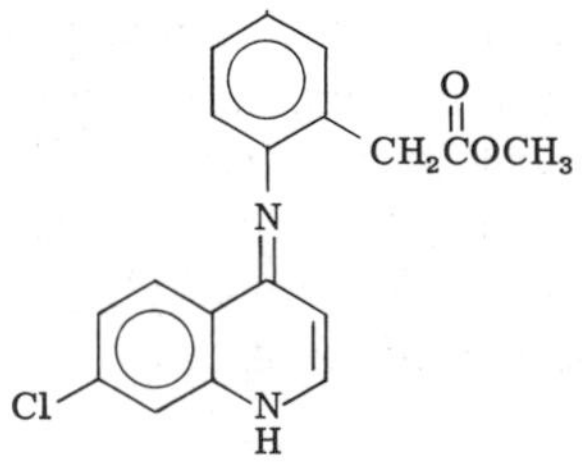

35

(35) described in the imino form, has moderate antiinflammatory activity (80% protection at 100 mg/kg in the UV-erythema assay).

B. Other Homologs

1. CINNAMIC AND PROPIONIC ACIDS

A series of 2-anilinocinnamic acids is disclosed by Sallmann and Pfister (1971b). The preferred substitution pattern corresponds to that of the N-arylanthranilic acids. The same cinnamic acids and some hydrocinnamic acids are described by Yamamoto et al. (1972). These compounds appear to be about a tenth as active in the UV assay as the corresponding anthranilic acids. These homologs have the potential for inherent activity as well as metabolic conversion (β-oxidation) to the anthranilic acid.

2. GLYCINE CONJUGATE

The pseudohomolog (36), a glycine conjugate of niflumic acid, is about as active on carrageenan and kaolin edema assays as niflumic acid (tested at 80 and 180 mg/kg, respectively; Hoffmann, 1970). Claims of advantage in acute toxicity and of clinical efficacy are reported in the reference cited.

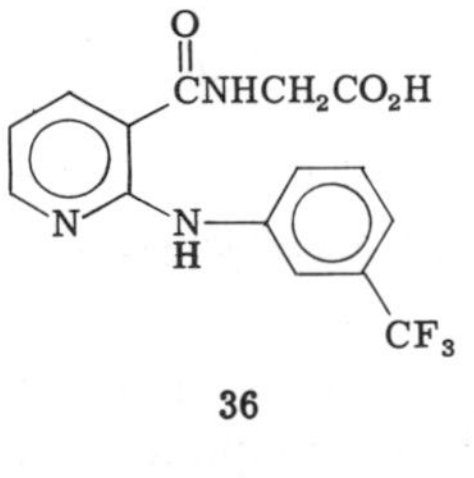

36

IV. FIXED-PLANAR ARYLCARBOXYLIC ACIDS

A. Phenothiazine- and Phenoxazinecarboxylic Acids

The relatively high activity of the benzothiophene, flutiazin (37), a sulfur "tied-back" flufenamic, acid, is unexpected in view of earlier evidence favoring the action of these agents in an antiplanar configuration. This is discussed further in Section V. Flutiazin is about as active as flufenamic acid on the UV-erythema assay (Sutton and Birnie, 1966), is antipyretic at 10 mg/kg, and has an ED_{50} against carrageenan paw edema of 25 mg/kg (Sutton, 1971). It is reported effective in man and in veterinary use (Sutton, 1971).

The isomeric acid (38) is inactive, and the oxygen analog (39) (Blank and Baxter, 1968) has only moderate activity, about one tenth of (37).

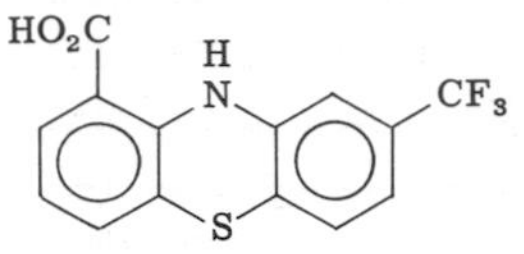

Flutiazin

37   38 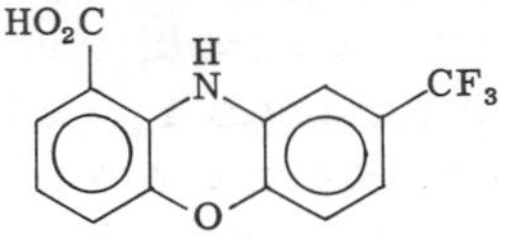   39

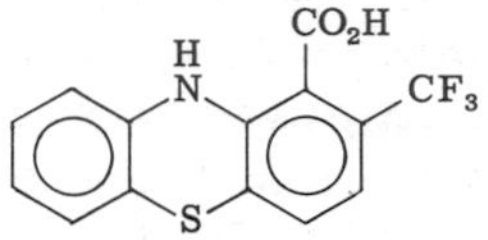

B. Acridonecarboxylic Acids

Fujihira *et al.* (1971) reported the acridone (40) as the most potent of a series against carrageenan rat paw edema (52% at 30 mg/kg), about the same activity as phenylbutazone in their laboratory. Some acridine mono- and dicarboxylic acids were less active.

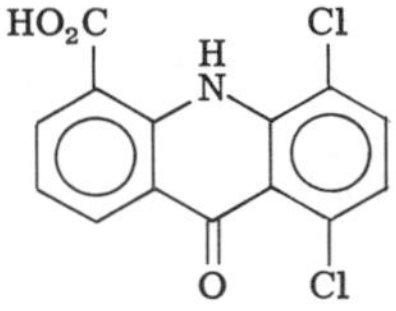

40

V. THE ANTIINFLAMMATORY RECEPTOR SITE

The evidence seems quite strong that some very potent nonsteroidal antiinflammatory agents have nonplanar configurations in their lowest energy levels, e.g., in *N*-(2,6-dichloro-3-tolyl)anthranilic acid (3) and 3-chloro-4-cyclohexylphenylacetic acid. It seems reasonable to postulate that an antiinflammatory receptor will be highly complementary to these potent compounds and therefore will have a cavity, trough, or right-angle surfaces to accomodate them (a proposed receptor site design is presented in Chapter 2).

The presence of relatively high activity in planar structures, such as (37), raises the question of the requirement for a trough. More precisely, the question might be whether the trough must be occupied to obtain anti-inflammatory activity. There may be more than one receptor, although I prefer the simplifying assumption that those compounds with properties of classical antiinflammatory agents are acting at the same receptor site. There are two ways to accommodate planar molecules to the proposed receptor. The trough may not be utilized, or, if the planar molecule occupies the trough, the flat area for the carboxyl-bearing ring cannot be used.

Westby and Barfknecht (1973) approached the question of the importance of conformation to activity by preparing three series of compounds
(41) to (43). These were selected to minimize complications in interpreta-
tion of activity changes on cyclization, e.g., A-ring substitution effects
and the introduction of additional groups in (2) → (37). They found that
for the series Y = CH$_3$ one antiplanar form (41) and the semiplanar (43)
were both poorly active. They conclude that factors other than conformation
are more important for activity. C. F. Barfkneckt points out (personal communication) that the 3^A-methyl can interfere with the attainment of the
antiplanar conformation (44).

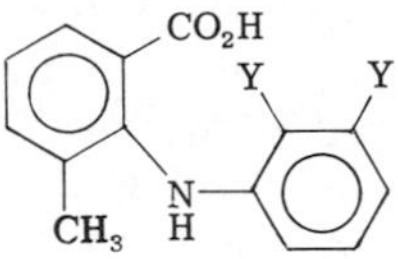

41

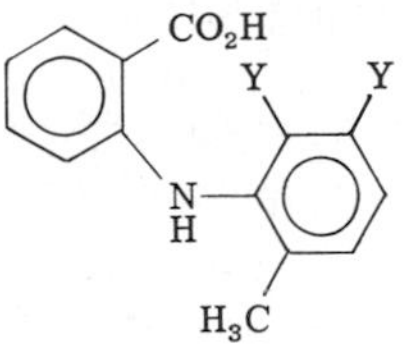

42

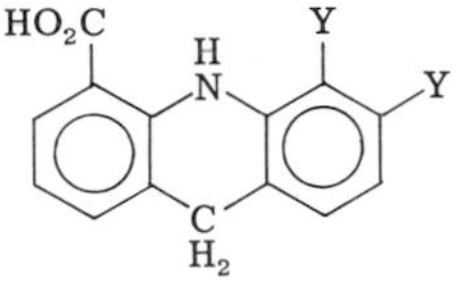

43

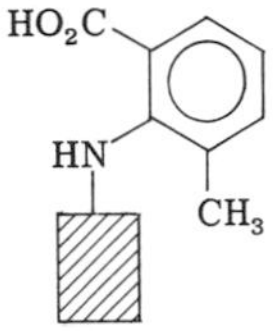

44

Compound	UV-erythema, ED$_{50}$ (mg/kg)	
	Y = CH$_3$	Y = H
41	> 100	> 100
42	6	> 100
43	100	100

VI. SALICYLIC ACIDS

A. Introduction

The oldest antiinflammatory agent, salicylic acid, is still the first agent
of choice, in one form or other, for treating rheumatic conditions. The story
of the development of the use of aspirin is told as well as anywhere by Collier
(1963).

The use of willow bark and other salicylic acid-containing natural products to relieve pain and fever was apparently known to the Greeks of
Hippocrates' time. This use of willow bark was rediscovered in England in
1763. A series of false assumptions and chance observations, mixed with
a little medicinal chemistry, led to the demonstrated efficacy of acetylsalicylic acid in 1899.

B. Acetylsalicylic Acid

Aspirin must be the most studied of all antiinflammatory agents in
terms of its biological and biochemical properties. Many of these properties are discussed in detail in Volume II. Most of the acidic nonsteroidal antiinflammatory agents are referred to as "aspirinlike" when
they exhibit a similarity of action in a few of the well-accepted models.
I feel it can be useful to consider aspirin as belonging to a larger group
of classical antiinflammatory agents (as discussed in Chapter 2) that includes
some nonacidic agents with the same pharmacological profile.

Two major questions have received attention regarding the pharmacology
of aspirin: its analgesic activity, as distinct from its antiinflammatory activity,
and the activity of aspirin versus salicylic acid. Collier (1969) discusses
these points in a highly documented pharmacological analysis of aspirin.
The concensus is that aspirin is more potent as an antiinflammatory agent
than salicylic acid and that the analgesic activity is almost all from
intact aspirin. Reviews of this class of agents are available in the proceedings of a salicylate symposium (Dixon et al., 1963) and a comprehensive
work edited by Smith and Smith (1966).

More recently attention has been directed toward structure–activity
relationships for fibrinolytic activity (Hansch and Von Kaulla, 1970), the
effects of aspirin on platelets and thrombosis (Fields and Hass, 1971), the
hypoglycemic activity of aspirin (Fang et al., 1968), and the capacity of
aspirin to acetylate proteins (Farr, 1972). The pharmacokinetics of absorption, hydrolysis, distribution, metabolism, and elimination are of special
interest with the introduction of long-acting formulations (Davison, 1970;
Tsuchiya and Levy, 1972; Rowland et al., 1972). Much more sophisticated
pharmacokinetic analyses are being brought to bear on all aspects of the
problem (discussed by Ober in Chapter 10, Volume II). About 30% of an oral
aspirin dose in man enters the peripheral circulation as salicylic acid
(Rowland et al., 1972).

By direct injections into the lateral cerebral ventrical of febrile rabbits,
Cranston et al. (1971) determined that antipyretic structure–activity
relationships were specific for aspirin and the ortho isomer of sodium

hydroxy benzoate. Neither salicylamide nor sodium benzoate was active at the dose examined (0.4 ml, 8.6 μM).

The proposal by Vane (1971) that aspirin exerts its antiinflammatory and antipyretic activity by inhibiting the synthesis of prostaglandin is very attractive. This is discussed in detail by Hichens (Chapter 8, Volume II). In *in vitro* assays aspirin is almost 10 times as active as salicylic acid in inhibiting prostaglandin synthetase. Vane (1971, 1972) postulates that the differential antiinflammatory *vis-à-vis* antipyretic activity for these two may be caused by a difference in their ability to reach the central nervous system (see also Hichens, Chapter 8, Volume II).

C. Carboxylic and Phenolic Derivatives

Adams and Cobb (1967) have critically reviewed the earlier literature on derivatives, substitution products, and analogs of salicylic acid. Little of this is repeated here. Their excellent survey also illustrates the frequency with which negative clinical reports can follow earlier favorable ones.

The main objective sought by modifying the carboxylic or phenolic function of salicylic acid is to reduce occult blood loss and gastric ulceration by minimizing direct contact of active drug forms with the stomach. This is a definite problem with aspirin, in contrast to many other classical antiinflammatory agents.

1. BENORYLATE

A derivative attracting considerable attention currently is (45), benorylate, an ester of acetylsalicylic acid with *N*-acetyl-*p*-aminophenol (acetaminophen). Because the latter is an analgesic and antipyretic, *in vivo* hydrolysis leads to compounds with complementary activity in different drug classes. Benorylate is reported to cause less gastrointestinal (GI) bleeding than aspirin (Croft *et al.*, 1972) but still allows attainment of desired levels of plasma salicylate (Beales *et al.*, 1972). In the latter study 4 gm of benorylate twice daily was comparable to 1.2 gm four times daily of soluble aspirin (8 gm versus 4.8 gm daily total). One tends to overlook the lack of placebo

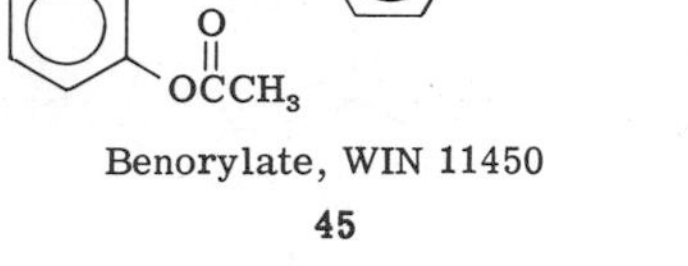

Benorylate, WIN 11450

45

control in these studies when salicylate plasma levels are demonstrable, and the common salicylate side effect tinnitus occurs in about a third of both patient groups. A recent paper (Khalili-Varasteh *et al.*, 1972) attributes some beneficial effects to the intact molecule.

2. POTENTIAL PRECURSORS OF ACETYLSALICYLIC ACID

There continues to be a constant slow stream of new salicylic acid derivatives in the patent literature about which nothing is heard subsequently. Of recent interest are the alkylcarbonate anhydrides (**46a**) (Kallianos *et al.*, 1972). There is potential for metabolic conversion to acetylsalicylic acid and indications of prolonged blood levels of free salicylate. The conversions of a derivative to aspirin instead of salicylic acid should be advantageous for therapeutic effects. This possibility is present in the glyceryl ester (**46b**) (Sherlock, 1972a), the hydroxyalkyl esters (**46c**) (Chiego, 1971), and the acetoxymethyl esters (**46d**) (Borrows and Johnson, 1971).

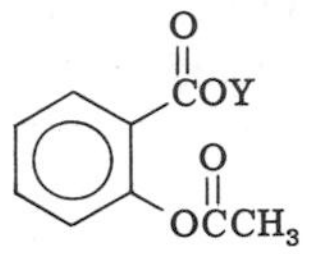

Compound	Y
46a	$-\overset{\overset{\text{O}}{\|\|}}{\text{C}}\text{OC}_2\text{H}_5$
46b	$-\text{CH}_2\overset{\overset{\text{OH}}{\|}}{\text{CH}}\text{CH}_2\text{OH}$
46c	$-\text{CH}_2\overset{\overset{\text{OH}}{\|}}{\text{CH}}-\text{alkyl}$
46d	$-\text{CH}_2\text{O}\overset{\overset{\text{O}}{\|\|}}{\text{C}}\text{CH}_3$

46a–d

3. OTHERS

Some phenolic derivatives of salicylic acid that have recently appeared are (**47**) (Diamond and Martin, 1972), (**48**) (Cross *et al.*, 1969), and (**49**) (Misher *et al.*, 1968). The latter is about equal to aspirin in the adjuvant arthritis assay on a molar basis and affords comparable levels of free

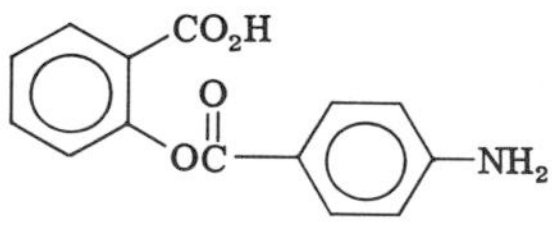

47 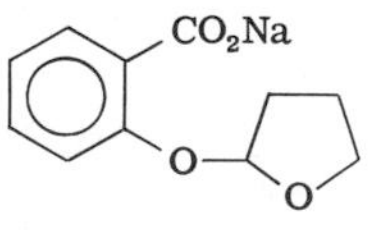   48 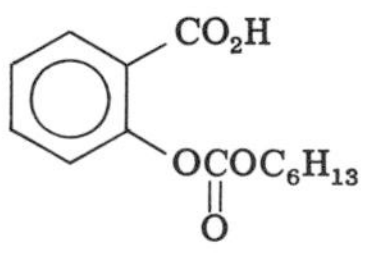   49

salicylate in rat plasma, with reduced gastric irritation. The acetal (**48**) has been shown to undergo a rapid intramolecular carboxyl-catalyzed hydrolysis (Fife and Anderson, 1971). That compounds such as (**47**) may have inherent activity is not ruled out.

A cyclic derivative of salicylic acid, seclazone (**50**), is discussed in Chapter 7 by Shen.

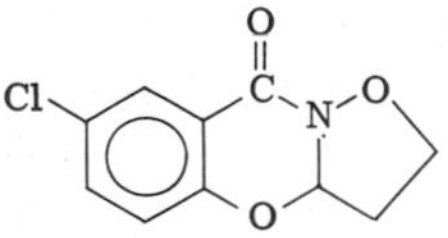

Seclazone

50

D. Ring-Substituted Salicylic Acids

With few other early "lead" compounds in evidence, substituted salicylic acids have naturally attracted attention over the years. Some have even reached the stage of claimed clinical activity (reviewed by Adams and Cobb, 1967). A disadvantage to earlier workers was the lack of good assay models, especially for inflammation. I have to agree with Adams and Cobb that one should be wary if an "aspirinlike" agent being studied is not like aspirin to the point of being active in the UV-erythema assay. A high percentage of these early claimed-active hydroxybenzoic acids are not active in the UV-erythema assay. It is probably also true that the same high percentage are noted for their low GI toxicity.

1. FLUFENISAL

a. DEVELOPMENT AND ACTIVITY. Earlier efforts to find a superior aspirin analog were dwarfed by the major systematic effort of the Merck laboratories toward this objective. The goals were to find a more potent, better tolerated, and longer acting derivative (Shen, 1972a). Four hundred and fifty related compounds were submitted over several years to carrageenan

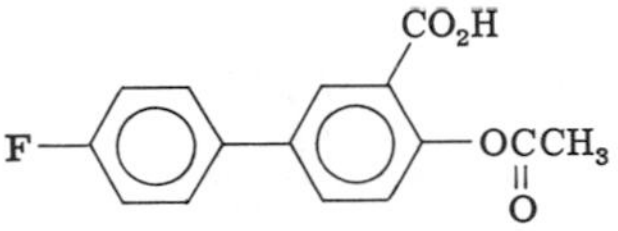

Flufenisal

51

and cotton pellet granuloma testing (Sarett, 1971). The results confirmed and extended the earlier findings that simple substitution of aspirin with Cl, Br, OH, OCH_3, $N(CH_3)_2$, $NHCOCH_3$, methyl, and acetyl produced compounds no better than aspirin (Hannah et al., 1970). A 3- or 5-F, 4-CF_3, or 4- or 5-phenyl substituent did have beneficial effects.

From this work, flufenisal, the 5-(p-fluorophenyl) derivative, was selected for development and eventual clinical studies; it is four- to fivefold more active than aspirin in antiinflammatory assays but only one fifteenth as liable to produce gastric hemorrhage in rats (Shen, 1972a). Some details of structure–activity relationships in the series in comparison with prior-art compounds is available (Ruyle et al., 1972). Flufenisal is readily deacetylated in man so is predominantly present in the plasma as the phenol. An interesting differentiation of the series from aspirin is in the relative potencies of the acetyl and free phenol derivatives in the in vitro inhibition of prostaglandin synthetase, Table VIII (Ham et al., 1972).

Flufenisal was active against postpartum pain at one fourth to one half the dose of aspirin with a longer duration of action (Bloomfield et al., 1970). It was more recently reported, however (Sarett, 1971), that after 77 months of development work and clinical study, flufenisal was dropped for lack of sufficient superiority over aspirin. It is hoped that whatever factors went into this decision will become generally available to improve the selection procedure for future compounds—whether it be a particular toxicity or side effect to try to avoid; a general guide to the potency, blood levels, and half-

TABLE VIII

Flufenisal and Deacetylflufenisal

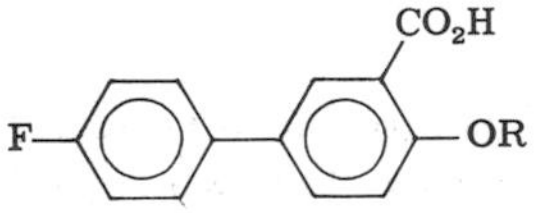

CO_2H

F—⟨◯⟩—⟨◯⟩—OR

	Carrageenan edema, ED_{50}[a]	Prostaglandin synthetase ID_{50} (μg/ml)[a]
Flufenisal	25	11
Deacetylflufenisal	25	0.8
Aspirin	75, 72[b]	15, 6.3[c]
Salicylic acid	98[b]	100[c]

[a] Ham et al. (1972).
[b] Niemegeers et al. (1964).
[c] Vane (1971).

life that should be strived for in future candidates; or a retrospective assessment of available animal models.

b. SYNTHESES.   Two indicated routes to flufenisal have some generality
(Scheme VI). One is Kolbe-Schmidt carbonation of a phenol and the other is
a buildup of the A ring (Schoenwaldt *et al.*, 1972).

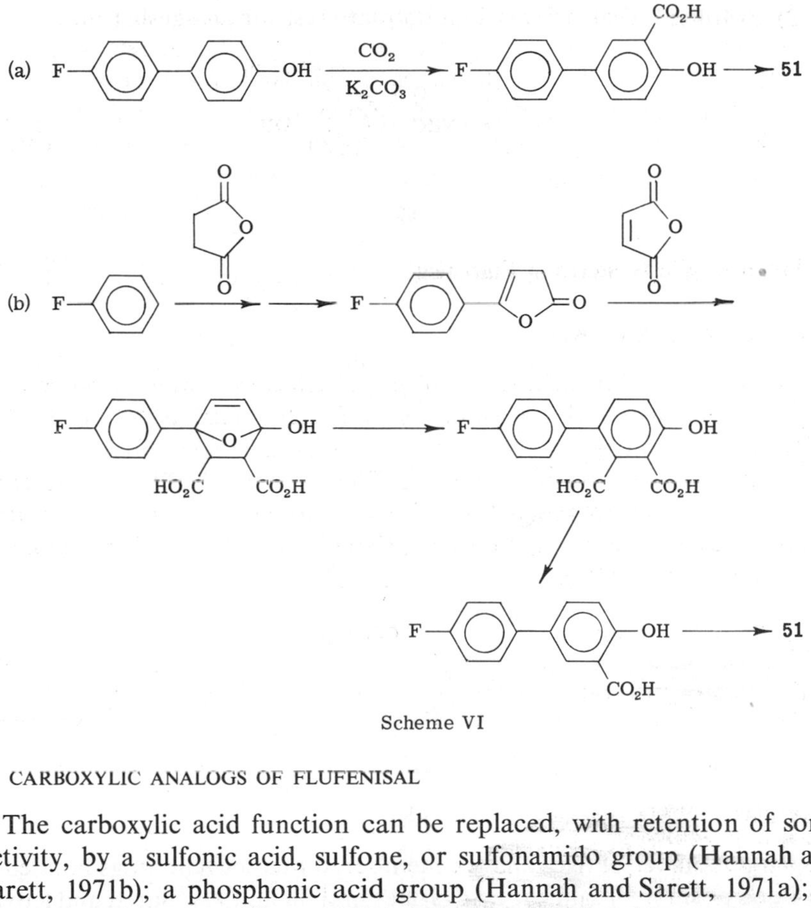

Scheme VI

2. CARBOXYLIC ANALOGS OF FLUFENISAL

The carboxylic acid function can be replaced, with retention of some
activity, by a sulfonic acid, sulfone, or sulfonamido group (Hannah and
Sarett, 1971b); a phosphonic acid group (Hannah and Sarett, 1971a); or
an acetic acid group (Shen, 1972c). The phosphonic acids are the first of
this class with antiinflammatory activity to my knowledge. More details of
activity and other biological properties are awaited with interest.

3. ARYL-γ-SALICYLIC ACID DERIVATIVES

The *p*-fluorophenyl group may be linked to salicylic acid by any one of
many one- and two-atom functions, including carbonyl (Shen *et al.*, 1972e),

methylene, vinylidene, ethylene, vinylene (Shen *et al.*, 1971b), oxy (Merck, 1971b), imino (Merck, 1971c), thio, sulfinyl, sulfonyl (Shen *et al.*, 1972f), —CH$_2$S—, —SCH$_2$—, —CH$_2$SO—, —CH$_2$SO$_2$—, —SO$_2$CH$_2$—, —SS— (Shen *et al.*, 1971c), —SO$_2$NH—, —NHSO$_2$— (Merck, 1971a),—NHCH$_2$—, —CH$_2$NH—, —N=CH—, —CH=N—, —NHCO—, and —CONH— (Shen *et al.*, 1972a).

A series of hydroxyisophthalic acid derivatives, e.g., (**52**), (Spano *et al.*, 1972), exhibited weak activity in a hotplate test for analgesia (mice).

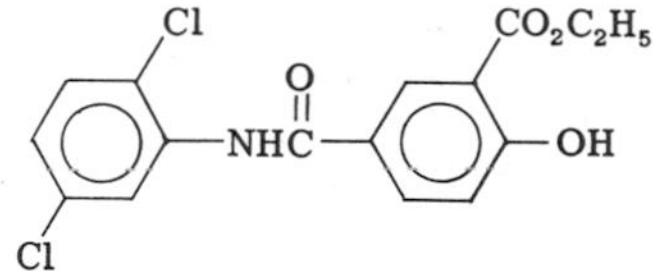

52

E. Heterocyclic Isosteres of Flufenisal

1. A-RING AZA DERIVATIVES

A 6-aza analog of flufenisal (**53**), approaches the latter in potency in animals, whereas the 4-aza isomer is essentially inactive (Walford *et al.*, 1971). The 2-hydroxy and acetoxy derivatives are apparently considered equivalent by omission of comment. The former should lack the complication of potential acetylation of body proteins. Other representative heterocycles include 2-arylpyrimidines (**54**) (Shen, 1972b) and arylpyrazines (**55**), (Shen *et al.*, 1971c).

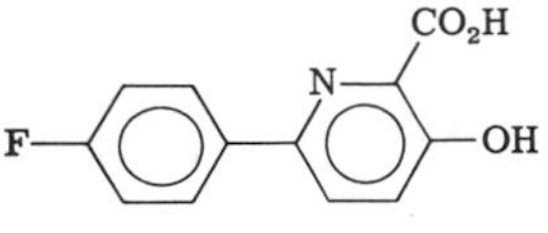

53 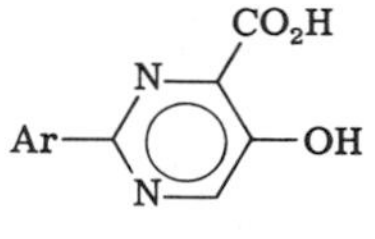   54 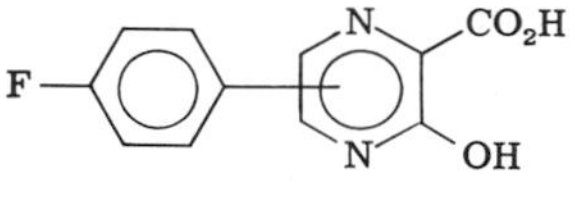   55

2. OTHERS

A large number of five- and six-membered heterocyclic rings bonded to the 4 or 5 position of salicylic acid (Jones and Shen, 1971; Sarett and Ruyle, 1969, 1971, 1972) or linked by a variety of atoms (Shen *et al.*, 1972g) have been described. Some examples are (**56**) and (**57**). No activity values are available.

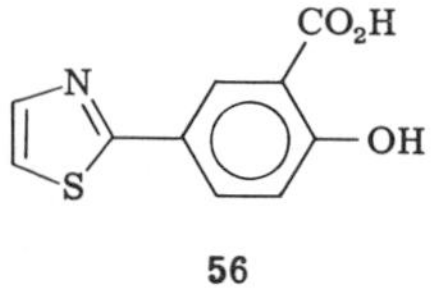

56 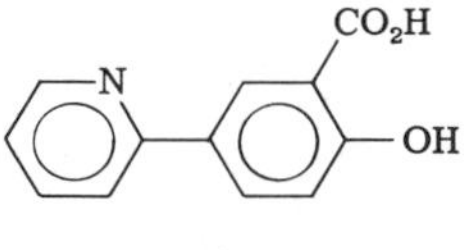   57

VII. o-HYDROXY"TRICYCLE"CARBOXYLIC ACIDS

Several series of tricyclic analogs round out this cursory listing of patent disclosures related to flufenisal. They include a central four-membered ring (Shen *et al.*, 1972b), a variety of central five-membered rings (Shen *et al.*, 1971a, 1972d), and six-membered rings (Shen *et al.*, 1972c). Some examples are (58)–(60).

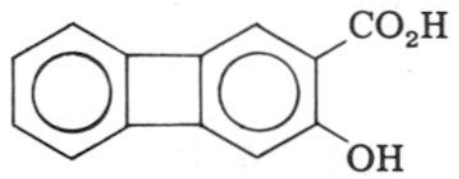

58 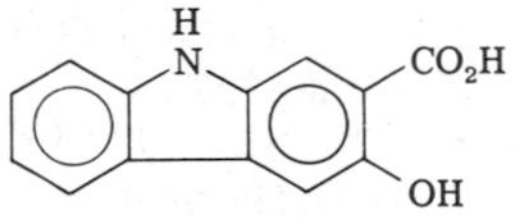   59 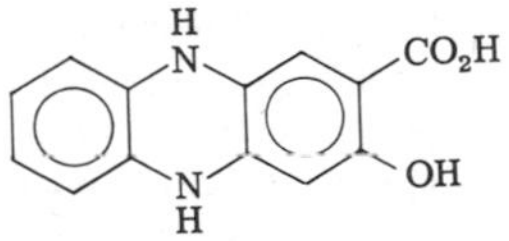   60

A phenothiazine derivative (61) (Saggiomo and Sutton, 1968) was one fourth as potent as phenylbutazone on a filter paper granuloma assay but inactive at five times the ED_{50} of phenylbutazone in the antierythema assay. The related 1-carboxyphenothiazine (37) (Section IV, A) is active in the latter test.

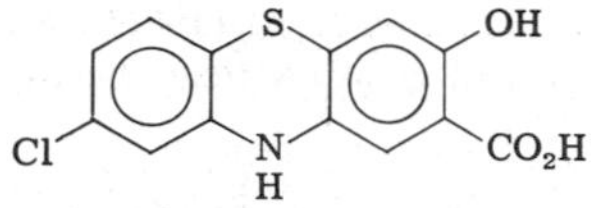

61

VIII. MISCELLANEOUS CARBOXYLIC ACIDS

A recent patent (Misaki *et al.*, 1971) describes carbostyril derivatives from diarylamine-2-carboxaldehydes and malonic acid. The derivative (62) has an ED_{50} against carrageenan paw edema of 150 mg/kg. The indazole (63) is reported active in the adjuvant arthritis screen at 25 mg/kg (Wajngurt, 1971).

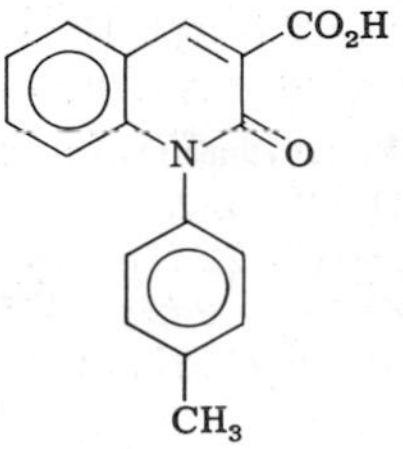

62 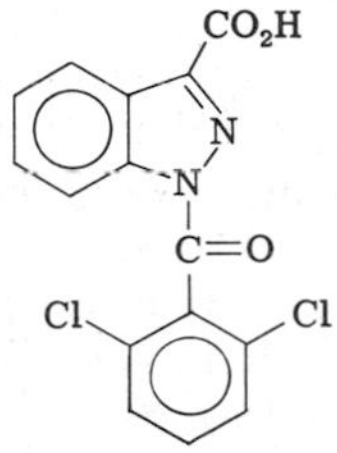   63

REFERENCES

Acheson, R. M. (1956). *In* "Acridines," pp. 122–165. Wiley (Interscience), New York.

Adams, S. S., and Cobb, R. (1967). *Progr. Med. Chem.* **5**, 59–138.

Albert, A. (1966). "The Acridines," pp. 56–77. Arnold, London.

Alkede, B., and Neuhold, K. (1969). South African Patent 68/4065 (to Aktieselskabet Gea); *Chem. Abstr.* **72**, 12408 (1970).

Allais, A., and Girault, P. (1970). U.S. Patent 3,502,680 (to Roussel-UCLAF).

Allais, A., and Meier, J. (1966). U.S. Patent 3,232,944 (to Roussel-UCLAF).

Allais, A., and Meier, J. (1972). U.S. Patent 3,644,368 (to Roussel-UCLAF).

Allais, A., Rousseau, G., Girault, P., Mathieu, J., Peterfalvi, M., Branceni, D., Azadian-Boulanger, G., Chifflot, L., and Jequier, R. (1966). *Chem. Ther.* p. 65.

Alpermann, H. G. (1970). *Arzneim.-Forsch.* **20**, 293.

Anonymous. (1972). *Med. Lett.* **14**, 31.

Basu, U. P., Sen Gupta, P. N., and Sikdar, J. (1946). *Ann. Biochem. Exp. Med.* **6**, 41.

Bauer, V. J., and Safir, S. R. (1972). *J. Med. Chem.* **15**, 440.

Beales, D. L., Burry, H. C., and Grahame, R. (1972). *Brit. Med. J.* **2**, 483.

Beringer, F. M., and Falk, R. A. (1964). *J. Chem. Soc., London* p. 4442.

Beringer, F. M., and Huang, S. J. (1964). *J. Org. Chem.* **29**, 445.

Blank, B., and Baxter, L. L. (1968). *J. Med. Chem.* **11**, 807.

Bloomfield, S. S., Barden, T. P., and Hille, R. (1970). *Clin. Pharmacol. Ther.* **11**, 747.

Blum, J. (1970). French Medicament Patent 7766M (to Roussel-UCLAF).

Blum, J. (1971). French Patent 2,068,429.

Boissier, J. R., and Fichelle-Pagny, J. (1967). *Therapie* **22**, 149–155.

Boissier, J. R., Lwolf, J. M., and Hertz, F. (1970). *Therapie* **25**, 43.

Boissier, J. R., Tillement, J. P., and Larousse, C. (1971). *Therapie* **26**, 211.

Boltze, K. H., and Lorenz, D. (1970). South African Patent 70/07385 (to Tropon G.m.b.H.); *Chem. Abstr.* **76**, 140225 (1972).

Boltze, K. H., Brendler, O., and Lorenz, D. (1971a). German Patent 1,939,111 (to Tropon Werke Dinklage); *Chem. Abstr.* **74**, 76185(1971).

Boltze, K. H., Brendler, O., and Lorenz, D. (1971b). German Patent 1,939,112 (to Tropon Werke Dinklage); *Chem. Abstr.* **74**, 76186 (1971).

Borrows, E. T., and Johnson, J. M. (1971). British Patent 1,220,447 (to John Wyeth and Brother, Ltd.); *Chem. Abstr.* **75**, 35462(1971).

Camus, J. P. (1968). *Presse Med.* **76**, 1071.

Carrano, R. A., and Malbica, J. O. (1972). *J. Pharm. Sci.* **61**, 1450.

Chausse, L. (1971). French Patent 2,068,411; *Chem. Abstr.* **77**, 34531 (1972).

Chiego, B. (1971). German Patent 2,037,017; *Chem. Abstr.* **76**, 24921 (1972).

Ciofalo, V. B., Patel, J., and Taber, R. I. (1972). *Jap. J. Pharmacol.* **22**, 749.

Collier, H. O. J. (1963). *Sci. Amer.* **209**(5), 97–108.

Collier, H. O. J. (1967). *Ann. Phys. Med., Suppl.* pp. 50–54.

Collier, H. O. J. (1969). *Advan. Pharmacol. Chemother.* **7**, 333–405.

Collier, H. O. J., Dinneen, L. C., Johnson, C. A., and Schneider, C. (1968a). *Brit. J. Pharmacol. Chemother.* **32**, 295.

Collier, H. O. J., James, G. W. L., and Piper, P. J. (1968b). *Brit. J. Pharmacol.* **34**, 76–87.

Cranston, W. I., Luff, R. H., and Rawlins, M. D. (1971). *J. Physiol. (London)* **216**, 81p.

Croft, D. N., Cuddigan, J. H. P., and Sweetland, C. (1972). *Brit. Med. J.* **2**, 546.

Cross, A. D., Edwards, J. A., and Berkoz, B. (1969). U.S. Patent 3,429,899 (to Syntex).

Cummings, J. R., Ronsberg, M. A., Stokey, E. H., and Gussin, R. Z. (1968). *Pharmacologist* **10**, 162.

Davison, C. (1970). *Ann N. Y. Acad. Sci.* **179**, 249–268.

De Marchi, F., Torrielli, M. V., and Tamagnone, G. F. (1968). *Chim. Ther.* **3**, 433.

de Salcedo, I., Carrington, M. D., Santos, J. A., and Silva, J. L. (1970). *Hormones* **1**, 193.

Diamond, J., and Martin, G. J. (1972). U.S. Patent 3,642,865 (to W. H. Rorer, Inc.).

Dixon, A. St. J., Martin, B. K., Smith, M. J. H., and Wood, P. H. N., eds. (1963). "Salicylates." Little, Brown, Boston, Massachusetts.

Egyesult Gyogyszer es Tapszergyar. (1968). French Patent 1,525,428; *Chem. Abstr.* **71**, 80908 (1969).

Evans, D., Hallwood, K. S., Cashin, C. H., and Jackson, H. (1967). *J. Med. Chem.* **10**, 428.

Falch, E., Weis, J., and Natvig, T. (1968). *J. Med. Chem.* **11**, 608.

Fang, V., Foye, W. O., Robinson, S. M., and Jenkins, H. J. (1968). *J. Pharm. Sci.* **57**, 2111.

Farr, R. S. (1972). *In* "Proceedings of the Symposium on Mechanisms of Toxicity," pp. 87–102. St. Martin's Press, New York.

"Fenamates in Medicine." (1967). *Ann. Phys. Med.*, *Suppl.* pp. 7–134.

Fields, W. S., and Hass, W. K. (1971). "Aspirin, Platelets and Stroke." Green, St. Louis, Missouri.

Fife, J. H., and Anderson, E. (1971). *J. Amer. Chem. Soc.* **93**, 6610.

Finch, J. S., and De Kornfeld, J. J. (1971). *J. Clin. Pharmacol. New Drugs* **11**, 371.

Flower, R., Gryglewski, R., Herbaczyńska-Cedro, K., and Vane, J. R. (1972). *Nature (London)*, *New Biol.* **238**, 104.

Fujihira, E., Otomo, S., Sota, K., and Nakazawa. M. (1971). *Yakugaku Zasshi* **91**, 143.

Galvez, C., and Balasch, J. (1971). *Quim. Ind. (Madrid)* **1**, 129; *Chem. Abstr.* **75**, 48973 (1971).

Gittos, M. W., and James, J. W. (1970). U.S. Patent 3,531,493 (to Aspro-Nicholas Ltd.).

Gryglewski, R. J., Panczenko, B., Górka, Z., Chytkowski, A., and Zmuda, A. (1969). *Diss. Pharm. Pharmacol.* **21**, 1.

Gupta, K. C., Rupawalla, E. N., Sheth, V. K., Sisodia, P., and Kandlikar, R. P. (1970). *Indian J. Med. Res.* **58**, 110.

Ham, E. A., Cirillo, V. J., Zanetti, M., Shen, T. Y., and Kuehl, F. A., Jr. (1972). *In* "Prostaglandins in Cellular Biology" (P. W. Ramwell and B. B. Pharriss, eds.), pp. 345–352. Plenum, New York.

Hannah, J., and Sarett, L. H. (1971a). French Patent Appl. 2,053,018 (to Merck and Co.); *Chem. Abstr.* **76**, 113372 (1972).

Hannah, J., and Sarett, L. H. (1971b). French Patent Appl. 2,053,027 (to Merck and Co.); *Chem. Abstr.* **76**, 112895 (1972).

Hannah, J., Ruyle, W. W., Kelly, K., Matzuk, A., Hoitz, W. J., Witzel, B. E., Winter, C. A., Silber, R. H., and Shen, T. Y. (1970). *Joint Conf. Chem. Inst. Can. Amer. Chem. Soc.*, *1970* Abstract, Medi 18.

Hansch, C., and Von Kaulla, K. N. (1970). *Biochem. Pharmacol.* **19**, 2193.

Hinman, R. L., and Hoogenboom, B. E. (1961). *J. Org. Chem.* **26**, 3641.

Hoffmann, C. (1970). U. S. Patent 3,538,106 (to Labs. U. P. S. A., Gennevilliers, Hauts-de-Seine, France).

Izard-Verchere, C., Cavier, R., Morin, R., Manuel-Menillet, C., and Viel, C. (1971). *Chim. Ther.* **6**, 346.

Jamison, M. M., and Turner, E. E. (1937). *J. Chem. Soc.*, *London* p. 1954.

Jones, H., and Shen, T. Y. (1971). German Patent 2,130,709 (to Merck and Co.); *Chem. Abstr.* **76**, 113209 (1972).

Juby, P. F. (1967). *U. S. Patent* 3,300,496 (To Bristol-Myers).

Juby, P. F., Hudyama, T. W., and Brown, M. (1968). *J. Med. Chem.* **11**, 111.

Jutz, C., and Mueller, W. (1970). U. S. Patent 3,523,119 (to Byk-Gulden Lomberg Chemische Fabrik).

Kallianos, A. G., Mold, J. D., and Simpson, M. (1972). U. S. Patent 3,646,201 (to Liggett and Myers).

Kater, M. M. H. (1968). *Med. J. Aust.* **1**, 848.

Khalili-Varasteh, H., Rosner, I., Legros, J., and Mottot, G. (1972). *Int. Congr. Pharmacol. 5th, 1972* Abstr. No. 738.

Kinoshita, Y., Miyazawa, T., and Kato, H. (1971). Japanese Patent 71/27745 (to Hokuriku Pharm. Co.); *Chem. Abstr.* **75**, 140857 (1971).

Kirichek, L. M. (1971). *Farmakol. Toksikol.* (*Kiev*) No. 6, p. 118; *Chem. Abstr.* **76**, 121798 (1972).

Kirichek, L. M., and Trinus, F. P. (1971). *Farmakol. Toksikol.* (*Kiev*) No. 6, p. 111; *Chem. Abstr.* **76**, 121796 (1972).

Krupp, P. J., Jaques, R., Menassé, R., Wilhelmi, G., and Ziel, R. (1972). *Int. Congr. Pharmacol., 5th, 1972* Abstr. No. 782.

Le Goff, E. (1962). *J. Amer. Chem. Soc.* **84**, 3786.

Linari, G., and Spano, R. (1971). *Farmaco. Ed. Sci.* **26**, 303.

Littell, R., Smith, J. M., and Allen, D. S. (1969). U. S. Patent 3,454,587 (to American Cyanamid).

Lombardino, J. G. (1966). *J. Med. Chem.* **9**, 770.

Manghisi, E. (1972). U. S. Patent 3,642,864 (to Istituto Luso Farmaco d'Italia).

Marshall, W. S. (1972). U. S. Patent 3,644,641 (to Eli Lilly and Co).

Maruyama, H., Fujhira, E., and Nakazawa, M. (1969). *J. Med. Soc. Toho Univ.* **16**, 558.

Matter, M., and Staehelin, F. R. (1968). U. S. Patent 3,361,749 (to HACO A. G.).

Merck. (1971a). French Patent 2,053,014.

Merck. (1971b). French Patent 2,053,016.

Merck. (1971c). French Patent 2,053,019.

Misaki, A., Izumi, T., Koshiba, M., and Yamamoto, H. (1971). Japanese Patent 71/15097 (to Sumitomo Chem. Ind.); *Chem. Abstr.* **75**, 48925 (1971).

Misher, A., Adams, H. J., Fishler, J. J., and Jones, R. G. (1968). *J. Pharm. Sci.* **57**, 1128.

Moertel, C. G., Ahmann, D. L., Taylor, W. F., and Schwartau, N. (1972). *N. Engl. J. Med.* **286**, 813.

Mokhort, N. A. (1970). *Farm. Zh.* (*Kiev*) **25**, 76; *Chem. Abstr.* **74**, 15702 (1971).

Mokhort, N. A., and Korkhova, N. S. (1968). *Farmakol. Toksikol.* (*Kiev*) No. 4, p. 85–9; *Chem. Abstr.* **71**, 29080 (1969).

Moriyama, H., Nagata, H., and Tamaki, T. (1971). Japanese Patent 71/14656 (to Sumitomo Chem. Co.); *Chem. Abstr.* **75**, 48703 (1971).

Mörsdorf, K., and Wolf, G. (1972). *Arzneim.-Forsch.* **22**, 2105.

Nakanishi, M., Okada, T., and Kudo. A. (1967). Japanese Patent 67/9945 (to Yoshitomi Pharm. Ind., Ltd.); *Chem. Abstr.* **67**, 99879 (1967).

Nantka-Namirski, P. (1967). *Acta Pol. Pharm.* **24**, 111; *Chem. Abstr.* **67**, 108538 (1967).

Niemegeers, C. J. E., Verbruggen, F. J., and Janssen, P. A. J. (1964). *J. Pharm. Pharmacol.* **16**, 810.

Official Literature on New Drugs. (1968). *Clin. Pharmacol. Ther.* **9**, 540.

O'Mant, D. M., and Smith, S. C. (1972). German Patent 2,136,961 (to Imperial Chemical Industries Ltd.).

Panse, P., Zeiller, P., and Sensch, K. H. (1971). *Arzneim.-Forsch.* **21**, 1605.

Peterfalvi, M., Branceni, D., Azadian-Boulanger, G., Chifflot, L., and Jequier, R. (1966). *Med. Pharmacol. Exp.* **15**, 254.

Picciola, G., Gaggi, R., and Caliari, W. (1968). *Farmaco, Ed. Sci.* **23**, 502.

"Profile of an Antirheumatic Compound." (1969). *Therapie Woche* **19**, 1765–1811.

Queval, P. J., and Falconnet, R. L. M. (1972). U. S. Patent, 3,654,310 (to SERDEX Société d'Etudes de Recherches de Diffusion et d'Exploitation).

Rhone-Poulenc, (1966). Netherlands Patent Appl. 6,515,071; *Chem. Abstr.* **66**, 2379 (1967).

Robinson, R. G., and Radcliff, F. J. (1972). *Med. J. Aust.* **1**, 1079.

Ross, S. T., and Zirkle, C. L. (1970). U. S. Patent 3,513,199 (to Smith Kline and French).

Rowland, M., Riegelman, S., Harris, P. A., and Sholkoff, S. D. (1972). *J. Pharm. Sci.* **61**, 379.

Ruedy, J., and Bentley, K. C. (1969). *Clin. Pharmacol. Ther.* **11**, 718.

Ruschig, H., Meixner, W., and Alpermann, H. G. (1969). U. S. Patent 3,445,473 (to Farbwerke Hoechst).

Ruyle, W. V., Sarett, L. H., and Matzuk, A. R. (1972). U. S. Patent 3,674,870 (to Merck and Co.).

Saggiomo, A. J., and Sutton, B. M. (1968). *J. Med. Chem.* **11**, 1089.

Saksena, S. K., Radhakrishnan, A. V., Kartha, C. C., and Gokhale, S. V. (1971). *Indian J. Med. Res.* **59**, 1283.

Sallmann, A., and Pfister, R. (1971a). U. S. Patent 3,558,690 (to Geigy Chemical Co.).

Sallmann, A., and Pfister, R. (1971b). U. S. Patent 3,573,290 (to Geigy Chemical Co.).

Sallmann, A., and Pfister, R. (1971c). U. S. Patent 3,590,039 (to Geigy Chemical Co.).

Sarett, L. H. (1971). *Arzneim.-Forsch.* **21**, 1759.

Sarett, L. H., and Ruyle, W. V. (1969). German Patent, 1,801,303 (to Merck and Co.); *Chem. Abstr.* **71**, 70627 (1969).

Sarett, L. H., and Ruyle, W. V. (1971). U. S. Patent 3,558,641 (to Merck and Co.).

Sarret, L. H., and Ruyle, W. V. (1972). U. S. Patent 3,676,451 (to Merck and Co.).

Schardein, J. L., Blatz, A. T., Woosley, E. T., and Kaump, D. H. (1969). *Toxicol. Appl. Pharmacol.* **15**, 46.

Scherrer, R. A. (1963). U. S. Patent 3,107,263 (to Parke, Davis and Co.).

Scherrer, R. A. (1965a). German Patent 1,185,622 (to Parke, Davis and Co.); *Chem. Abstr.* **62**, 16138g (1965).

Scherrer, R. A. (1965b). German Patent 1,186,871 (to Parke, Davis and Co.); *Chem. Abstr.* **63**, 544c (1965).

Scherrer, R. A. (1965c). German Patent 1,190,951 (to Parke, Davis and Co.); *Chem. Abstr.* **63**, 4209d (1965).

Scherrer, R. A. (1965d). Netherlands Patent Appl. 6,507,783 (to Parke, Davis and Co.); *Chem. Abstr.* **64**, 19501c (1966).

Scherrer, R. A. (1966). U. S. Patent 3,238,201 (to Parke, Davis and Co.); *Chem. Abstr.* **64**, 17614b (1966).

Scherrer, R. A. (1968a). U. S. Patent 3,369,042 (to Parke, Davis and Co.); *Chem. Abstr.* **65**, 16904h (1966).

Scherrer, R. A. (1968b). U. S. Patent 3,390,172 (to Parke, Davis and Co.).

Scherrer, R. A. (1968c). U. S. Patent 3,413,313 (to Parke, Davis and Co.); *Chem. Abstr.* **68**, 2712 (1968).

Scherrer, R. A. (1968d). U. S. Patent 3,413,339 (to Parke, Davis and Co.); *Chem. Abstr.* **69**, 18818 (1968).

Scherrer, R. A. (1969a). U. S. Patent 3,458,519 (to Parke, Davis and Co.).

Scherrer, R. A. (1969b). U. S. Patent 3,471,559 (to Parke, Davis and Co.).

Scherrer, R. A. (1970). U. S. Patent 3,506,684 (to Parke, Davis and Co.).

Scherrer, R. A., and Beatty, H. R. (1972). *J. Org. Chem.* **37**, 1681.

Scherrer, R. A., and Richter, H. I. (1965). German Patent 1,190,952 (to Parke, Davis and Co.); *Chem. Abstr.* **63**, 6921e (1965).

Scherrer, R. A., and Short, F. W. (1965). British Patent 989,951 (to Parke, Davis and Co.); *Chem. Abstr.* **63**, 1669a (1965).

Scherrer, R. A., and Short, F. W. (1967). U. S. Patent 3,313,848 (to Parke, Davis and Co.); *Chem. Abstr.* **67**, 73368 (1967).

Scherrer, R. A., and Short, F. W. (1969). U. S. Patent 3,420,871 (to Parke, Davis and Co.).

Scherrer, R. A., Winder, C. V., and Short, F. W. (1964) *9th Nat. Med. Chem. Symp.*, *Amer. Chem. Soc.*, *1964* Abstr., pp. 11a–11i.

Schoenwaldt, E. F., Hazen, G. G., and Shuman, R. F. (1972). U. S. Patent 3,660,372 (to Merck and Co.).

Schulenberg, J. W., and Archer, S. (1965). *Org. Rct.* **14**, 1–51.

Shen, T. Y. (1972a). *Angew. Chem., Int. Ed. Engl.* **11**, 460.

Shen, T. Y. (1972b). U. S. Patent 3,660,403 (to Merck and Co.).

Shen, T. Y. (1972c). U. S. Patent 3,671,580 (to Merck and Co.).

Shen, T. Y., Walford, G. L., Witzel, B. E., and Ruyle, W. V. (1971a). German Patent 2,031,223 (to Merck and Co.); *Chem. Abstr.* **74**, 125270 (1971).

Shen, T. Y., Walford, G. L., Witzel, B. E., and Bugianesi, R. L. (1971b). German Patent 2,031,224 (to Merck and Co.); *Chem. Abstr.* **75**, 5499 (1971).

Shen, T. Y., Walford, G. L., and Witzel, B. E. (1971c). German Patent 2,031,228; *Chem. Abstr.* **74**, 88051 (1971).

Shen, T. Y., Walford, G. L., and Witzel, B. E. (1971d). German Patent 2,031,232 (to Merck and Co.); *Chem. Abstr.* **74**, 141309 (1971).

Shen, T. Y., Walford, G. L., and Witzel, B. E. (1972a). U. S. Patent 3,632,760 (to Merck and Co.).

Shen, T. Y., Witzel. B. E., and Walford, G. L. (1972b). U. S. Patent 3,641,134 (to Merck and Co.).

Shen, T. Y., Greenwald, R., Witzel, B. E., and Walford, G. L. (1972c). U. S. Patent 3,642,997 (to Merck and Co.).

Shen, T. Y., Witzel, B. E., and Walford, G. L. (1972d). U. S. Patent 3,655,697 (to Merck and Co.).

Shen, T. Y., Walford, G. L., Witzel, B. E., and Bugianesi, R. L. (1972e). U. S. Patent 3,657,430 (to Merck and Co.).

Shen, T. Y., Walford, G. L., and Witzel, B. E. (1972f). U. S. Patent 3,657,431 (to Merck and Co.).

Shen, T. Y., Walford, G. L., and Witzel, B. E. (1972g). U. S. Patent 3,657,432 (to Merck and Co.).

Sherlock, M. H. (1972a). U. S. Patent 3,644,424 (to Schering Corp.).

Sherlock, M. H. (1972b). U. S. Patent 3,681,394 (to Schering Corp.).

Sherlock, M. H., and Sperber, N. (1967). U. S. Patent 3,337,570 (to Schering Corp.).

Smith, M. J. H., and Smith, P. K., eds. (1966). "The Salicylates." Wiley (Interscience), New York.

Sota, K., Noda, K., Maruyama, H., Fujihira, E., and Nakazawa, M. (1969). *Yakugaku Zasshi* **89**, 1392.

Spano, R., and Linari, G. (1971). *Farmaco, Ed. Sci.* **26**, 844.

Spano, R., and Marri, R. (1968). *Boll. Chim. Farm.* **107**, 512–515.

Spano, R., Linari, G., and Marri, R. (1972). *J. Med. Chem.* **15**, 552.

Stepanov, F. N., Mokhort, N. A., Danilenko, G. I., Danilenko, V. F., Dikolenko, E. I., and Zosim, L. A. (1970). U.S.S.R. Patent 287,011; *Chem. Abstr.* **75**, 35440 (1971).

Stepanov, F. N., Mokhort, N. A., Danilenko, G. I., Danilenko, V. F., Dikolenko, E. I., and Zosim, L. A. (1971). *Khim-Farm. Zh.* **5**, 9; *Chem. Abstr.* **76**, 14029 (1972).

Sutton, B. M. (1971). U. S. Patent 3,591,692 (to Smith Kline and French).

Sutton, B. M., and Birnie, J. H. (1966). *J. Med. Chem.* **9**, 835.

Terada, H., and Muraoka, S. (1972). *Mol. Pharmacol.* **8**, 95.

Tsuchiya, T., and Levy, G. (1972). *J. Pharm. Sci.* **61**, 800.
Van Coller, P. E. (1970). *Med. Proc.* **16**, 340.
Vane, J. R. (1971). *Nature (London), New Biol.* **231**, 232.
Vane, J. R. (1972). *Hosp. Pract.* **7** (3), 61.
Van Riezen, H., and Bettink, E. (1968). *J. Pharm. Pharmacol.* **20**, 474.
Von Kaulla, K. N., and Thilo, D. (1970). *Klin. Wochenschr.* **48**, 668.
Wajngurt, A. (1971). U. S. Patent 3,567,721 (to Geigy Chem. Co.).
Walford, G. L., Jones, H., and Shen, T. Y. (1971). *J. Med. Chem.* **14**, 339.
Wasley, J. W. F., and Gruenfeld, N. (1972). U. S. Patent 3,637,710 (to Geigy Chem. Co.).
Watnick, A. S., Taber, R. I., and Tabachnick, I. I. A. (1971). *Arch. Int. Pharmacodyn. Ther.* **190**, 78.
Wax, J., Clinger, W. A., Varner, P., Bass, P., and Winder, C. V. (1970). *Gastroenterology* **58**, 772.
Westby, T. R., and Barfknecht, C. F. (1973). *J. Med. Chem.* **16**, 40.
Whitehouse, M. W. (1967). *Biochem. Pharmacol.* **16**, 753.
Winder, C. V., Wax, J., Scotti, L., Scherrer, R. A., Jones, E. M., and Short, F. W. (1962). *J. Pharmacol. Exp. Ther.* **138**, 1195.
Winder, C. V., Wax, J., Serrano, B., Jones, E. M., and McPhee, M. L. (1963). *Arthritis Rheum.* **6**, 36.
Winder, C. V., Wax, J., and Welford, M. (1965). *J. Pharmacol. Exp. Ther.* **148**, 422.
Winder, C. V., Kaump, D. H., Glazko, A. J., and Holmes, E. L. (1967). *Ann. Phys. Med. Suppl.* pp. 7–49.
Winder, C. V., Lembke, L. A., and Stephens, M. D. (1969). *Arthritis Rheum.* **12**, 472.
Winter, C. A. (1965). *Int. Symp. Non-Steroidal Anti-Inflammatory Drugs, Proc., 1964* pp. 190–206.
Winter, C. A., and Flataker, L. (1965a). *J. Pharmacol. Exp. Ther.* **148**, 373.
Winter, C. A., and Flataker, L. (1965b). *J. Pharmacol. Exp. Ther.* **150**, 165.
Yaburchi, T., Fujimura, H., Nakagawa, A., and Kimura, R. (1971). German Patent 2,120,663 (to Hisamitsu Pharm. Co.); *Chem. Abstr.* **76**, 72548 (1972).
Yagupolskii, L. M., Yufa, P. A., Fialkov, Y. A., Fadeicheva, A. G., Endelman, E. S., Butlerouskii, M. A., Trinus, F. P., and Mokhort, N. A. (1972). U.S.S.R. Patent 331,058; *Chem. Abstr.* **77**, 34156 (1972).
Yamamoto, H., Hirohashi, A., Izumi, T., and Koshiba, M. (1972). U. S. Patent 3,673,243 (to Sumitomo Chem. Co.).
Yonan, P. (1972). U. S. Patent 3,636,094 (to G. D. Searle and Co.).
Zoni, G., and Molinari, M. L. (1971). *Boll. Chim. Farm.* **110**, 105.
Zoni, G., Molinari, M. L., and Banfi, S. (1971). *Farmaco, Ed. Sci.* **26**, 525.

Chapter 4

Aryl- and Heteroarylalkanoic Acids and Related Compounds

PETER F. JUBY

Bristol Laboratories
Division of Bristol-Myers Company
Syracuse, New York

I. INTRODUCTION

Without doubt the aryl- and heteroarylalkanoic acids have been one of the most widely explored groups of nonsteroidal compounds for potential antiinflammatory activity. In fact, so many compounds have been described that it is impossible to include them all in a chapter of this size. Therefore, the development of this area is outlined through accounts of what I feel are the most significant agents. The emphasis is on the relationships between chemical structure and observed antiinflammatory activity. Accounts of the general biological properties and the possible modes of action of the agents appear in Volume II.

In preparation for the discussion of the overall structure–activity relationships of the aryl- and heteroarylalkanoic acids in Section XV, the antiinflammatory properties of each compound or series of compounds are presented individually in Sections II–XIV. The structures of the acids are drawn so as to bring out the greatest degree of similarity in the group as a whole.

In general, the chemistry involved in the syntheses of many of the compounds described in this chapter is of a routine nature. Apart from one typical sequence (Section V,B,1), therefore, only unusual synthetic schemes are included. Appropriate references are provided for many of the other syntheses.

For the purposes of this chapter, all 2-arylalkanoic acids are classified as arylacetic acids. For example, 2-(4-isobutylphenyl)propionic acid (**4**, ibuprofen) is considered an α-methylphenylacetic acid. An exception to the inclusion of all arylacetic acids in this chapter is that 2-anilinophenylacetic acids are found in the preceding chapter as homologs of the fenamic acids.

Unless otherwise indicated, all agents were administered orally in both the animal assays and the clinical trials covered in this survey.

II. PHENYLACETIC ACIDS

A. RD 10335

The origin of a significant proportion of the interest in aryl- and heteroarylalkanoic acid antiinflammatory agents can be traced to pioneering work in the early 1960's by the Boots Pure Drug Company in England. From a large group of 4-alkyl-, 4-cycloalkyl-, 4-alkoxy-, 4-phenylthio-, and 4-phenoxyphenylacetic acids (Boots Pure Drug Company Limited, 1962), the 4-*t*-butyl compound (**1**) was selected for clinical trials. This compound, RD 10335, proved to be active in rheumatoid arthritis at a daily dose of 2–4 gm, but a significant proportion of patients developed a skin rash and the compound was dropped (Buckler and Adams, 1968).

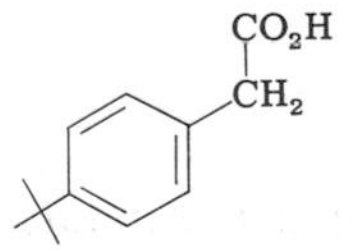

1

B. Ibufenac

The next compound to be studied by Boots was ibufenac (**2**). In the UV-erythema screen in the guinea pig, ibufenac had two to four times the potency of aspirin (Adams *et al.*, 1963, 1968) and was twice as potent as aspirin in an adjuvant-induced arthritis model in the rat (Adams *et al.*, 1968). In several clinical trials against rheumatoid arthritis (Chalmers,

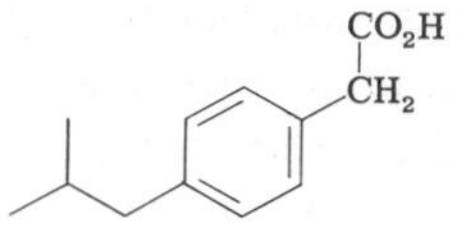

2

1963; Thompson *et al.*, 1964; Hart and Boardman, 1965), the compound was felt to have antiinflammatory and analgesic activities comparable to aspirin but at about half the dose. In spite of some evidence for the possibility of the compound causing liver dysfunction (Thompson *et al.*, 1964; Hart and Boardman, 1965), ibufenac was marketed in Great Britain in 1966 as Dytransin. The compound was eventually withdrawn in 1968 because of hepatotoxicity (Anonymous, 1968).

C. RD 10499

The next compound in the series to be studied clinically by Boots was the 4-cyclohexyl derivative (**3**), RD 10499. Like compound (**1**), compound (**3**) also produced a skin rash in a significant proportion of patients and was dropped from consideration (Buckler and Adams, 1968).

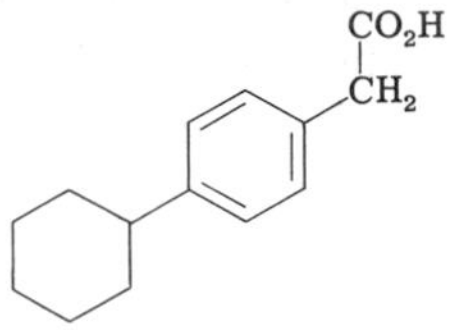

3

D. Ibuprofen

Boots next proceeded with an α-methyl derivative of ibufenac, ibuprofen (**4**). This racemic product was shown to have antiinflammatory, analgesic, and antipyretic properties with a potency of 16–32 times aspirin in a variety of animal screens (Adams *et al.*, 1969a). In a single-dose carrageenan-induced rat paw edema test, ibuprofen was more potent than phenylbutazone. In a multiple-dose established adjuvant-induced arthritis assay, however, the potency of (**4**) was only about 0.65 times that of phenylbutazone. It has been suggested that this relatively low activity can be explained, in part, by the fact that ibuprofen is less persistent in the blood of the rat than phenylbutazone. No evidence was found in rats for any adverse effects on hepatic function (Adams *et al.*, 1969b), and the only significant pathological effect in animals was gastric ulceration. The (+) and (−) isomers of (4) were found to be equipotent in the UV-erythema test in the guinea pig (Adams *et al.*, 1967).

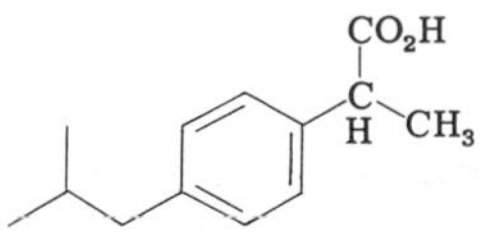

4 (±)

   Many clinical studies have been reported on ibuprofen, including a recent claim that about 70% of 983 patients with rheumatoid arthritis, osteoarthritis, and allied conditions have shown improvement on long-term therapy (Goldberg *et al.*, 1971). In a review of many of the clinical studies, however, it has been concluded that, although ibuprofen is an effective analgesic agent, it so far has not been shown to have anti-inflammatory effects in man (Huskisson *et al.*, 1971). A very thorough review has recently appeared (Davies and Avery, 1972). At the usual daily dose of 0.6–1.2 gm no serious side effects have been attributed to ibuprofen. The principal urinary metabolites in man have been identified (Adams *et al.*, 1967) as the two dextrorotatory products (5) and (6), which were inactive in the UV-erythema screen (Adams *et al.*, 1969a). Ibuprofen is now being sold in Great Britain as Brufen. Perseverance has been rewarded.

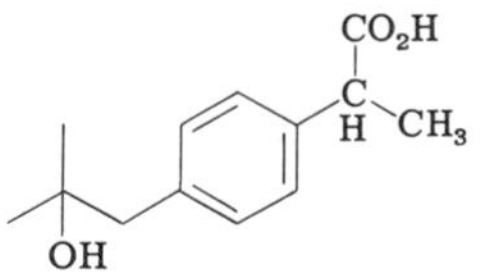

5 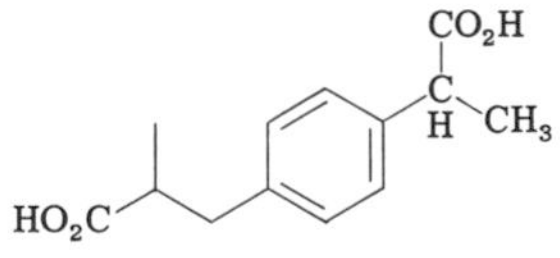 (+)   **6** (+)

E. MK-830

   Patent claims to a large series of phenylacetic acid antiinflammatory agents that were published in 1965 indicated that Merck and Company in the United States was also interested in this area (1965a,b). Brief reports (Anonymous, 1967; Shen, 1967a) on a series of biphenylylacetic acids of general structure (7) indicated that they showed high antiinflammatory activity in the rat. The potentiating effect of an α-methyl substituent was noted.

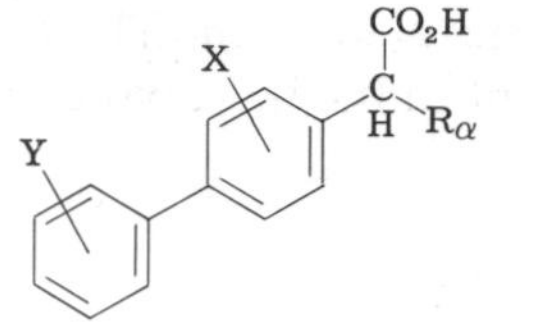

R_α = H, CH_3, =CH_2, C_2H_5 R_α = H, CH_3, =CH_2, C_2H_5

X, Y = H, Cl, F, CH_3O, HO   X = H, Cl, CH_3S, HO

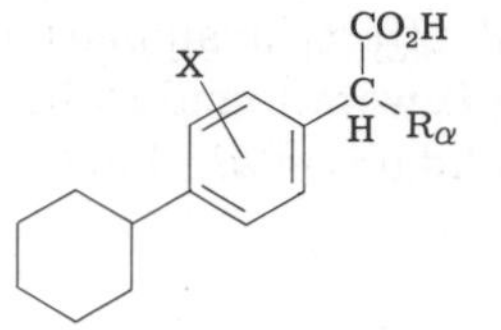

7   **8**

Antiinflammatory activity is also reported for an analogous series of 4-cyclohexylphenylacetic acids (**8**) (Anonymous, 1967; Shen, 1967a). A variety of syntheses that are applicable to arylacetic acids in general are described for these compounds (Merck and Company, 1966). The corresponding cyclopentyl, cycloheptyl, and 2-norbornyl analogs are less active. Once again, the preferred group at R_α is methyl. The potency of these acids is further enhanced by nuclear substitution, particularly in the 3 position. The most potent compound was found to be MK-830, the (S)-(+) isomer (**9**) of the 3-chloro analog. This is 10–20 times more potent than indomethacin in the carrageenan-induced paw edema assay in the rat, with an ED_{50} of about 0.3 mg/kg. Because its use results in both renal and gastrointestinal toxicity in animals, however, MK-830 has been withdrawn from clinical trial (Sarett, 1971).

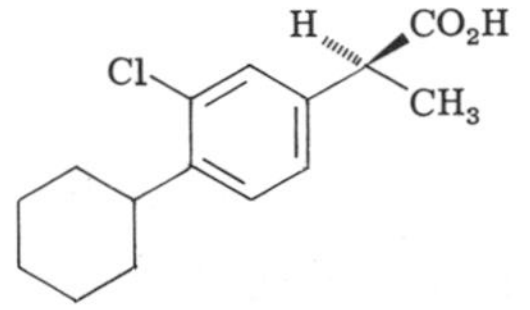

9 (S)-(+) 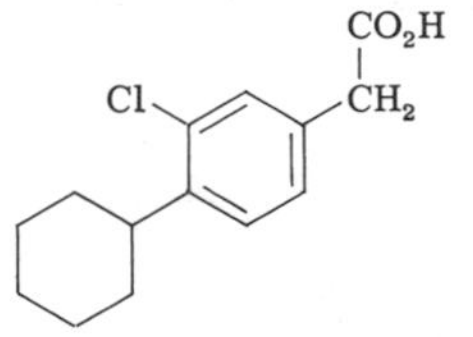   **10**

More recently some French workers have reported (Redel *et al.*, 1971) that the acid **10**, which does not have an α-methyl substituent, was only equipotent to indomethacin in the carrageenan edema screen.

Antiinflammatory activity has also been claimed for the corresponding carbinols (Merck, 1968a) and aldehydes (Merck, 1968b) of the 4-cyclohexylphenylacetic acids.

Of current clinical interest is another compound from Boots, flurbiprofen (**7**, R_α = CH_3, X = 3-F, Y = H). Significant antiarthritic activity was demonstrable at a daily dose of 45 mg (Chalmers *et al.*, 1972).

A planar analog of the biphenyl series is the fluorene-2-acetic acid (**7**, X, Y = 3, 2'-CH_2 bridge, R_α = CH_3) (Stiller *et al.*, 1972). It had an ED_{50}

in the carrageenan edema assay about the same as phenylbutazone (82 mg/kg).

F. Alclofenac

From Belgium came the 4-allyloxy acid alclofenac (11), which was found to be equipotent to phenylbutazone in an established adjuvant-induced arthritis assay in the rat (Lambelin *et al.*, 1970a). After toxicity (Lambelin *et al.*, 1970b) and metabolic (Roncucci *et al.*, 1970) studies, alclofenac (Mervan) was advanced to the clinic (Lambotte, 1970; Desproges-Gotteron *et al.*, 1971; Klemm *et al.*, 1971) for the treatment of such inflammatory conditions as osteoarthritis, rheumatoid arthritis, and ankylosing spondylitis. Effectiveness was claimed at daily doses of 1.5–3.0 gm, the drug being well tolerated. Clinical improvement was also noted in rheumatoid arthritics receiving the ethanolamine salt of (11) at 0.5–1.5 gm/day intramuscularly (Pavelka *et al.*, 1971).

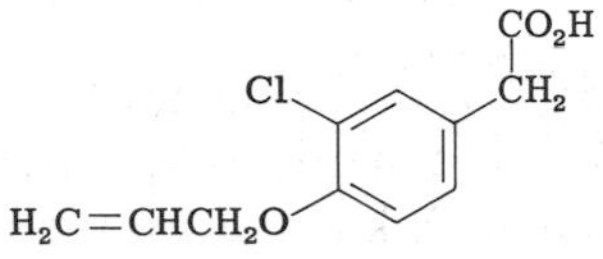

11

G. Bufexamac

Another 4-alkoxyphenylacetic acid derivative that has aroused some interest is bufexamac (12). Bufexamac, one of more than 200 arylacethydroxamic acids that show antiinflammatory, analgesic, antipyretic, and antispasmodic activities in varying degrees, has about one-half the potency of phenylbutazone in the carrageenan-induced abscess test in the rat (Lambelin *et al.*, 1968). The observation of greatly reduced antiinflammatory activity of the parent 4-butoxyphenylacetic acid, both in acute and chronic screens (Lambelin *et al.*, 1968) is of interest, pointing to a specific role for the hydroxylamine function in bufexamac. Contrary to previous reports (Buu-Hoï *et al.*, 1966; Lambelin *et al.*, 1966), the antiinflammatory activity of (12) in the rat is not related to adrenocortical stimulation (Lambelin *et*

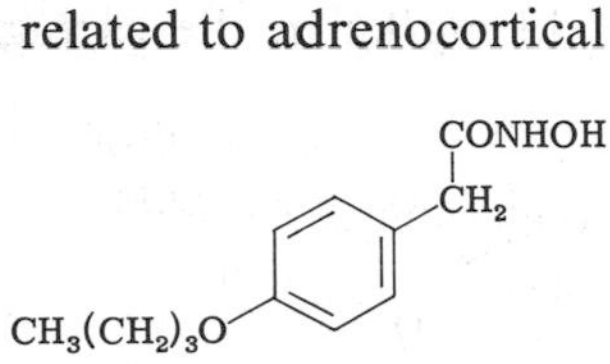

12

al., 1969). Reports have appeared (Lambelin *et al.*, 1968); Van Cauwenberge and Franchimont, 1968; Rose *et al.*, 1970; Pavelka and Wagenhauser, 1970; Bloch-Michel and Parrot, 1970) on the clinical efficacy of bufexamac (Droxaryl) at daily doses of 1.0–1.5 gm in rheumatoid arthritis and osteo-arthritis.

H. Fenoprofen

The racemic α-methyl-3-phenoxyphenylacetic acid (**13**), fenoprofen, was reported by workers at Eli Lilly and Company to be active in the carra-geenan-induced paw edema assay in both normal and adrenalectomized rats, to inhibit adjuvant-induced arthritis in the rat, and to have an ED_{50} of 0.5–1.0 mg/kg in the UV-erythema assay in the guinea pig (Nickander *et al.*, 1971). Significant analgesic and antipyretic activities were also observed. The (+) and (−) isomers appeared to be equipotent. The major urinary metabolites in the rat and the rabbit were free and conjugated 4′-hydroxy derivatives, whereas the major product from the dog was con-jugated fenoprofen (Culp, 1971).

In a clinical trial, patients with rheumatoid arthritis who were treated with fenoprofen obtained symptomatic relief after 4 days (Ridolfo *et al.*, 1971). Absorption and elimination kinetics for the sodium and calcium salts were determined in man (Rubin *et al.*, 1971). Fenoprofen was 99% bound to plasma proteins and had a half-time for elimination of about 2 hours.

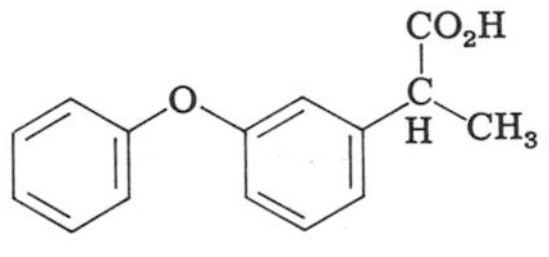

13 (±)

I. Leo-1028

To date, only a pharmacological paper has appeared (Rohte, 1971) describing the antiinflammatory, analgesic, and antipyretic properties of the methylenedioxyphenylacetic acid (**14**), Leo-1028. Leo-1028 has a minimal effective dose of 13 mg/kg in the carrageenan-induced rat paw

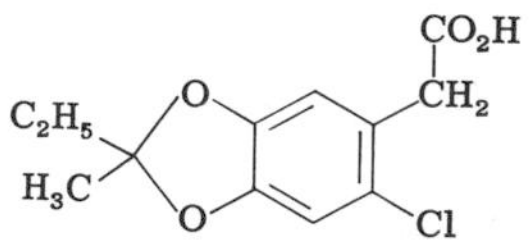

14

edema test and shows significant activity at daily doses of 32 mg/kg in an adjuvant-induced arthritis assay in the rat.

J. Ketoprofen

Molecular modifications of known phenothiazinealkanoic acid anti-inflammatory agents (Section IX) eventually led (Julou *et al.*, 1971) to the synthesis of the racemic 3-benzoyl-α-methylphenylacetic acid (**15**) keto-profen, 19,583 R.P. This product showed potency comparable to indo-methacin in the carrageenan-induced rat paw edema assay and significant activity at daily doses of 2.5 mg/kg in nonestablished adjuvant-induced arthritis in the rat. In chronic toxicity studies in rats and dogs, the ulcero-genic effect of (**15**) was clearly less than that of indomethacin. Ketoprofen was found to be equivalent to the same dosage of indomethacin (100 mg/day) in a study against rheumatoid arthritis and osteoarthrosis of the hip (Gyory *et al.*, 1972).

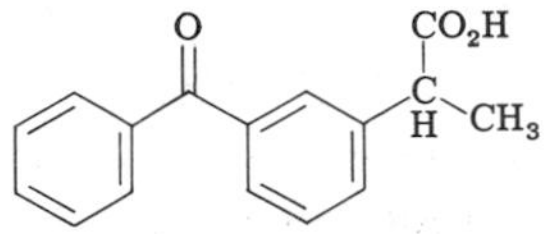

15 (±)

K. Namoxyrate

The dimethylaminoethanol salt of an old compound, 2-(*p*-biphenylyl)-butyric acid, was taken to the clinic as the antiinflammatory–analgesic agent namoxyrate (**16**). This α-ethylphenylacetic acid provided sympto-matic relief to geriatric arthritics at daily doses of 1.2–1.8 gm (Denko *et al.*, 1965; Cohen *et al.*, 1965). As an analgesic agent, namoxyrate was reported to be similar to codeine in clinical effectiveness (Cohen and DeFelice, 1965; Corgill *et al.*, 1965). The pharmacology was reported by Emele and Shanaman (1967). Namoxyrate is believed to be no longer under clinical study.

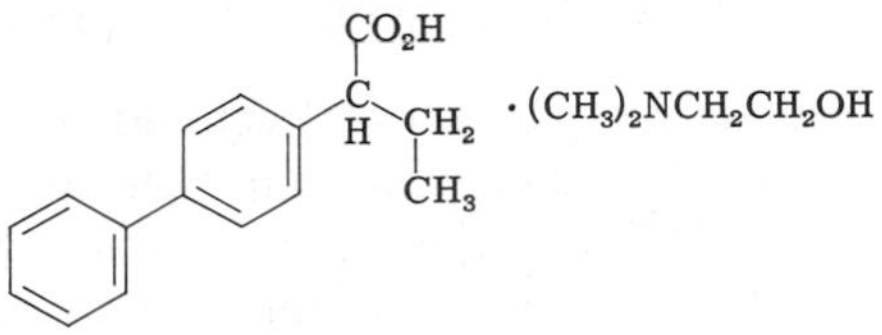

16 (±)

L. (±)-2-(4-Cyclohexylcyclohexen-1-yl)propionic Acid

Of some interest is a recent report (Vincent *et al.*, 1972) describing the antiinflammatory properties of some racemic 2-(4-cycloalkylcyclohexen-1-yl)propionic acids in which the usual phenyl ring is partially reduced. The most potent of these compounds is (±)-2-(4-cyclohexylcyclohexen-1-yl)propionic acid (**21**), which is synthesized as outlined in Scheme I. The endocyclic nature of the double bond has been ascertained by infrared and ultraviolet spectroscopy. Compound (**21**) has about one-half the potency

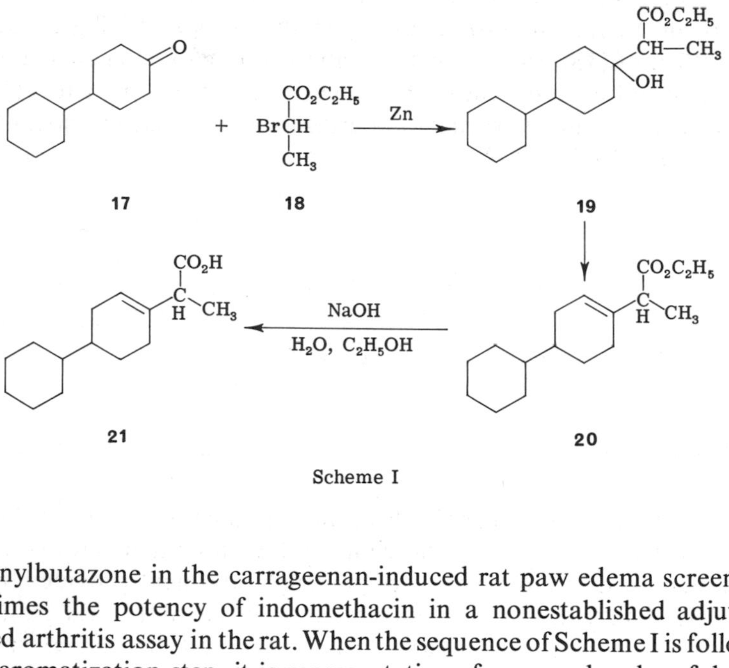

Scheme I

of phenylbutazone in the carrageenan-induced rat paw edema screen and 0.05 times the potency of indomethacin in a nonestablished adjuvant-induced arthritis assay in the rat. When the sequence of Scheme I is followed by an aromatization step, it is representative of a general and useful route to arylacetic acids.

III. 3-PHENYLPROPIONIC ACIDS

A series of compounds with the general structure (**22**) was found (Redel *et al.*, 1970) to be active in the carrageenan-induced rat paw edema test, but inactive in rat pellet and granuloma assays. Where X = Cl and R = H, compound (**22**) gave 62% inhibition of edema at a dose of 25 mg/kg (cf. **9**).

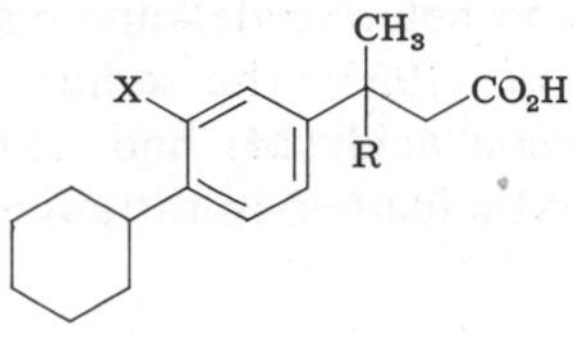

X = H, Cl
R = H, HO

22

IV. 4-PHENYLBUTYRIC ACIDS

BDH 7538 (MJ-1983)

On examination of the antiinflammatory properties of about 30 4-aryl-3-hydroxybutyric acids, it was found (Barron *et al.*, 1968a) that the highest order of activity was associated with the unsubstituted *p*-biphenylyl nucleus. BDH 7538 (**23**) was found to be 2.5 times more potent than phenylbutazone in the carrageenan-induced rat paw edema test, and rather more potent than phenylbutazone in a nonestablished adjuvant-induced arthritis assay in the rat (Barron *et al.*, 1968b). BDH 7538 (MJ-1983) was 4 times more potent than phenylbutazone in the UV-erythema screen in the guinea pig, with a longer duration of action (Brown, 1967). The main side effect observed in chronic toxicity studies in the rat and the dog was gastrointestinal irritation (Barron *et al.*, 1968b). No clinical trials were reported. This compound is no longer under investigation in the United States.

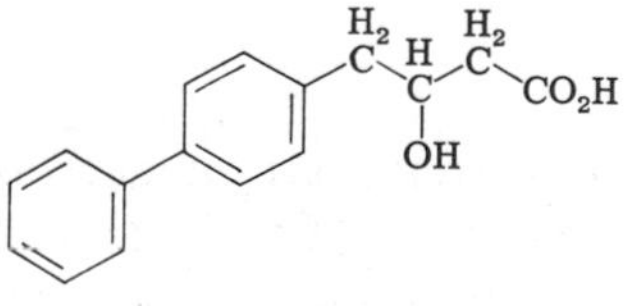

23 (±)

V. NAPHTHALENEACETIC ACIDS

A. 1-Naphthaleneacetic Acids

1. SODIUM α-(2-FURFURYL)-1-NAPHTHALENEACETATE

Not long after the early revelations of the antiinflammatory properties of the phenylacetic acids, reports began to appear on the antiinflammatory activities of other aryl- and heteroarylalkanoic acids and their derivatives. According to Durant *et al.* (1965), the sodium salt of the racemic α-(2-furfuryl)-l-naphthaleneacetic acid (24) had nearly twice the potency of ibufenac (2) in the UV-erythema test in the guinea pig.

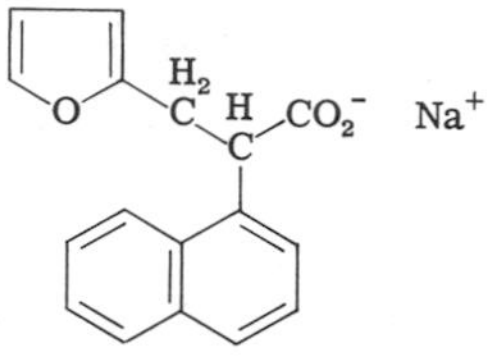

24 (±)

2. NAPHTHYPRAMIDE

From observations (Pala *et al.*, 1965) on the antiinflammatory and analgesic activities of a series of racemic l-naphthylacetamides and l-naphthylacetonitriles it was concluded that the skeletal structure (25) is required for high potency. The most potent antiinflammatory compound of the series is naphthypramide (26), with a potency slightly less than that

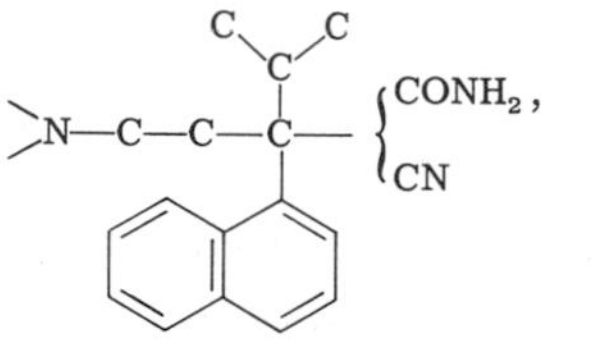

25 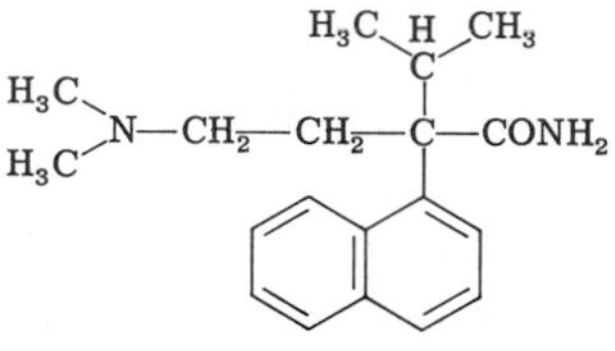   **26**

of phenylbutazone in the carrageenan-induced paw edema model in the rat (Marazzi-Uberti and Turba, 1966). The compound is not metabolized in the rat, the rabbit, or man (Coppi, 1966), and little toxicity has been observed in chronic studies in animals (Marazzi-Uberti and Coppi, 1967; Noel, 1968). Claims for clinical efficacy in acute stages of osteoarthritis (Camarri *et al.*, 1970) and other rheumatic conditions (Klare, 1966) have been made for naphthypramide.

The corresponding α-substituted l-naphthaleneacetic acids display somewhat lower antiinflammatory activity than the nitriles and amides (Pala *et al.*, 1966). This is discussed further in Section XV. This series is unusual in that ordinarily at least one α hydrogen is required for good antiinflammatory activity.

3. 4(5)-PHENYL-1-NAPHTHALENEACETIC ACIDS

Parke–Davis and Company (1965) has claimed antiinflammatory activity for a series of 1-naphthaleneacetic acids (**27** and **28**) that in structure closely resemble the phenylacetic acid agents (see Section II).

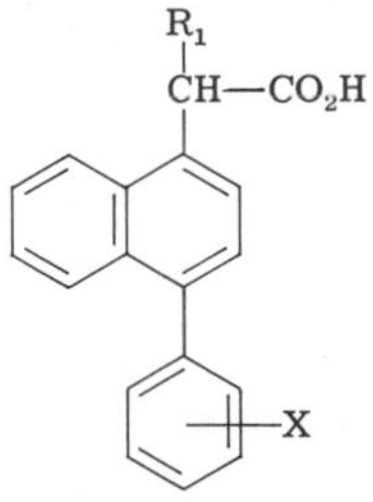

R₁ = H, CH₃
X = H, Cl
27

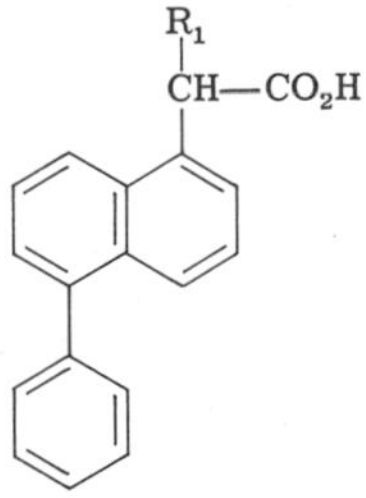

R₁ = H, CH₃
28

B. 2-Naphthaleneacetic Acids

1. NAPROXEN

More recently, a series of 2-naphthaleneacetic acids was found (Harrison *et al.*, 1970) to possess antiinflammatory, analgesic, and antipyretic activities. The lead compound was 2-naphthaleneacetic acid itself, the antiinflammatory activity of which was enhanced by substitution of small lipophilic groups at position 6 and by an α-methyl substituent. Naproxen (**34**), the (+) isomer of the 6-methoxy analog, which was prepared as outlined in Scheme II, was selected for further study. This sequence is typical of the approaches used in the syntheses of many of the arylacetic acids described in this chapter. Naproxen had a potency of 11 times phenylbutazone in the carrageenan-induced rat paw edema assay (Harrison *et al.*, 1970; Roszkowski *et al.*, 1971) and significantly reduced hind paw inflammation in an established adjuvant-induced arthritis assay after 14 daily doses of 0.2 mg per rat (Rooks, 1971). The corresponding aldehyde and carbinol (naproxol) were found to be biologically equivalent to naproxen (Harrison *et al.*, 1970). In a clinical trial, naproxen was claimed to be effective against rheumatoid arthritis at daily doses of 300–500 mg (Lussier *et al.*, 1972). The absorption, distribution, metabolism, and excretion in animals and man were reported by Runkel *et al.*, (1972).

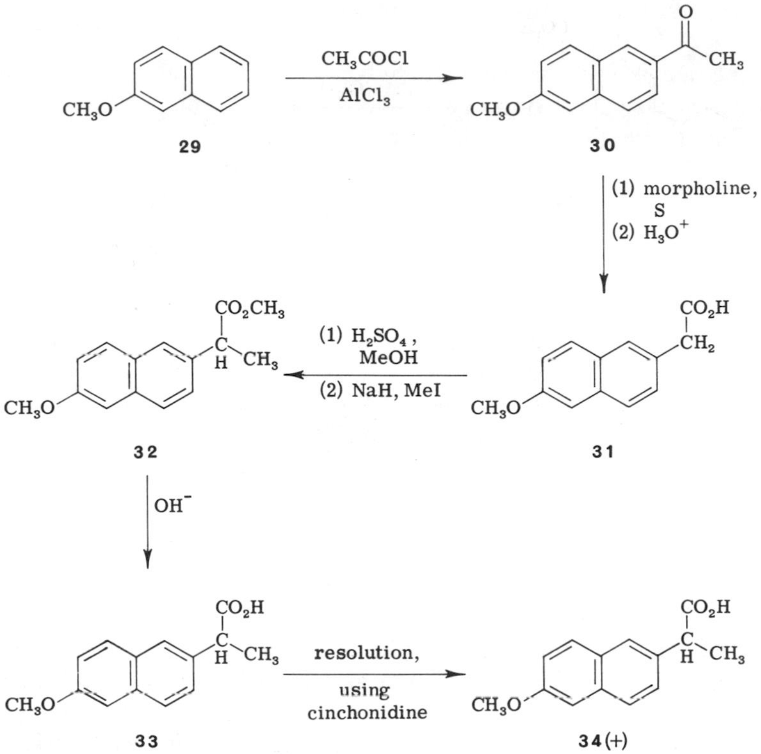

Scheme II

VI. INDANCARBOXYLIC ACIDS

A. Indan-l-carboxylic Acids

A series of 5-cyclohexylindan-l-carboxylic acids with the general structure (35) were reported (Bristol-Myers Company, 1970) to show high anti-inflammatory activity in the carrageenan-induced rat paw edma test.

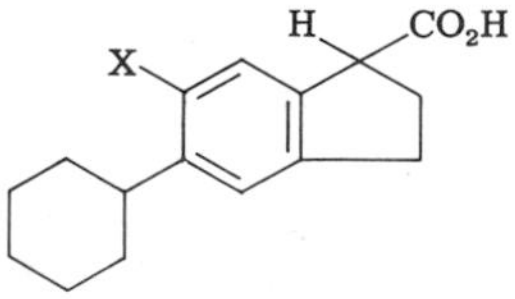

X = H, Cl, F, NO$_2$,
NH$_2$, HO, CH$_3$O

35

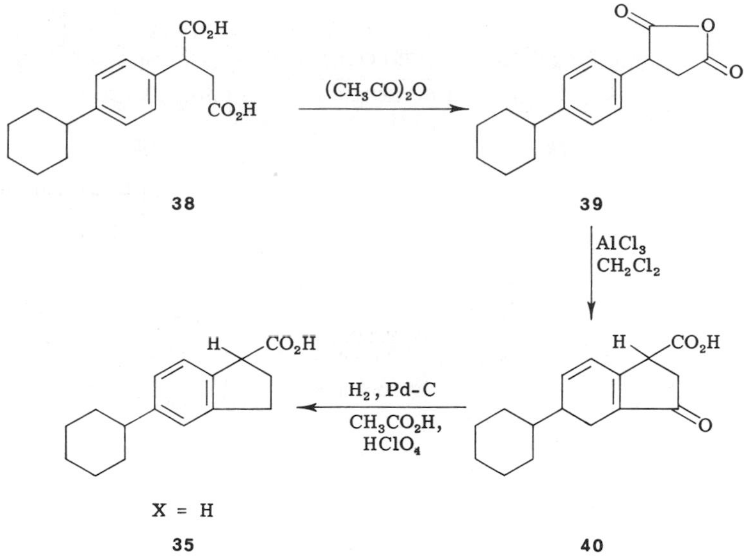

Scheme III

($\pm$)-5-Cyclohexylindan-1-carboxylic acid (35, X = H), which is synthesized as outlined in Scheme III, has an ED_{30} of 3.7 mg/kg and a LD_{50} of 287 mg/kg in the rat. Most of the activity resides in the ($-$) isomer (36), which has since been assigned the S configuration (Juby et al., 1972b). Detailed pharmacological studies have been reported for (36) (Pircio et al. 1972), as well as studies on the inhibition of platelet aggregation (Fleming et al., 1972).

($\pm$)-6-Chloro-5-cyclohexylindan-1-carboxylic acid (35, X = Cl), prepared (Juby et al., 1972b) by the treatment of (35), X = H, with N-chlorosuccinimide in DMF, has an ED_{30} of 1.2 mg/kg and a LD_{50} of 41 mg/kg. Most of the activity resides in the (S)-($+$) isomer (37), which has an ED_{30} of 0.85 mg/kg. These indan-1-carboxylic acids incorporate a phenylacetic acid moiety, with the carboxyl group being held in an essentially rigid, out-of-plane conformation.

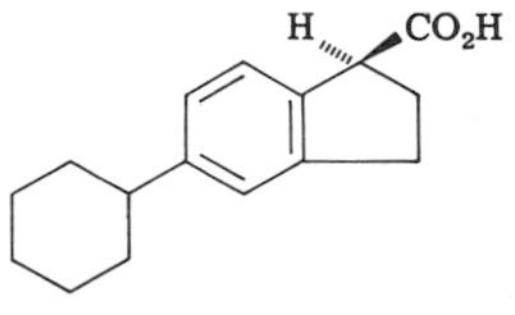

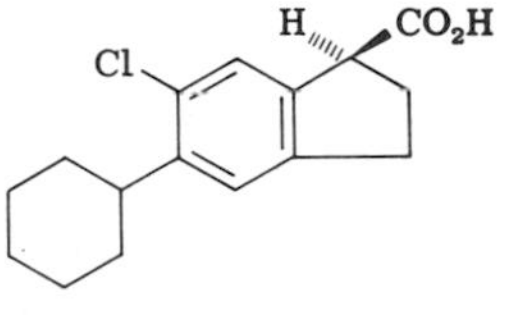

Independent disclosures from Takeda Chemical Industries, Ltd. indicated that the racemic acid (35), X = Cl, (TAI-284) shows potency comparable to indomethacin in a wide variety of acute and chronic antiinflammatory animal screens (Kawai *et al.*, 1971). Most of the activity resides in the (*S*)-(+) isomer (37) (Noguchi *et al.*, 1971). Contrary to the findings of the Bristol Laboratories group (Bristol-Myers Company, 1970), however, only slight activity was reported (Noguchi *et al.*, 1971) for (35), X = H.

It will be remembered that the potency of the phenylacetic acids (8) was enhanced by chlorine substitution in one of the two equivalent positions meta to the acetic acid side chain. Illustrating the nonequivalence of the 4 and 6 positions in the indan nucleus was the lack of activity shown by (±)-4-chloro-5-cyclohexylindan-1-carboxylic acid (41) (Noguchi *et al.*, 1971; Juby *et al.*, 1972b).

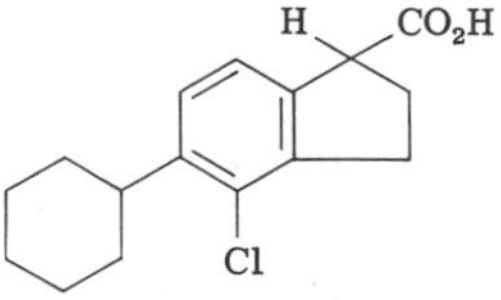

41 (±)

More recently it has been claimed (Juby *et al.*, 1972a) that (±)-5-phenyl-lindan-1-carboxylic acid has an ED_{30} of 4.5 mg/kg in the carrageenan-induced rat paw edema test, with most of the activity residing in the (−) isomer.

B. Indan-2-carboxylic Acids

Antiinflammatory activity at a dose of 30 mg/kg in a paw edema screen has been reported (Minssen-Guetté *et al.*, 1968) for the indan-2-carboxylic acid (42) which incorporates a 3-phenylpropionic acid moiety.

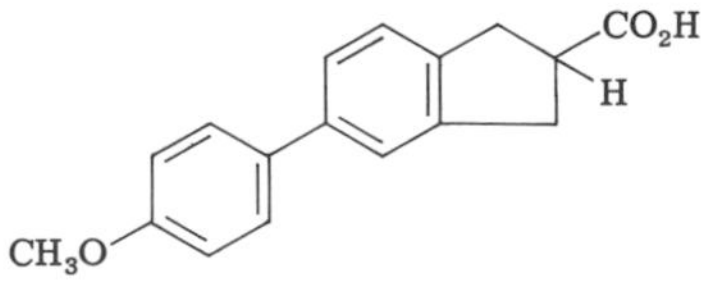

42

VII. 1,2,3,4-TETRAHYDRO-l-NAPHTHOIC ACIDS

Moderate antiinflammatory activity in animal screens is claimed (Ciba, S. A., 1970; Juby *et al.*, 1971) for 1,2,3,4-tetrahydro-l-naphthoic acids of the general structure (**43**).

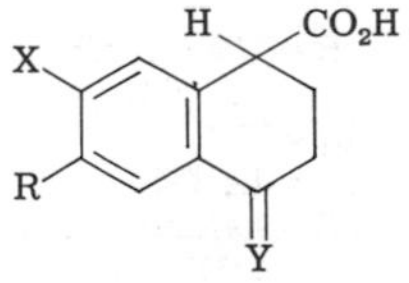

X = H, Cl
Y = H_2, O
R = cyclohexyl,
     phenyl

43

Like the indan-l-carboxylic acids (Section VI,A), these 1,2,3,4-tetrahydro-l-naphthoic acids incorporate a phenylacetic acid moiety but, this time, it is held within a more flexible framework. Both racemic (**44**) and (**45**) had an ED_{30} of about 64 mg/kg in the carrageenan-induced rat paw edema test (Juby *et al.*, 1972c).

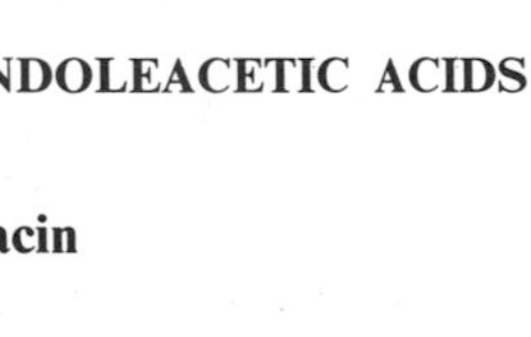

44 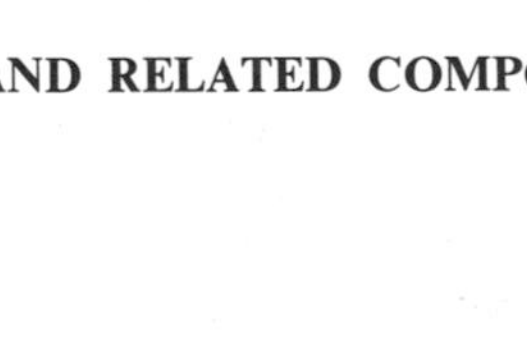 (±)   45 (±)

VIII. INDOLEACETIC ACIDS AND RELATED COMPOUNDS

A. Indomethacin

In the late 1950's chemists at Merck and Company (Shen, 1965) began synthesizing indole derivatives as potential antagonists of serotonin, 3-(2-aminoethyl)-5-hydroxyindole, which was then erroneously believed to play an important role as an inflammatory mediator in man. A few compounds, however, were found to have significant antiinflammatory activity in the cotton pellet granuloma assay in the rat. In the process of modifying the lead compounds to enhance this activity, Merck prepared over 350

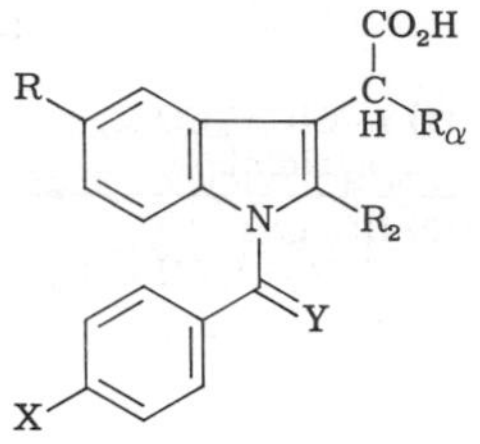

R = CH_3O, $(CH_3)_2N$,
   F, CH_3
R_2 = CH_3
R_α = H, CH_3
X = halogen, CF_3,
   CH_3S
Y = O, H_2

46

indoles, the optimal structural features of which are indicated by (**46**).
l-(4-Chlorobenzoyl)-5-methoxy-2-methylindole-3-acetic acid (**50**), indomethacin, was selected for further study.

Although many patents have now been issued describing a variety of
syntheses for indomethacin, only the original Merck synthesis (Shen *et al.*,
1963; Shen, 1964) (Scheme IV) and an elegant Japanese variation (Yamamoto, 1968; Yamamoto *et al.*, 1968) (Scheme V) are outlined here.

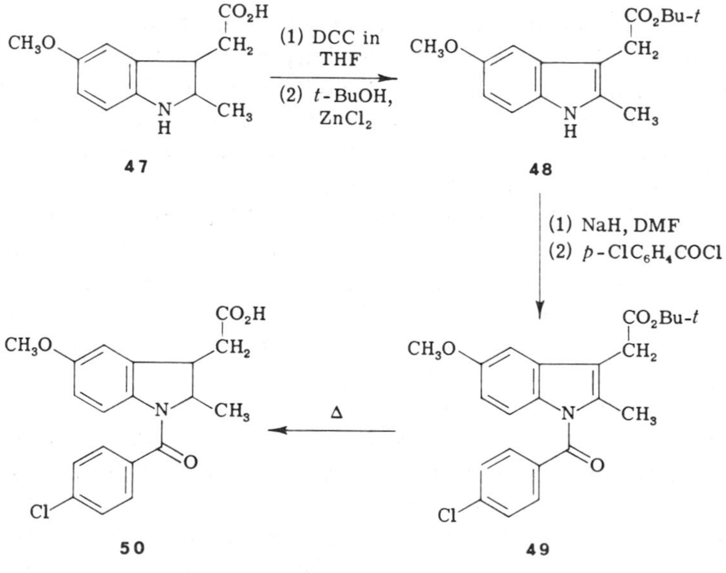

Scheme IV

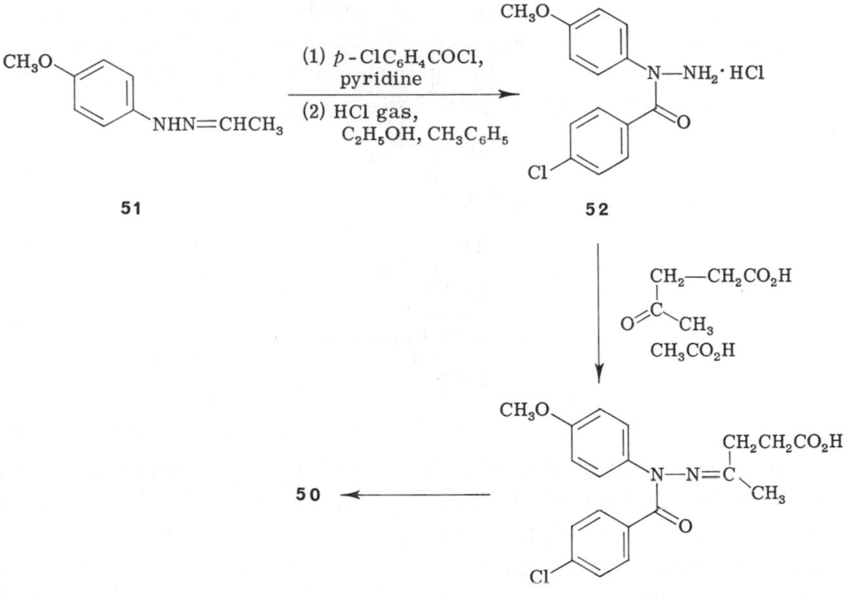

CH₃O — ⟨benzene ring⟩ — NHN=CHCH₃

51

$\xrightarrow{\text{(1) } p\text{-ClC}_6\text{H}_4\text{COCl, pyridine} \quad \text{(2) HCl gas, } C_2H_5OH, CH_3C_6H_5}$

CH₃O — ⟨benzene ring⟩ — N—NH₂·HCl
⟨C=O⟩
Cl — ⟨benzene ring⟩

52

↓

$\underset{\displaystyle CH_3CO_2H}{\overset{\displaystyle \underset{O}{\overset{\displaystyle CH_2-CH_2CO_2H}{\underset{\parallel}{C}}}-CH_3}{}}$

CH₃O — ⟨benzene ring⟩ — N—N=C(CH₂CH₂CO₂H)(CH₃)
⟨C=O⟩
Cl — ⟨benzene ring⟩

50 ⟵ ——————— **53**

Scheme V

In the Merck procedure it was necessary to protect the carboxyl function of (**47**) from acylation by means of a t-butyl group. Because of the lability of the amide linkage of indomethacin (**50**) toward either acid- or base-catalyzed hydrolysis, the protecting group was removed thermally. The Japanese scheme obviated the need for a protecting group and gave an overall yield of about 90% based on (**51**).

All available evidence (Shen, 1965; 1967b; Kistenmacher and Marsh, 1972) suggests that, at a hypothetical *in vivo* receptor site, the preferred conformation of the 4-chlorophenyl group of indomethacin is cis to the methoxyphenyl moiety of the indole ring (see Section VIII,B,1). Anti-inflammatory activity is invariably associated with the enantiomer having the S absolute configuration for those analogs of indomethacin in which $R_\alpha = CH_3$ in (**46**) (Shen, 1967b).

In the cotton pellet granuloma assay in the rat, indomethacin had 85 times the potency of phenylbutazone, with effectiveness in the absence of the adrenals (Winter *et al.*, 1963). In the carrageenan-induced rat paw edema test indomethacin had 20 times the potency of phenylbutazone. Antipyretic (Winter *et al.*, 1963) and analgesic (Winter, 1965) activities, the latter in an inflamed paw screen, were also demonstrated for indomethacin. Indomethocin was found to be 25 times more potent than phenylbutazone in its ability to inhibit the incidence of adjuvant-induced arthritis in the rat (Glenn, 1964). Gastrointestinal lesions resulted from both single-dose and chronic administration of indomethacin to rats, although at doses that were claimed to be well above those required for minimal antiinflammatory activity (Phelps et al., 1968; Brodie et al., 1970).

In contrast to earlier reports (Harman et al., 1964), indomethacin is now found to be extensively O-demethylated and N-deacylated in man (Duggan et al., 1972). The glucuronide (54) is a major but not the sole urinary metabolite as previously believed. In the rabbit, rat, guinea pig, and monkey the N-deacylated derivative, the O-demethyl derivative, and the corresponding acylglucuronides are the major urinary metabolites. In the dog indomethacin is excreted almost exclusively as the glucuronide (54) in the feces (Hucker et al., 1966). All the metabolites have been synthesized (Strachan et al., 1964) and shown to be devoid of antiinflammatory activity (Shen, 1967b). The increasing use of pharmacokinetics in drug evaluation is excellently illustrated by the work of Duggan et al. Indomethacin metabolism is further discussed by Ober (Chapter 10, Volume II).

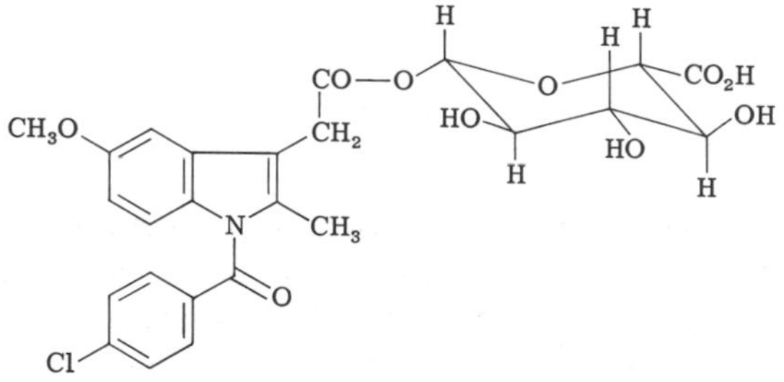

54

Space limitations prevent the complete documentation of the many articles that have appeared since clinical testing of indomethacin began in late 1961. Two good sources of papers, however, are the proceedings (Garattini and Dukes, 1965) of a symposium in Milan, Italy, 1964, on nonsteroidal antiinflammatory drugs, and the Proceedings (1971) of a symposium in Florence, Italy on inflammation and its treatment with indomethacin. The latter also includes a comprehensive bibliography, with titles, on indomethacin through 1970. In summary, indomethacin has been found to be of use in inflammatory diseases, such as osteoarthritis, ankylosing spondylitis, gout, and rheumatoid arthritis, at daily doses of 50–200 mg. Side effects that have been observed, particularly at the higher doses, include headaches, dizziness, and gastrointestinal disturbances. Indomethacin (Indocin, Indocid, Amuno) was approved for marketing in the United States in 1965, and its immediate commercial success has provided a powerful impetus to research in the area of aryl- and heteroarylalkanoic acid antiinflammatory agents.

B. l-Arylideneindene-3-acetic Acids

1. *CIS*-1-(4-CHLOROBENZYLIDENE)-5-METHOXY-2-METHYLINDENE-3-ACETIC ACID

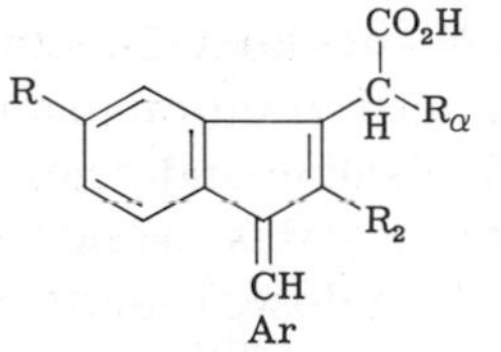

Ar = phenyl, substituted
phenyl, heteroaryl
R = CH_3O, CH_3, F, H, etc.
R_2, R_α = H, CH_3

55

The isosteres (**55**) of the indole-3-acetic acids are synthesized by the base-catalyzed condensation of an indene-3-acetic acid with an aromatic aldehyde (Shen *et al.*, 1966; Winter and Shen, 1967). A representative synthesis is outlined in Scheme VI. The predominant product is the thermodynamically more stable isomer (**58**), which has the 4-chlorophenyl group cis to the methoxyphenyl moiety of the indole ring (Shen, 1967a).

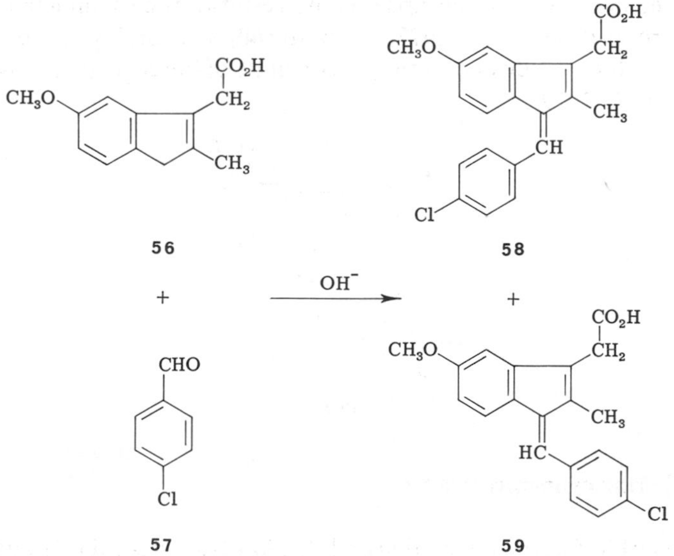

Scheme VI

The structure–activity relationships of the arylideneindene-3-acetic acids closely parallel those of the corresponding indole-3-acetic acids (Shen, 1967a). Furthermore, the preferred compound (58), which is about one half as active as indomethacin in the carrageenan-induced rat paw edema and cotton pellet granuloma assays, has 5 times the potency of (59). It is largely on the basis of the above evidence that a preferred *in vivo* conformation is assigned to indomethacin (Section VIII,A).

cis-l-(4-Chlorobenzylidene)-5-methoxy-2-methylindene-3-acetic acid (58) caused much less gastrointestinal irritation in animals than did indomethacin and is stable under both alkaline and acidic conditions (Shen, 1967a). This promising agent, however, was withdrawn from the clinic after crystalluria was observed at high doses (Sarett, 1971).

2. (±)-*CIS*-5-FLUORO-2-METHYL-1-(4-METHYLSULFINYLBENZYLIDENE) INDENE-3-ACETIC ACID

According to a very recent report, the desirable *in vivo* solubility that was lacking in (58) was attained by the synthesis of (±)-*cis*-5-fluoro-2-methyl-l-(4-methylsulfinylbenzylidene)indene-3-acetic acid (60) (Shen *et al.*, 1972). Compound (60) had an ED_{50} of 3.6 mg/kg in the carrageenan-induced rat paw edema test and was effective at a dose of 0.42 mg/kg/day in the adjuvant-induced arthritis assay in the rat (Van Arman *et al.*, 1972). Like (58), (60) caused less gastrointestinal disturbance than did indomethacin. No significant differences in biological activities were observed for the separate enantiomers, which arise as the result of the asymmetric methyl-sulfinyl group (Shen *et al.*, 1972). In man (60) was largely excreted in the urine as its glucuronide and as the glucuronide of the corresponding sulfone (Hucker *et al.*, 1972).

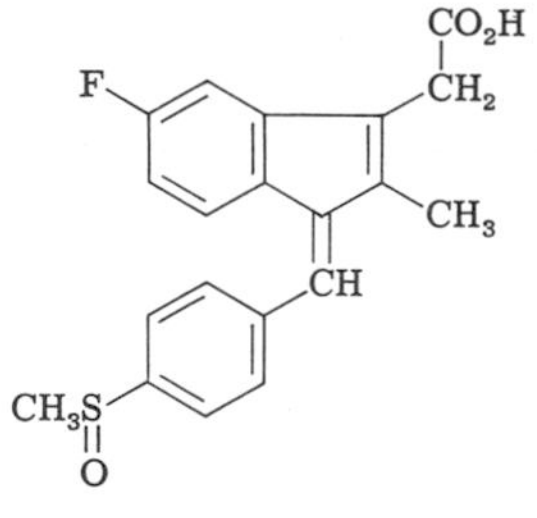

60 (±)

C. 3-(5-Tetrazolylmethyl)indoles

A series of 3-(5-tetrazolylmethyl)indoles has been described in which the carboxyl group of indomethacin and other indole-3-acetic acid antiinflammatory agents (Section VIII,A) has been replaced by the comparably acidic 5-tetrazolyl group (Juby and Hudyma, 1969). Structure–activity relationships in this series do not parallel those of the acetic acids. The most active compound was intrazole (BL-R743) (61), which was one sixteenth as potent as indomethacin in the carrageenan-induced rat paw edema test. The main advantage claimed for intrazole over other available antiinflammatory agents was its lower level of toxicity in both single- and multiple-dose animal studies (Fleming et al., 1969). Brief reports have appeared on the clinical efficacy of intrazole in rheumatoid arthritis (Rakic et al., 1969; Englund and Roth, 1969; Roth and Englund, 1969). The compound was judged less effective than indomethacin in the treatment of acute gout and pseudogout (Steele and Phelps, 1971).

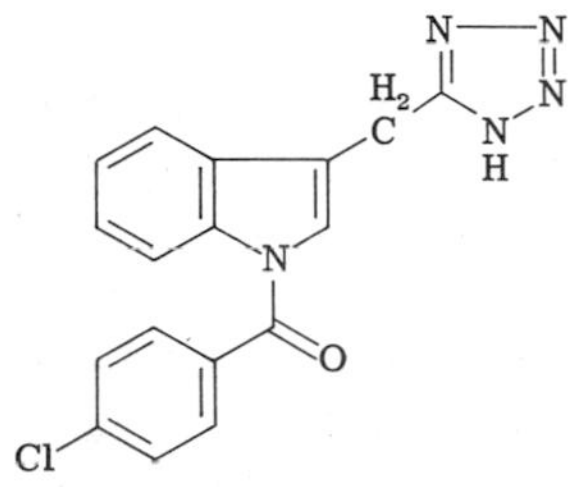

61

D. Indolizineacetic Acids

The indolizine analogs, 3-(4-chlorobenzoyl)-7-methoxy-2-methylindolizine-1-acetic acid (62) and 1-(4-chlorobenzoyl)-6-methoxy-2-methylindolizine-3-acetic acid (63), both had about 0.2 times the potency of indomethacin in the carrageenan-induced rat paw edema test (Casagrande et al., 1971).

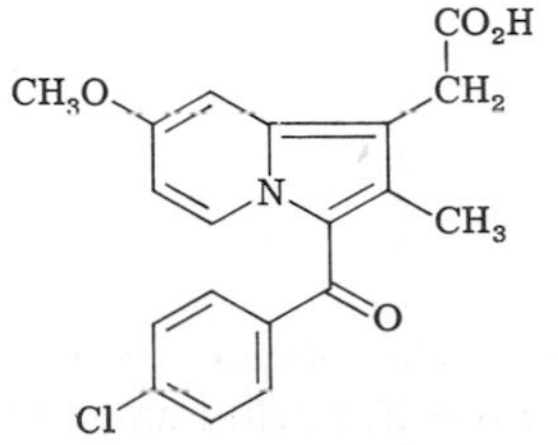

62

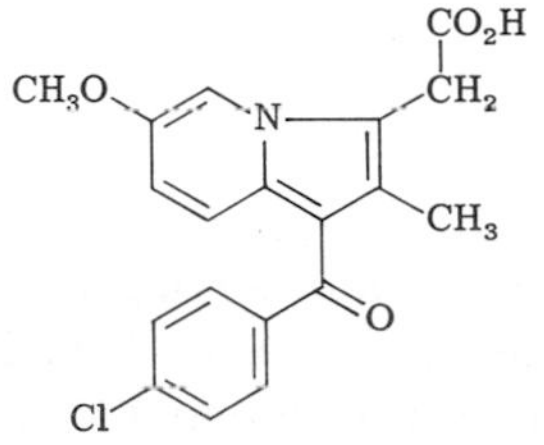

63

IX. PHENOTHIAZINE-2-ACETIC ACIDS

Metiazinic Acid (16,091 R.P.)

Metiazinic acid, 10-methylphenothiazine-2-acetic acid (**64**), emerged as the most potent compound of a large series of phenothiazinealkanoic acids that were examined for antiinflammatory activity in animal screens (Messer and Farge, 1967; Messer et al., 1969). Metiazinic acid had an ED_{50} of 35 mg/kg in the carrageenan-induced abscess assay in the rat (Messer et al., 1969) and was 3 times more potent than phenylbutazone in the carrageenan-induced foot edema test (Julou et al., 1969a). It should be noted that among the straight chain homologs of (**64**), the propionic acid was inactive, whereas the butyric acid had an ED_{50} of 90 mg/kg in the carrageenan abscess assay (Messer et al., 1969).

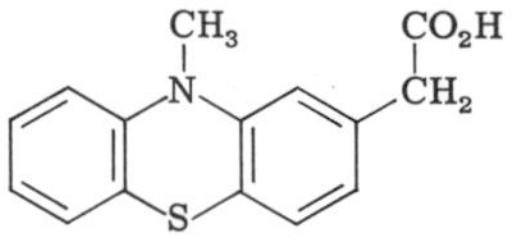

$$CH_3 \qquad CO_2H$$

64

In further studies metiazinic acid showed antipyretic and analgesic properties as well as a pronounced protective effect at 100 mg/kg/day in the adjuvant-induced arthritis assay in the rat (Julou et al., 1969a). Gastrointestinal disturbances were observed in rats and dogs receiving (**64**) at daily doses of 120–180 mg/kg for 3 months (Julou et al., 1969b). In the rabbit and man the major metabolites were found to be nuclear hydroxylated derivatives, in both free and conjugated forms (Populaire et al., 1969).

In the clinic, metiazinic acid (Soripal) at daily doses of 0.75–1.5 gm has been judged to be of benefit to patients suffering from a variety of arthritic afflictions (Deshayes and Gogny, 1970; Gross, 1971).

X. PYRROLEALKANOIC ACIDS

A. Pyrroleacetic Acids

1. TOLMETIN

A group of 5-benzoyl-1-methyl-2-pyrroleacetic acids modeled after indomethacin was found to possess marked antiinflammatory activity (Carson et al., 1971). Tolmetin (**65**) had 0.38 times the potency of indomethacin in the carrageenan-induced rat paw edema test and was reported to be active in the adjuvant-induced arthritis assay in the rat.

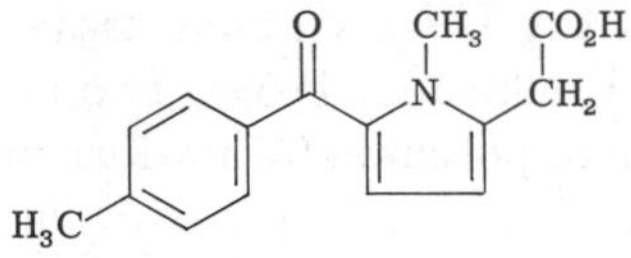

65

B. Pyrrolepropionic Acids

Antiinflammatory activity has been claimed for compounds with the general structure (**66**) (Short, 1965).

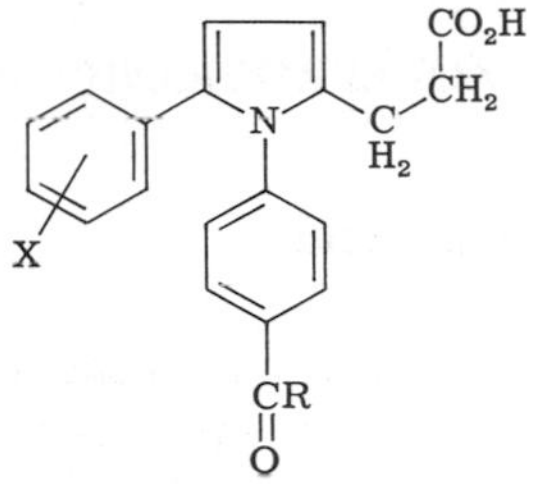

R = alkyl
X = H, halogen, alkyl,
    alkoxy, alkylthio, etc.

66

XI. FURANALKANOIC ACIDS

A. Furanacetic Acids

A series of 5-aryl-2-furanacetic acids was prepared and tested for anti-inflammatory activity in the UV-erythema assay in the guinea pig (Kalten-bronn and Rhee, 1968). Compound (**67**) had 1.7 times the potency of phenyl-butazone.

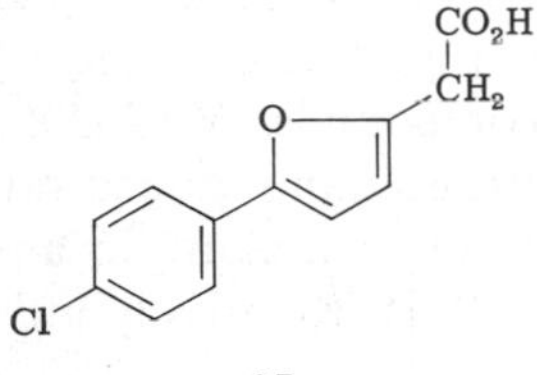

67

B. Furanpropionic Acids

3-(5-Aryl-2-furan)propionic acids were found to be less potent anti-inflammatory agents in the UV-erythema assay than the corresponding acetic acids (Short and Rockwood, 1969). The best of the propionic acids (**68**), was only one fourth as potent as (**67**), with a minimum effective dose of 12.5 mg/kg.

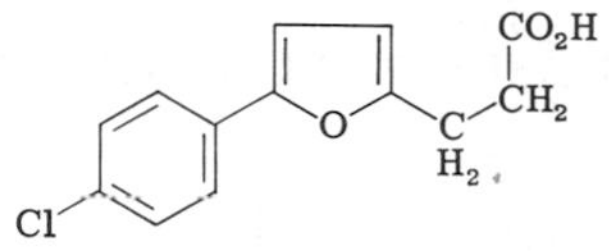

68

XII. OXAZOLEPROPIONIC ACIDS

A. 3-(5-Aryl-2-oxazole)propionic Acids

Antiinflammatory activity comparable to the analogous furanpropionic acids (Section XI,B) was found for some 3-(5-aryl-2-oxazole)propionic acids (Short and Long, 1969). Minimum effective doses of 12.5 mg/kg and 25 mg/kg were established for compounds (**69**), X = Br, and (**69**), X = Cl, respectively, in the UV-erythema assay in the guinea pig.

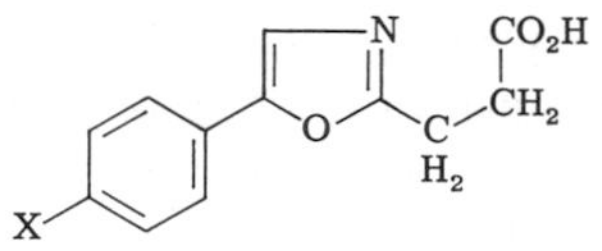

69

B. 3-(4,5-Diaryl-2-oxazole)propionic Acids

Brief reports (Brown et al., 1968; Green and Green, 1971) have appeared on the antiinflammatory properties of some 3-(4,5-diaryl-2-oxazole)propionic acids. One of these compounds, Wy 23205, (**70**), was twice as potent as phenylbutazone in the carrageenan-induced rat paw edema test and 8–20 times more potent than phenylbutazone in an adjuvant-induced arthritis assay (Green and Green, 1971). Relatively little gastrointestinal irritation was observed.

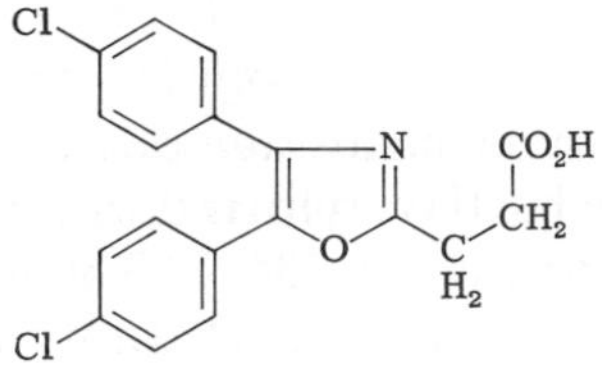

70

XIII. THIAZOLEACETIC ACIDS

A. Fenclozic Acid

Several points of interest arose from the studies on fenclozic acid, 2-(4-chlorophenyl)-4-thiazoleacetic acid (**72**), which was synthesized by the treatment of 4-chlorothiobenzamide (**71**) with ethyl ω-bromoacetoacetate, followed by hydrolysis of the intermediate ester (Hepworth and Stacey, 1966; Hepworth et al., 1969).

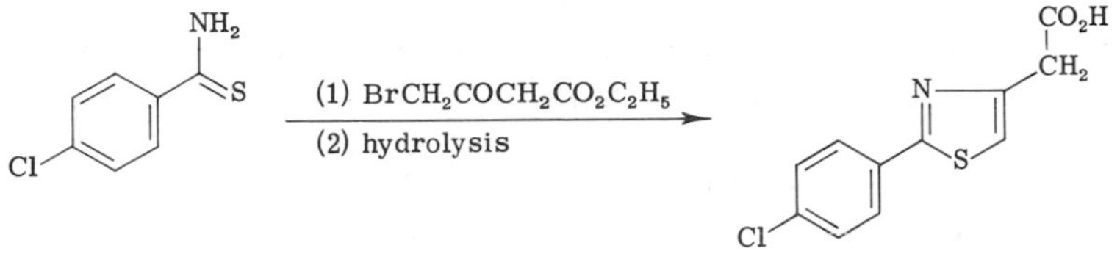

71   **72**

In the single-dose carrageenan-induced rat paw edema test, fenclozic acid had a potency equal to phenylbutazone (Newbould, 1969). In the multiple-dose established and nonestablished adjuvant-induced arthritis assays of longer duration, however, fenclozic acid was several times more potent than phenylbutazone (Newbould, 1969). This variation was attributed to the much longer serum half-life of fenclozic acid in rats (about 30 hours) as compared to phenylbutazone (about 6 hours). A correlation was observed between the serum levels and the therapeutic effect of fenclozic acid in the adjuvant-induced arthritis assay (Platt, 1971).

Chronic toxicity studies indicated that rats could tolerate a daily dose of fenclozic acid in excess of 10 times the minimum effective dose in the adjuvant-induced arthritis assay (Newbould, 1969). Deaths occurred at higher doses from peptic ulceration. Antipyretic activity in rats and analgesic activity in a mouse squirm test were also observed.

In the monkey, fenclozic acid is largely excreted in the urine as the acyl-glucuronide (Foulkes, 1970). In the rat and the dog, however, fenclozic acid undergoes the NIH shift (Foulkes, 1969, 1970). Hydroxylation occurs at position 4 of the benzene ring, with both loss and migration of the chloro group originally present at that position. The two resulting metabolites, (73) and (74), are excreted in the urine as their acylglucuronides and in the feces in unconjugated form.

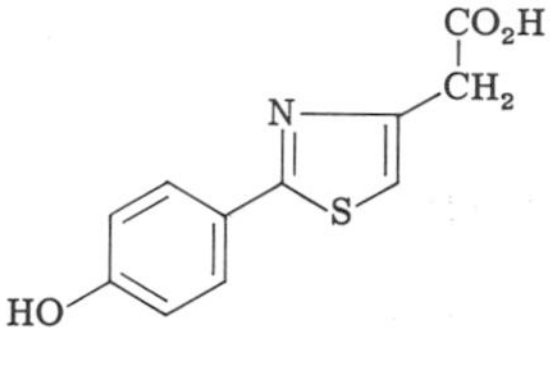

73 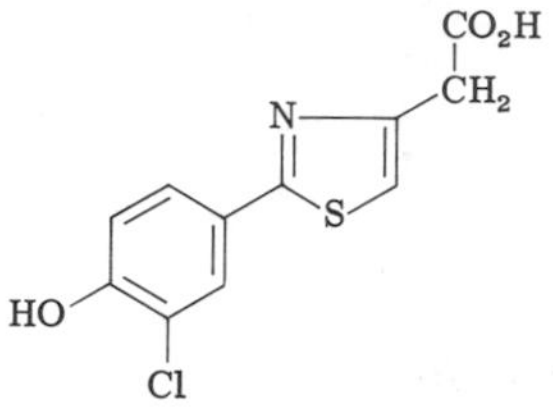   74

After preliminary serum concentration studies (Chalmers *et al.*, 1969a), fenclozoic acid (Myalex) (200–400 mg/day) was compared with aspirin (3.6 gm/day) in a double-blind, crossover trial in patients with rheumatoid arthritis (Chalmers *et al.*, 1969b). It was concluded that fenclozic acid afforded symptomatic relief and was comparable to aspirin. Unfortunately, hepatotoxicity was observed in subsequent trials and the drug was withdrawn from the clinic (Hart *et al.*, 1970).

B. 2,4-Diaryl-5-thiazoleacetic Acids

The most potent antiinflammatory agent in a series of 2,4-diaryl-5-thiazoleacetic acids was (75), which had 5 times the potency of phenylbutazone in the carrageenan-induced rat paw edema test (Brown *et al.*, 1968). It was claimed that gastrointestinal disturbances with (75) and related compounds were less than with equally effective doses of aspirin, phenylbutazone, or indomethacin.

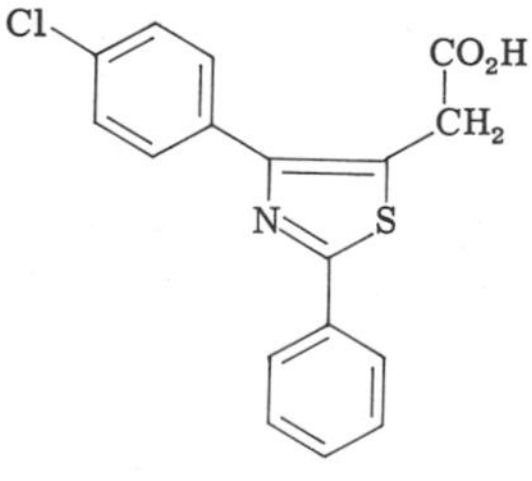

75

XIV. TETRAZOLEALKANOIC ACIDS

From structure–activity studies on a large group of aryltetrazolealkanoic acids it was established that, for optimum antiinflammatory activity, a halogenated phenyl group should be attached at position 5 and a propionic acid residue at position 2 of the tetrazole ring (Buckler *et al.*, 1970). A Hansch analysis of the data led to an equation containing π values as the only variable (Buckler, 1972). The most active compound was (**76**), which had 6.2 times the potency of phenylbutazone in the carrageenan-induced abscess assay and 3.6 times the potency of phenylbutazone in the adjuvant-induced arthritis assay (both in the rat). Gastrointestinal irritation in the rat was observed at high doses of some of the more active compounds.

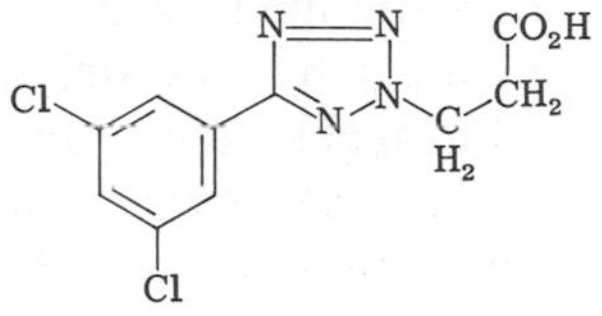

76

XV. OVERALL STRUCTURE–ACTIVITY RELATIONSHIPS

A. Potency

There is little evidence in Sections II–XIV to indicate that, at its optimum dose, any one of the aryl- and heteroarylalkanoic acids is much more effective than the others in its ability to influence the inflammatory process. The compounds do, however, vary widely in their relative potencies. In this section an attempt is made to define those structural features which appear in compounds endowed with particularly high potency in animal screens. Too few compounds have reached the clinic for there to be a meaningful discussion based on activity data from human studies.

There are two reasons why it is difficult, if not impossible, to rank all the compounds in order of their antiinflammatory potencies. First, the same animal assays were not used for each compound. Second, where the same assays were used, variations in the methodology and animal strains in different laboratories have resulted in divergent results even for the same compound.

The majority of the molecular structures that are described in this chapter have a carboxyl group, or its equivalent, separated by one carbon atom from a flat, aromatic nucleus. Increasing this separation usually results in lower potency. There are, however, important exceptions to this latter generalization. BDH 7538 (23) is somewhat more potent than might be expected of a 4-phenylbutyric acid. In this case it is tempting, even without experimental evidence, to propose that BDH 7538 is converted to the corresponding phenylacetic acid by an *in vivo* β oxidation. Does *in vivo* β oxidation also explain why metiazinic acid (64) and the corresponding straight chain butyric acid (Section IX,A) show significant antiinflammatory activity, whereas the corresponding 3-substituted propionic acid (Section IX) is inactive? Substantial antiinflammatory activity is also observed among several of the smaller five-ring heteroarylpropionic acids (compounds 66, 69, and 70) and in the case of the tetrazolealkanoic acids (Section XIV) a two-carbon separation is preferred.

Partial reduction of the aromatic nucleus, as exemplified by compound (21), appears to be accompanied by lowered potency, although more examples are needed before a firm generalization can be made.

The potent activity of the indan-l-carboxylic acids (35), with their out-of-plane carboxyl groups, may give an indication of the preferred *in vivo* conformation of the acetic acid side chains of the aryl- and heteroarylacetic acids.

The potentiating effect of an α-methyl substituent has been observed for a number of the arylacetic acids. Increasing the size of this substituent usually results in progressively lower activity, although sodium α-(2-furfuryl)-l-naphthaleneacetate (24) and naphthypramide (26) are two notable exceptions to this rule. This deviation on the part of naphthypramide, coupled with the fact that the corresponding carboxylic acid is less active (see Section V,A,2), may be grounds enough for not grouping naphthypramide with the aryl- and heteroarylalkanoic acid antiinflammatory agents.

The α-substituted aryl- and heteroarylalkanoic acids contain an asymmetric carbon atom. In several cases it has been observed that one optical isomer is more active than the other (See Sections II,E; V,B; VI,A; VIII,A). Where the stereochemistry has been determined, the more active isomer has the S absolute configuration (compounds 9, 36, 37, and 46).

Most of the compounds that have been described have one or more large, lipophilic groups attached to a carbon of the aromatic nucleus that is two or three carbon or heteroatoms removed from the point of attachment of the alkanoic acid side chain. In addition, the potentiating effect of a small group, preferably chlorine, in a position meta to the alkanoic acid side chain has been observed for many of the phenylacetic acids. Combinations of these two features are noted in fused systems, such as Leo-1028 (14) and naproxen (34). Once again, naphthypramide (26) does not conform to the pattern.

Although few pharmacological data have appeared in the general literature, ester and amide derivatives of the aryl- and heteroarylalkanoic acids are often claimed in patents as being potent antiinflammatory agents in animals. These derivatives are probably hydrolyzed *in vivo* to the acids. Corresponding carbinols and aldehydes appear to be biologically equivalent to the acids (Sections II,E; V,B), probably by being oxidized *in vivo* to the acids. Whether or not the hydroxamic acid group functions as a carboxyl equivalent is open to question. Many structural features of bufexamac (12) are similar to those of potent arylacetic acid compounds, but 4-butoxyphenylacetic acid itself had very weak antiinflammatory activity (Section II,G).

B. Toxicity

As is the case for many of the nonsteroidal antiinflammatory agents, the main side effect associated with the aryl- and heteroarylalkanoic acids is gastrointestinal disturbance. In the rat, death in LD_{50} determinations is usually caused by peritonitis resulting from perforated intestinal ulceration. Although it has not been possible to completely dissociate this side effect from antiinflammatory activity, higher toxic dose/therapeutic dose ratios have been obtained by molecular modification (e.g., see Section VI, A).

Hepatotoxicity has doomed at least two compounds, ibufenac (2) and fenclozic acid (72), but this does not seem to be too serious a problem because a close analog of ibufenac, ibuprofen (4), appears to be free of adverse effects on the liver.

XVI. CONCLUSION

It is hoped that after reading this chapter and Chapter 2, by Scherrer, the reader will find it easier to envision the possibility of a hypothetical *in vivo* receptor site, and that this concept will prove useful in the design of new and improved aryl- and heteroarylalkanoic acid antiinflammatory agents.

XVII. ADDENDUM

In the time that has elapsed since completion of this chapter and receipt of the proofs, several of the agents that have been discussed have advanced to the marketing stage and several new, potent compounds have been reported. This addendum is a brief update.

In man, fenoprofen (Section II, H) is eliminated mainly in the urine as the glucuronide (45%) and as the glucuronide of the 4'-hydroxy metabolite (45%) (Rubin et al., 1972). Fenoprofen calcium (1.6–2.4 gm/day acid equivalent) was compared with aspirin (4–6 gm/day) in a double-blind crossover study in patients with rheumatoid arthritis (Fries and Britton, 1973). The aspirin appeared to be slightly more effective. Fenoprofen is being readied for the market (Anonymous, 1973).

A double-blind crossover clinical trial with ketoprofen (Section II, J) in patients with rheumatoid arthritis suggested that ketoprofen had superior antiinflammatory activity to ibuprofen (Section II, D) (Mills et al., 1973). Significant difference in favor of ketoprofen (100 mg/day) over placebo was claimed in another study (Cathcart et al., 1973). Ketoprofen was marketed as Orudis in Britain in late 1973 by May and Baker.

Further clinical studies with naproxen (Section V,B,1) at daily doses of 300–500 mg in patients with rheumatoid arthritis have been reported (Katona et al., 1971; Lussier et al., 1973a,b). Naproxen has been on sale in Mexico as Naxen since September 1972 and was launched in Britain in the fall of 1973 as Naprosyn.

Further elaboration of the 2-pyrroleacetic acid series (Section X, A, 1) has led to 4-methyl substituted compounds with potencies comparable to indomethacin in animal screens (Carson and Wong, 1973). 5-p-Chlorobenzoyl-1,4,α-trimethyl-pyrrole-2-acetic acid (McN-2891) had an ID_{50} of 1.1 mg/kg in a nonestablished adjuvant-induced arthritis assay in the rat (Wong et al., 1973).

Toxicological (Kawai et al., 1973) and metabolic (Tanayama et al., 1973; Kanai et al., 1973; Tanayama, 1973) studies have now been reported for the indan-1-carboxylic acid TAI-284 (Section VI, A). The relatively weak antiinflammatory activity for two 5-cyclohexyl-1-hydroxyacetylindans in the carrageenin screen as compared to the corresponding indan-1-carboxylic acids (Juby et al., 1972d) does not lend support for the idea (Noguchi et al., 1971) that the antiinflammatory activity of the indan-l-carboxylic acids is due to a steroidlike mechanism.

Among some newer agents are 2-[4-(1-oxo-2-isoindolinyl)phenyl] propionic acid (K 4277) and 2-[3-chloro-4-(3-pyrrolin-1-yl) phenyl] propionic acid (Su-21524). Racemic K 4277, which is now in clinical trial, was found to be the most active of a series of 62 1-oxo-2-substituted isoindoline derivatives (Nannini et al., 1973; Buttinoni et al., 1973), with 19 times the potency of phenylbutazone in the carrageenan-induced rat paw edema test. Racemic Su-21524 had a potency of 1.56 times indomethacin in the carrageenan-induced rat paw edema screen, with little difference in activity between the two optical isomers (Carney et al., 1973). Daily doses of 400 mg of Su-21524 were found to give improvement comparable to that given by indomethacin at 100 mg/day in patients with rheumatoid arthritis (Proctor et al., 1973).

REFERENCES

Adams, S. S., Cliffe, E. E., Lessel, B., and Nicholson, J. S. (1963). *Nature (London)* **200**, 271.
Adams, S. S., Cliffe, E. E., Lessel, B., and Nicholson, J. S. (1967). *J. Pharm. Sci.* **56**, 1686.
Adams, S. S., Hebborn, P., and Nicholson, J. S. (1968). *J. Pharm. Pharmacol.* **20**, 305.
Adams, S. S., McCullough, K. F., and Nicholson, J. S. (1969a). *Arch. Int. Pharmacodyn. Ther.* **178**, 115.
Adams, S. S., Bough, R. G., Cliffe, E. E., Lessel, B., and Mills, R. F. N. (1969b). *Toxicol. Appl. Pharmacol.* **15**, 310.
Anonymous. (1967). *Chem. Eng. News* **45**(7), 10.
Anonymous. (1968). *Drug Ther. Bull.* **6**, 48.
Anonymous. (1973). *FDC Reports* **35** (42), T & G-2.
Barron, D. I., Bysouth, P. T., Clarke, R. W., Copley, A. R., Stephenson, O., Vallance, D. K., and Wild, A. M. (1968a). *J. Med. Chem.* **11**, 1139.
Barron, D. I., Copley, A. R., and Vallance, D. K. (1968b). *Brit. J. Pharmacol. Chemother.* **33**, 396.
Bloch-Michel, H., and Parrot, M. (1970). *Therapie* **25**, 969.
Boots Pure Drug Company Limited. (1962). South African Patent 62/294.
Bristol-Myers Company. (1970). Belgian Patent 745,177.
Brodie, D. A., Cook, P. G., Bauer, B. J., and Dagle, G. E. (1970). *Toxicol. Appl. Pharmacol.* **17**, 615.
Brown, J. H. (1967). *Abstr. Pap. 154th Meet. Amer. Chem. Soc. 1967*, p. 13P.
Brown, K., Cavalla, J. F., Green, D., and Wilson, A. B. (1968). *Nature (London)* **219**, 164.
Buckler, J. W., and Adams, S. S. (1968). *Med. Proc.* **14**, 574.
Buckler, R. T. (1972). *J. Med. Chem.* **15**, 578.
Buckler, R. T., Hayao, S., Lorenzetti, O. J., Sancilio, L. F., Hartzler, H. E., and Strycker, W. G. (1970). *J. Med. Chem.* **13**, 725.
Buttinoni, A., Cuttica, A., Franceschini, J., Mandelli, V., Orsini, G., Passerini, N., Turba, C., and Tommasini, R. (1973). *Arzneim.-Forsch.* **23**, 1100.
Buu-Hoï, N. P., Lambelin, G., Gillet, C., Lepoivre, C., Thiriaux, J., and Mees, G. (1966). *Nature (London)* **211**, 752.
Camarri, E., D'Alonzo, D., and Zaccherotti, L. (1970). *Curr. Ther. Res., Clin. Exp.* **12**, 1.
Carney, R. W. J., Chart, J. J., Goldstein, R., Howie, N., and Wojtkunski, J. (1973). *Experientia* **29**, 938.
Carson, J. R., and Wong, S. (1973). *J. Med. Chem.* **16**, 172.
Carson, J. R., Mckinstry, D. N., and Wong, S. (1971). *J. Med. Chem.* **14**, 646.
Casagrande, C., Invernizzi, A., Ferrini, R., and Miragoli, G. (1971). *Farmaco, Ed. Sci.* **26**, 1059.
Cathcart, B. J., Vince, J. D., Gordon, A. J., Bell, M. A., and Chalmers, I. M. (1973). *Ann. Rheum. Dis.* **32**, 62.
Chalmers, T. M. (1963). *Ann. Rheum. Dis.* **22**, 358.
Chalmers, T. M., Pohl, J. E. F., and Platt, D. S. (1969a). *Ann. Rheum. Dis.* **28**, 590.
Chalmers, T. M., Kellgren, J. H., and Platt, D. S. (1969b). *Ann. Rheum. Dis.* **28**, 595.
Chalmers, I. M., Cathcart, B. J., Kumar, E. B., Dick, W. C., and Buchanan, W. W. (1972). *Ann. Rheum. Dis.* **31**, 319.
Ciba, S. A. (1970). Belgian Patent 740,314.
Cohen, A., and DeFelice, E. A. (1965). *J. New Drugs* **5**, 153.
Cohen, A., DeFelice, E. A., Beber, C. R., Shaffer, J. W., and Forbes, J. A. (1965). *Curr. Ther. Res., Clin. Exp.* **7**, 759.
Coppi, G. (1966). *Arch. Int. Pharmacodyn. Ther.* **162**, 422.

Corgill, D. A., Ligon, C. W., and DeFelice, E. A. (1965). *Curr. Ther. Res., Clin. Exp.* **7**, 263.

Culp, H. W. (1971). *Fed. Proc., Fed. Amer. Soc. Exp. Biol.* **30**, 564.

Davies, E. F., and Avery, G. S. (1972). *Drugs* **2**, 416.

Denko, C. W., DeFelice, E. A., and Shaffer, J. (1965). *Curr. Ther. Res., Clin. Exp.* **7**, 749.

Deshayes, P., and Gogny, J.-C. (1970). *Rhumatologie (Paris)* **22**, 29.

Desproges-Gotteron, R., Leroy, V., and Comte, B. (1971). ʿ*Curr. Ther. Res., Clin. Exp.* **13**, 393.

Duggan, D. E., Hogans, A. F., Kwan, K. C., and McMahon, F. G. (1972). *J. Pharmacol. Exp. Ther.* **181**, 563.

Durant, G. J., Smith, G. M., Spickett, R. G. W., and Szarvasi, E. (1965). *J. Med. Chem.* **8**, 598.

Emele, J. F., and Shanaman, J. E. (1967). *Arch. Int. Pharmacodyn. Ther.* **170**, 99.

Englund, D. W., and Roth, S. H. (1969). *Int. Cong. Rheumatol. 12th, 1969* Abstract. No. 807.

Fleming, J. S., Bierwagen, M. E., Pircio, A. W., and Pindell, M. H. (1969). *Arch. Int. Pharmacodyn. Ther.* **178**, 423.

Fleming, J. S., Bierwagen, M. E., Campbell, J. A. L., and King, S. P. (1972). *Arch. Int. Pharmacodyn. Ther.* **199**, 164.

Foulkes, D. M. (1969). *Nature (London)* **221**, 582.

Foulkes, D. M. (1970). *J. Pharmacol. Exp. Ther.* **172**, 115.

Fries, J. F., and Britton, M. C. (1973). *Arthritis Rheum.* **16**, 629.

Garattini, S., and Dukes, M. N. G., eds. (1965). "Non-Steroidal Anti-Inflammatory Drugs." Exerpta Med. Found., Amsterdam.

Glenn, E. M. (1964). *Abstr. Pap. Nat. Med. Chem. Symp., Amer. Chem. Soc., 1964.*, p. 10a.

Goldberg, A. A. J., Hall, J. E., Buckler, J. W., Dodsworth, P. G., and Agar, J. (1971). *Practitioner* **207**, 343.

Green, A. Y., and Green, D. (1971). *Brit. J. Pharmacol.* **42**, 638P.

Gross, D. (1971). *Praxis* **60**, 1334.

Gyory, A. N., Bloch, M., Burry, H. C., and Grahame, R. (1972). *Brit. Med. J.* **4**, 398.

Harman, R. E., Meisinger, M. A. P., Davis, G. E., and Kuehl, F. A., Jr. (1964). *J. Pharmacol. Exp. Ther.* **143**, 215.

Harrison, I. T., Lewis, B., Nelson, P., Rooks, W., Roszkowski, A., Tomolonis, A., and Fried, J. H. (1970). *J. Med. Chem.* **13**, 203.

Hart, F. D., and Boardman, P. L. (1965). *Ann. Rheum. Dis.* **24**, 61.

Hart, F. D., Bain, L. S., Huskisson, E. C., Littler, T. R., and Taylor, R. T. (1970). *Ann. Rheum. Dis.* **29**, 684.

Hepworth, W., and Stacey, G. J. (1966). British Patent 1,099,389.

Hepworth, W., Newbould, B. B., Platt, D. S., and Stacey, G. J. (1969). *Nature (London)* **221**, 582.

Hucker, H. B., Zacchei, A. G., Cox, S. V., Brodie, D. A., and Cantwell, N. H. R. (1966). *J. Pharmacol. Exp. Ther.* **153**, 237.

Hucker, H. B., Stauffer, S. C., Bower, R. J., Umbenhauer, E. R., and McMahon, F. G. (1972). *Fed. Proc., Fed. Amer. Soc. Exp. Biol.* **31**, 577.

Huskisson, E. C., Hart, F. D., Shenfield, G. M., and Taylor, R. T. (1971). *Practitioner* **207**, 639.

Juby, P. F., and Hudyma, T. W. (1969). *J. Med. Chem.* **12**, 396.

Juby, P. F., Partyka, R. A., and Hudyma, T. W. (1971). U.S. Patent 3,565,904.

Juby, P. F., Hudyma, T. W., and Partyka, R. A. (1972a). U.S. Patent 3,644,479.

Juby, P. F., Goodwin, W. R., Hudyma, T. W., and Partyka, R. A. (1972b). *J. Med. Chem.* **15**, 1297.

Juby, P. F., Goodwin, W. R., Hudyma, T. W., and Partyka, R. A. (1972c). *J. Med. Chem.* **15**, 1306.

Juby, P. F., Hudyma, T. W., and Partyka, R. A. (1972d). *J. Med. Chem.* **15**, 120.

Julou, L., Guyonnet, J. C., Ducrot, R., Bardone, M. C., Detaille, J. Y., and Laffargue, B. (1969a). *Arzneim.-Forsch.* **19**, 1198.

Julou, L., Ducrot, R., Fournel, J., Ganter, P., Populaire, P., Durel, J., Myon, J., Pascal, S., and Pasquet, J. (1969b). *Arzneim.-Forsch.* **19**, 1207.

Julou, L., Guyonnet, J.-C., Ducrot, R., Garret, C., Bardone, M.-C., Maignan, G., and Pasquet, J. (1971). *J. Pharmacol.* **2**, 259.

Kaltenbronn, J. S., and Rhee, T. O. (1968). *J. Med. Chem.* **11**, 902.

Kanai, Y., Kobayashi, T., and Tanayama, S. (1973). *Xenobiotica* **3**, 657.

Katona, G., Ortega, E., and Robles-Gil , J. (1971). *Clin. Trials J.* **8**, 3.

Kawai, K., Kuzuna, S., Morimoto, S., Ishii, H., and Matsumoto, N. (1971). *Jap. J. Pharmacol.* **21**, 621.

Kawai, K., Kuzuna, S., Matsumoto, N., Murata, Y., Nomura, M., and Katsumata, Y. (1973). *Pharmacometrics* **7**, 333.

Kistenmacher, T. J., and Marsh, R. E. (1972). *J. Amer. Chem. Soc.* **94**, 1340.

Klare, V. (1966). *Wien. Med. Wochenshr.* **116**, 930.

Klemm, C., Fricke, R., Schattenkirchner, M., Treiber, W., and Mathies, H. (1971). *Z. Rheumaforsch.* **30**, 17.

Lambelin, G., Mees, G., and Buu-Hoï, N. P. (1966). *Naturwissenschaften* **53**, 157.

Lambelin, G., Buu-Hoï, N. P., Brouilhet, H., Gautier, M., Gillet, C., Roba, J., and Thiriaux, J. (1968). *Arzneim.-Forsch.* **18**, 1404.

Lambelin, G., Roba, J., Parmentier, R., and Buu-Hoï, N. P. (1969). *Arch. Int. Pharmacodyn. Ther.* **180**, 241.

Lambelin, G., Roba, J., Gillet, C., and Buu-Hoï, N. P. (1970a). *Arzneim.-Forsch.* **20**, 610.

Lambelin, G., Roba, J., Gillet, C., Gautier, M., and Buu-Hoï, N. P. (1970b). *Arzneim.-Forsch.* **20**, 618.

Lambotte, F. (1970). *Arzneim.-Forsch.* **20**, 569.

Lussier, A., MacCannell, K. L., Alexander, S. J., Multz, C. V., Boost, G., and Segre, E. J. (1972). *Clin. Pharmacol. Ther.* **13**, 146.

Lussier, A., Regoli, D., Gysling, E., Boost, G., and Varady, J. C. (1973a). *Int. J. Clin. Pharmacol.* **7**, 6.

Lussier, A., Segre, J., Multz, C. V., MacCannell, K. L., Alexander, S. J., Howard, D. L. G., Boost, G., Varady, J., and Strauss, W. (1973b). *Clin. Pharmacol. Ther.* **14**, 434.

Marazzi-Uberti, E., and Coppi, G. (1967). *Arzneim.-Forsch.* **17**, 1451.

Marazzi-Uberti, E., and Turba, C. (1966). *Arch. Int. Pharmacodyn. Ther.* **162**, 378.

Merck and Company. (1965a). Netherlands Patent Appl. 65,07505.

Merck and Company. (1965b). Belgian Patent 664,187.

Merck and Company. (1966). Netherlands Patent Appl. 66,08311.

Merck and Company. (1968a). Eire Patent 704/68.

Merck and Company. (1968b). Eire Patent 705/68.

Messer, M., and Farge, D. (1967). *C. R. Acad Sci., Ser. C* **265**, 758.

Messer, M., Farge, D., Guyonnet, J. C., Jeanmart, C., and Julou, L. (1969). *Arzneim.-Forsch.* **19**, 1193.

Mills, S. B., Bloch, M., and Bruckner, F. E. (1973). *Brit. Med. J.* **4**, 82.

Minssen-Guetté, M., Dvolaitzky, M., and Jacques, J. (1968). *Bull. Soc. Chim. Fr.* p. 2111.

Nannini, G., Giraldi, P. N., Molgora, G., Biasoli, G., Spinelli, F., Logemann, W., Dradi, E., Zanni, G., Buttinoni, A., and Tommasini, R. (1973). *Arzneim.-Forsch.* **23**, 1090.

Newbould, B. B. (1969). *Brit. J. Pharmacol.* **35**, 487.

Nickander, R. C., Kraay, R. J., and Marshall, W. S. (1971). *Fed. Proc., Fed. Amer. Soc. Exp. Biol.* **30**, 563.

Noel, P. R. B. (1968). *Arzneim.-Forsch.* **18**, 356.

Noguchi, S., Kishimoto, S., Minamida, I., Obayashi, M., and Kawakita, K. (1971). *Chem. Pharm. Bull.* **19**, 646.

Pala, G., Casadio, S., Bruzzese, T., Crescenzi, E., and Marazzi-Uberti, E. (1965). *J. Med. Chem.* **8**, 698.

Pala, G., Bruzzese, T., Marazzi-Uberti, E., and Coppi, G. (1966). *J. Med. Chem.* **9**, 603.

Parke, Davis and Company. (1965). British Patent 1,009,288.

Pavelka, K., and Wagenhauser, F. (1970). *Curr. Ther. Res., Clin. Exp.* **12**, 69.

Pavelka, K., Kaňková, D., Wagenhäuser, F., and Böni, (1971). *Z. Rheumaforsch.* **30**, 50.

Phelps, A. H., Bagdon, W. J., Mattis, P. A., Winter, C. A., and Zwickey, R. E. (1968). *Fed. Proc., Fed. Amer. Soc. Exp. Biol.* **27**, 598.

Pircio, A. W., Bierwagen, M. E., Strife, W. E. and Nicolosi, W. D. (1972). *Arch. Int. Pharmacodyn. Ther.* **199**, 151.

Platt, D. S. (1971). *J. Pharm. Sci.* **60**, 366.

Populaire, P., Terlain, B., Pascal, S., Lebreton, G., and Decouvelaere, B. (1969). *Arzneim.-Forsch.* **19**, 1214.

Proceedings of an International Symposium on Inflammation and its Treatment with Indomethacin. (1971). *Arzneim.-Forsch.* **21**, 1757.

Proctor, J. D., Evans, E. F., Velandia, J., and Wassermann, A. J. (1973). *Clin Pharmacol. Ther.* **14**, 143.

Rakic, M., Gross, L., and Agre, K. (1969). *Int. Congr. Rheumatol. 12th 1969* Abstract No. 325.

Redel, J., Brouilhet, H., Bazely, N., Jouanneau, M., and Delbarre, F. (1970). *C. R. Acad. Sci., Ser. D* **270**, 224.

Redel, J., Brouilhet, H., Delbarre, F., Bazely, N., and Jouanneau, M. (1971). *C. R. Acad. Sci., Ser. D* **273**, 911.

Ridolfo, A. S., Gruber, C. M., and Mikulascheck, W. M. (1971). *Clin. Pharmacol. Ther.* **12**, 300.

Rohte, O. (1971). *Acta Pharmacol. Toxicol.* **29**, Suppl. 4, 47.

Roncucci, R., Simon, M.-J., Lambelin, G., Gillet, C., Staquet, M., and Buu-Hoï, N. P. (1970). *Arzneim.-Forsch.* **20**, 631.

Rooks, W. H., II. (1971). *Fed. Proc., Fed. Amer. Soc. Exp. Biol.* **30**, 386.

Rose, B. S., Isdale, I. C., and Conlon, P. W. (1970). *Curr. Ther. Res., Clin. Exp.* **12**, 150.

Roszkowski, A. P., Rooks, W. H., II, Tomolonis, A. J., and Miller, L. M. (1971). *J. Pharmacol. Exp. Ther.* **179**, 114.

Roth, S. H., and Englund, D. W. (1969). *Arthritis Rheum.* **12**, 328.

Rubin, A., Rodda, B. E., Warrick, P., Ridolfo, A., and Gruber, C. M. (1971). *J. Pharm. Sci.* **60**, 1797.

Rubin, A., Warrick, P., Wolen, R. L., Chernish, S. M., Ridolfo, A. S., and Gruber, C. M., Jr. (1972). *J. Pharmacol. Exp. Ther.* **183**, 449.

Runkel, R., Chaplin, M., Boost, G., Segre, E., and Forchielli, E. (1972). *J. Pharm. Sci.* **61**, 703.

Sarett, L. H. (1971). *Arzneim.-Forsch.* **21**, 1759.

Shen, T. Y. (1964). U.S. Patent 3,161,654.

Shen, T. Y. (1965). *Int. Symp. Non-Steroidal Anti-Inflammatory Drugs, Proc., 1964* pp. 13–20.

Shen, T. Y. (1967a). *Chim. Ther.* **2**, 459.

Shen, T. Y. (1967b). *Top. Med. Chem.* **1**, 29–78.

Shen, T. Y., Windholz, T. B., Rosegay, A., Witzel, B. E., Wilson, A. N., Willett, J. D., Holtz, W. J., Ellis, R. L., Matzuk, A. R., Lucas, S., Stammer, C. H., Holly, F. W., Sarett, L. H., Risley, E. A., Nuss, G. W., and Winter, C. A. (1963). *J. Amer. Chem. Soc.* **85**, 488.

Shen, T. Y., Ellis, R. L., Witzel, B. E., and Matzuk, A. R. (1966). *Abst. Pap. 152nd Meet. Amer. Chem. Soc. 1966* p. 3P.

Shen, T. Y., Witzel, B. E., Jones, H., Linn, B. O., McPherson, J., Greenwald, R., Fordice, M., and Jacobs, A. (1972). *Fed. Proc., Fed. Amer. Soc. Exp. Biol.* **31**, 577.

Short, F. W. (1965). U.S. Patent 3,168,529.

Short, F. W., and Long, L. M. (1969). *J. Heterocycl. Chem.* **6**, 707.

Short, F. W., and Rockwood, G. M. (1969). *J. Heterocycl. Chem.* **6**, 713.

Steele, A. D., and Phelps, P. (1971). *Arthritis Rheum.* **14**, 415.

Stiller, E. T., Diassi, P. A., Gerschutz, D., Meikle, D., Moetz, J., Principe, P. A., and Levine, S. D. (1972). *J. Med. Chem.* **15**, 1029.

Strachan, R. G., Meisinger, M. A. P., Ruyle, W. V., Hirschmann, R., and Shen, T. Y. (1964). *J. Med. Chem.* **7**, 799.

Tanayama, S. (1973). *Xenobiotica* **3**, 671.

Tanayama, S., Tsuchida, E., and Suzuoki, Z. (1973). *Xenobiotica* **3**, 643.

Thompson, M., Stephenson, P., and Percy, J. S. (1964). *Ann. Rheum. Dis.* **23**, 397.

Van Arman, C. G, Risley, E. A., and Nuss, G. W. (1972). *Fed. Proc., Fed. Amer. Soc. Exp. Biol.* **31**, 577.

Van Cauwenberge, H., and Franchimont, P. (1968). *J. Belge. Rhumatol. Med. Phys.* **23**, 133.

Vincent, M., Remond, G., and Poignant, J.-C. (1972). *J. Med. Chem.* **15**, 75.

Winter, C. A. (1965). *Int. Symp. Non-Steroidal Anti-Inflammatory Drugs, Proc, 1964*, pp. 190–202.

Winter, C. A., and Shen, T. Y. (1967). U.S. Patent 3,312,730.

Winter, C. A., Risley, E. A., and Nuss, G. W. (1963). *J. Pharmacol. Exp. Ther.* **141**, 369.

Wong, S., Gardocki, J. F., and Pruss, T. P. (1973). *J. Pharmacol. Exp.* Ther. **185**, 127.

Yamamoto, H. (1968). *Chem. Pharm. Bull.* **16**, 17.

Yamamoto, H., Nakao, M., and Kobayashi, A. (1968). *Chem. Pharm. Bull.* **16**, 647.

Chapter 5

Enolic Acids with Antiinflammatory Activity

JOSEPH G. LOMBARDINO

Pfizer Central Research
Pfizer, Inc.
Groton, Connecticut

I. INTRODUCTION

Many nonsteroidal organic compounds of diverse structure have been synthesized in a continuing search for drugs effective in suppressing some phase of the complex series of events leading to an inflammatory reaction in man. Most of the clinically useful nonsteroidal antiinflammatory agents reported to date are acidic (reviewed by Shen, 1967; Coyne, 1970; Weiner and Piliero, 1970; and Rosenthale, 1973), and the great majority of this class of compounds are carboxylic acids (e.g., aspirin, indomethacin, ibuprofen, niflumic acid, flufenamic acid) with acidity constants (pK_a) in the range of 3.5–6.5 (Unterhalt, 1970). This chapter discusses another class of antiinflammatory agents also possessing ionizable protons, i.e., enolic, or potentially enolic, β-diketones. The ionization process for the acidic proton in carboxylic and enolic acids may be compared by examining Eqs. (1) and (2).

Carboxylic acids: $RCOOH \rightleftharpoons RCOO^- + H^+$ $\hspace{4cm}$ (1)

Enolic acids:

$$R-\underset{\underset{O}{\|}}{C}-CH=\underset{HO}{\underset{|}{C}}R' \rightleftharpoons R-\underset{\underset{O}{\|}}{C}-CH_2-\underset{\underset{O}{\|}}{C}-R' \rightleftharpoons R-\underset{\underset{O}{|}}{C}-\underset{\ominus}{CH}-\underset{\underset{O}{|}}{C}-R' + H^+$$

$$\hspace{0.5cm} \text{Enol} \hspace{3cm} \text{Diketo} \hspace{3cm} \text{Enolate}$$

$\hspace{14cm}$ (2)

Although simple β-diketones, such as benzoylacetone or acetoacetic ester, are usually very weak acids (pK_a 9–12), the acidity of certain β-diketones can be markedly enhanced (i.e., to pK_a 4–7) so that they are significantly ionized *in vivo* to the anionic (enolate) species. This latter form appears to assist drug absorption, to increase protein binding, and often to enhance pharmacological activity in this class of drugs.

A number of animal models are available for assessing antiinflammatory activity, the most widely used being the rat paw edema test, the granuloma deposition test, the UV-erythema test, and the adjuvant arthritis test. Unfortunately, it is often difficult to establish accurate comparisons among various series of antiinflammatory agents when such data are published from different laboratories. For example, many reports do not indicate the effect of adrenalectomy on antiinflammatory activity, leaving open the possibility that observed antiinflammatory activity may result from the effects of adrenal steroids or catecholamines released *in vivo* by virtue of some peripheral or direct adrenal-stimulating mechanism (Domenjoz, 1966). In many cases, statements of comparative potency are made in the absence of dose–response comparisons between the test drug and a standard agent. In this review, an attempt is made to indicate the type of testing employed for the particular compounds discussed and to critically evaluate the more thoroughly described antiinflammatory enolic acids reported from 1968 through June 1973. Earlier literature is thoroughly reviewed by Winter (1967) and Whitehouse (1965). Incomplete reports are omitted, and only those series in which accurate comparisons can be made within the series and with standard drugs are discussed.

II. PYRAZOLIDINEDIONES

A. Phenylbutazone and Close Analogs

The oldest and most thoroughly studied antiinflammatory β-diketonic acid is the pyrazolidinedione, phenylbutazone (1). Since the serendipitous discovery of the clinically useful antiinflammatory activity of phenyl-

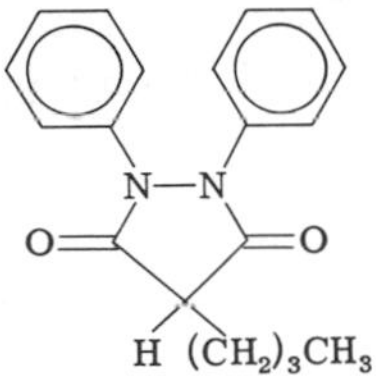

1

butazone more than 22 years ago, it has been widely used for treating a number of human inflammatory diseases. Phenylbutazone and one of its metabolites in man, oxyphenbutazone (2), are presently among the most widely used drugs for the treatment of inflammation. Of the various synthetic routes to phenylbutazone and closely related analogs, the condensation of hydrazobenzene with diethyl n-butylmalonate has achieved industrial importance Eq. (3).

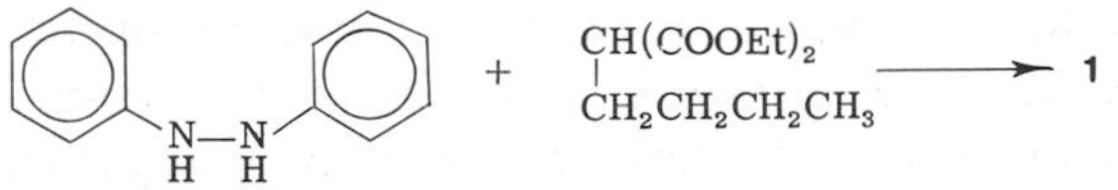

Von Rechenberg (1962), in his monograph on phenylbutazone, cites 1690 references through 1960, and publications by Whitehouse (1965), Burns et al. (1960), Seegmiller et al. (1960), Yü et al. (1958), Domenjoz (1960), and Randall (1963) provide detailed accounts of the history of phenylbutazone through 1965. A great many publications continue to appear, dealing mainly with the clinical effects of phenylbutazone or with the use of phenylbutazone as a positive control in some pharmacological screen. This review will survey only the highlights of the history of phenylbutazone and then will proceed to discuss recent reports on closely related antiinflammatory pyrazolidinediones.

In the course of determining structure–activity relationships for phenylbutazone analogs, biochemical pharmacology and pharmacokinetics have been utilized quite successfully as aids in the selection of clinical candidates from animal testing results. An excellent review of the physicochemical properties of phenylbutazone analogs (Perel *et al.*, 1964) presents correlations of acidity, partition coefficient, plasma binding, solubility, half-life, and tissue distribution for a number of analogs. In man, phenylbutazone is rapidly and completely absorbed from the gastrointestinal tract (Shulert *et al.*, 1952) and a portion is slowly metabolized in the liver by hydroxylation of both the side chain butyl group and of the para position of the phenyl ring (Burns *et al.*, 1955), Eq. (4). Although only a trace of unchanged phenylbutazone appears in the urine, not all of the ingested drug is accounted for as distinct metabolic products. Oxyphenbutazone, metabolite (2), is comparable in pK_a (4.7) and half-life (72 hours in man) to phenylbutazone and

$$1 \longrightarrow \quad \text{(structure 2)} \quad + \quad \text{(structure 3)} \quad + \quad \begin{array}{c} \text{Other} \\ \text{metabolites} \end{array} \quad (4)$$

accumulates in the body after chronic phenylbutazone administration. Metabolite (3) has a lower pK_a (4.0), a shorter half-life (12 hours), and much weaker clinical antirheumatic activity than phenylbutazone. Although many factors influence the metabolic disposition of a drug, there is a striking correlation between pK_a and half-life in man among several phenylbutazone analogs. Table I abstracts some of the data of Perel *et al.* (1964) and of Burns *et al.* (1958). Note that the incorporation into a pyrazolidine ring has enhanced the acidity of the β-diketonic function by more than 6 pK_a units (e.g., **1** has $pK_a = 4.5$) as compared, for example, to 3-methyl-2,4-pentanedione ($pK_a = 11$). The inductive effects of two phenyl-substituted nitrogen atoms in the pyrazolidine ring probably contribute to this enhanced acidity. However, too low a pK_a value can sometimes be detrimental. Not only does a very low pK_a usually shorten drug half-life in man, probably because of more rapid renal

TABLE I

Correlation of pK_a's of Phenylbutazone Analogs with
Their Half-Lives in Man

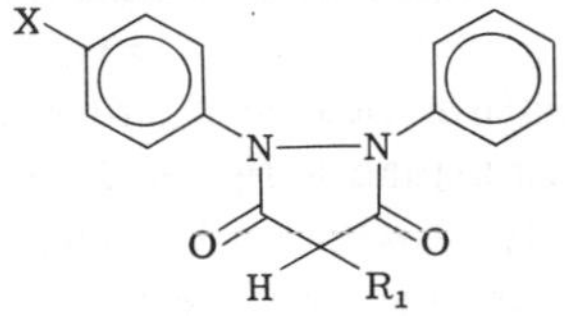

Compound	X	R_1	pK_a	$T_{1/2}$ (hours)
2	HO	$CH_3(CH_2)_3$	4.7	72
1	H	$CH_3(CH_2)_3$	4.5	72
4	HO	$PhS(CH_2)_2$	4.1	17
3	H	$CH_3CHOH(CH_2)_2$	4.0	12
5	H	$PhS(CH_2)_2$	3.9	3
6	H	$PhSO(CH_2)_2$	2.8	3
7	H	$CH_3(CH_2)_2CO$	2.0	1–3
8	HO	$CH_3(CH_2)_2CO$	2.3	8
9	H	$(CH_3)_3C$	7.0	1

tubular excretion of the drug, but a pK_a value of less than 3 actually diminishes antiinflammatory activity and favors uricosuric activity. The latter
activity probably arises from blocking of resorption and increasing urinary
excretion of uric acid. Thus, sulfinpyrazone, marketed as Anturane (6, Table
I), is a potent uricosuric agent (Burns et al., 1957) but is only weakly antiinflammatory. As an exception to the rule, 4-(butyryl)oxyphenbutazone (8),
although it has a comparatively low pK_a and exhibits uricosuric activity
(Seegmiller et al., 1960), has a longer half-life than sulfinpyrazone (6). Another notable exception to the lower pK_a/shorter half-life rule is the 4-t-butyl
analog (9). The short half-life of (9) has been explained by Perel et al. (1964)
as caused by two factors: that (9) has a high lipophilicity as measured by a
high partition coefficient ($K_p = 3.4$) in a peanut oil/pH 7 buffer system and
that (9) exhibits a relatively high pK_a of 7.0 because of the steric bulk of the
t-butyl group, which prevents coplanarity in the enolate ion. These properties combine to allow (9) to rapidly enter liver cells where conjugation to
the glucuronide takes place; facile excretion of the acidic glucuronide
metabolite (pK_a approximately 3) then explains the rapid clearance (i.e.,
short half-life) of (9).

Phenylbutazone has a broad spectrum of antiinflammatory activity in
acute tests, such as rat paw edema induced by carrageenan or by kaolin, and

in UV erythema in guinea pigs (ED_{50} 18 mg/kg, p.o.). Although several authors have suggested adrenal stimulation to be a factor in the antiinflammatory action of phenylbutazone, Feeney and Carlo (1955) found this effect to be insignificant. In another animal model, phenylbutazone inhibits granuloma deposition around a foreign body, such as a cotton pellet, at oral doses of 33 mg/kg or higher. The antiinflammatory effect of phenylbutazone is manifested even when drug is applied locally at the site of inflammation and the drug is known to accumulate in inflamed tissue after parenteral administration (Wilhelmi *et al.*, 1959).

Oxyphenbutazone (Tandearil, **2**) is similar to phenylbutazone in most of its pharmacological properties. Their activities are similar in formalin-induced rat paw edema; however, oxyphenbutazone is three times as effective as phenylbutazone in the kaolin-induced edema test (Wagner-Jauregg *et al.*, 1962). Granuloma deposition is more strongly inhibited by oxyphenbutazone than by phenylbutazone (Domenjoz, 1960).

A great variety of analogs of phenylbutazone have been made in an effort to improve activity and toleration and this work has led to several equally active pyrazolidinediones. Substitution in one or both of the phenyl rings of phenylbutazone by 4'-methyl, 4'-carboxy, 4'-nitro, or 4'-chloro (Bavin *et al.*, 1955; Yü *et al.*, 1958) produces active inhibitors of UV erythema when the drugs are administered intraperitoneally. 4'-Nitrophenylbutazone (pK_a = 3.2) has been studied in man (Yü *et al.*, 1959) and is uricosuric, antirheumatic, and causes retention of sodium. Replacement of the 4-*n*-butyl group of phenylbutazone by allyl or propyl also produces compounds as active as phenylbutazone when tested in the UV-erythema test (Bavin *et al.*, 1955). Replacement of the acidic proton at position 4 by a methyl group or preparation of the enol ether of phenylbutazone removes all antiinflammatory activity. The latter results emphasize the critical role played by the acidic proton in the activity of phenylbutazone. Carbocyclic analogs of phenylbutazone, where both nitrogen atoms of the pyrazolidinedione ring are replaced by carbon atoms to produce a cyclopentene system, are ineffective in inhibiting UV erythema (Bavin *et al.*, 1955). The possibility of a much higher pK_a for the latter carbocyclic compounds must be considered as a possible explanation for their lack of activity.

A remarkable amount of data on the pharmacokinetics of phenylbutazone and its many close analogs in man has been reported by Brodie, Burns, Dayton, Gutman, and their co-workers. The results of these workers have been efficiently tabulated by Bloom and Laubach (1962); Table II, with only minor modifications, is reproduced here with the kind permission of these authors and of *Annual Reviews*, Inc.

Compounds in Table II are arranged in order of increasing acidity (decreasing pK_a). As has been observed in a number of medicinal compounds in other structural classes, relatively small changes in substituents are found to dramatically alter the physical and biological properties of the resulting compounds. For example, compare in Table II the isomeric compounds *1* and *5*; they have pK_a values differing by 2.3 units because of a possible steric effect of the *t*-butyl group in *1*, which has already been discussed. Also compare compounds *6* and *7*, where the presence of a hydroxyl group in the side chain of *7* reduces oral absorption, decreases plasma half-life, and perhaps as a result of these abolishes antirheumatic activity. Correlation of low pK_a with short plasma half-life (e.g., compounds *12–17*) has already been discussed and facile metabolic degradation can explain the comparatively short half-life of such compounds as *7* and *8*. Compounds *3* and *9* are highly insoluble in water (less than 0.2 mg/ml at pH 7) and this probably leads to poor oral absorption and consequent lack of activity.

At plasma levels that produce therapeutic effects in man, phenylbutazone is 98% bound to serum proteins. This tight binding of phenylbutazone, mostly to serum albumin, is a characteristic of many acidic antiinflammatory agents and has been shown (Solomon *et al.*, 1968) to be competitive with binding of warfarin to the same site on albumin. As a consequence, simultaneous administration of both drugs will increase the unbound form of each drug and thereby potentiate its biological effects (O'Reilly and Aggeler, 1967a,b; O'Reilly and Levy, 1970). Other drugs, including sulfonamides, tolbutamide, and indomethacin, also compete with phenylbutazone for binding sites on human serum albumin. Plasma levels of phenylbutazone in man are found to plateau in the 80–140 μg/ml range with wide individual variations, whereas no further increases in serum levels are observed with oral doses above 800 mg/day (Burns *et al.*, 1953).

A balanced view of the role of phenylbutazone in the therapy of rheumatic diseases has been presented by Steinbrocker and Argyros (1960). Clinical side effects of phenylbutazone have been discussed in articles by von Rechenberg (1962), Mauer (1955), McCarthy and Chalmers (1964), Strandberg (1965), Hart (1953), and Siegmeth (1971). Other discussions of specific phenylbutazone side effects are given by Fowler (1967), Stevenson *et al.* (1971), Wissmuller (1971), Fraumeni (1967), Bloch *et al.* (1966), and Brodie *et al.* (1954).

Relatively minor structural modifications in the phenylbutazone molecule have led to new compounds that also exhibit antiinflammatory activity. For example, the effect of joining the two phenyl rings in phenylbutazone has been examined. Table III, summarizing the results of this work, illustrates the types of bridging functions that have been employed.

Although the activity of these bridged analogs is poorly documented, some antiinflammatory activity appears to be retained when the phenyl rings

TABLE II

Physical and Pharmacological (Man) Properties of Phenylbutazone Analogs[a]

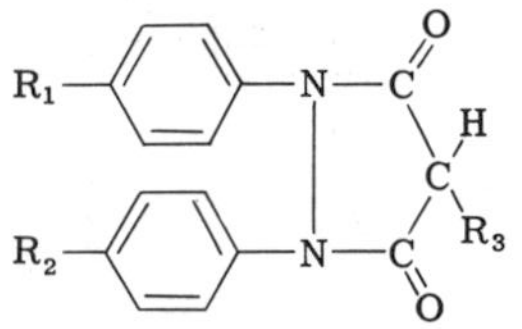

Compound	R_1	R_2	R_3	pK_a	Plasma half-life (hour)	Solubility (mg/ml) at pH 7.4	Plasma binding at (24 hour, pH 7.4)	Oral absorption	Disposition (% of dose recovered unchanged in 24 hour urine)	Anti-rheumatic activity	Uricosuric[b] potency	References[c]
1	HO	H	$C(CH_3)_3$	7.0	1				[d]			a
2	H	H	$CH(CH_3)_2$	5.5	72		At least 95%		<1		>1200	b,c
3	CH_3	CH_3	$CH_2CH_2CH_2CH_3$	4.9	24	0.12	At least 95%	I[e]			>1200	b,d,f
4	Cl	Cl	$CH_2CH_2CH_2CH_3$	4.8	20	0.09		I	<1		1000	d,b

136

No.												Ref.
5	HO	H	CH₂CH₂CH₂CH₃	4.7	72	10	98%	C	<2	+	800–1000	d,b,e
6	H	H	CH₂CH₂CH₂CH₃	4.5	72	2.2	98%	C	<1	+	800–1000	d,b,e,g
7	H	H	CH₂CH₂CHOHCH₃	4.0	8(10)		93%	I	8	–	150–300	b,e,f
8	H	H	CH₂CH₂SC₆H₅	3.9	3	1.6		C	<3		150–300	d,b
9	H	H	CH₂CH₂CH₂C₆H₅			0.14		I				d
10	CH₃SO₂	H	CH₂CH₂CH₂CH₃	3.4	24							h
11	NO₂	H	CH₂CH₂CH₂CH₃	3.2	24							b,i
12	H	H	CH₂CH₂SOC₆H₅	2.8	3		At least 95%	C	<2	+	30–100	b,c,i
13	CH₃SO₂	CH₃SO₂	CH₂CH₂CH₂CH₃	2.6	1		At least 95%		43	–	30–70	b,c
14	H	H	CH₂CH₂SO₂C₆H₅	2.7	1–3		At least 95%		40		100–150	b,c
15	HO	H	COCH₂CH₂CH₃	2.3	8				35			b,c
16	HO	H	COCH₂C₆H₅	2.0	3			C	41	–	30–70	b,j
17	H	H	COCH₂CH₂CH₃	2.0	1–3	0.12	At least 95%	I	25–50			b
												d,c

[a] Reproduced from *Annual Review of Pharmacology* **2**, 92 (1962) with the permission of Annual Reviews, Inc. and B. M. Bloom and G. D. Laubach
[b] I. V. infusion dose (mg) required for 100% increase in uric acid in gouty subjects (Gutman et al., 1960; Burns et al., 1958).
[c] a, Dayton et al. (1960); b, Gutman et al. (1960); c, Dayton et al. (1959); d, Brodie and Hogben (1957); e, Yü et al. (1958); f, Burns et al. (1960); g, Burns et al. (1953); h, Yü et al. (1960); i, Yü et al. (1959); j, Seegmiller et al. (1960).
[d] Rapidly metabolized and cleared as *p*-glucuronide (Dayton et al., 1960).
[e] I, Slow and incomplete; C, rapid and complete.

TABLE III

Phenyl-Bridged Analogs of Phenylbutazone

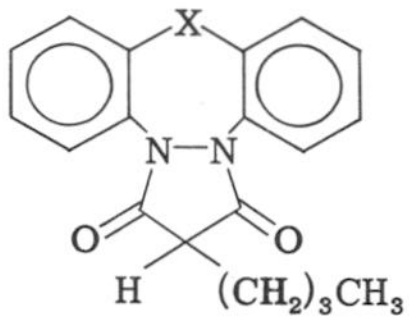

X	Antiinflammatory activity	Reference
—	Not reported	Kuhne and Erlenmeyer (1955)
CH_2	[a]	Lowrie (1962)
CH_2CH_2	[a]	Lowrie (1962)
O	[a]	Lowrie (1962)
S	[a]	Lowrie (1962)
SO_2	Not reported	Michel and Matter (1961)
NCH_3	[a]	Lowrie (1962)

[a]No quantitative data were reported; however, antiinflammatory activity for these bridged compounds was said to be "not as great as phenylbutazone" and the "most active" compounds, using the yeast-induced rat paw edema test, had X = S.

in phenylbutazone are connected by various atoms. It seems clear, however, that all of these compounds are less active than phenylbutazone.

A number of workers have studied still further variations in substituents in the pyrazolidine nucleus in attempts to improve antiinflammatory potency and to minimize toxicity. Thus, removal of one phenyl group from (**1**) produces monophenylbutazone (mobutazone), which has been employed clinically and is claimed (Thune, 1967) to produce equal antiinflammatory effects but to be less toxic than phenylbutazone. Monophenylbutazone causes ulceration of the rabbit stomach (Larsen and Bredahl, 1966). A double-blind comparison of monophenylbutazone (750 mg/day) with phenylbutazone (300 mg/day) (Woodbury et al., 1969) showed the latter drug to be more effective.

By replacing the 4-n-butyl group in (**1**) by the 3-ketobutyl substituent, compound (**10**), kebuzone, is obtained and it is reported (Horakova et al., 1958) to be less toxic and more potent than phenylbutazone in formalin- or kaolin-induced edema in rats. One clinical study of kebuzone (Nyfos and Lunding, 1968), however, reveals efficacy similar and side effects comparable to those observed with phenylbutazone, whereas another (Gibson and Burry, 1971) reports hepatoxic effects with this drug.

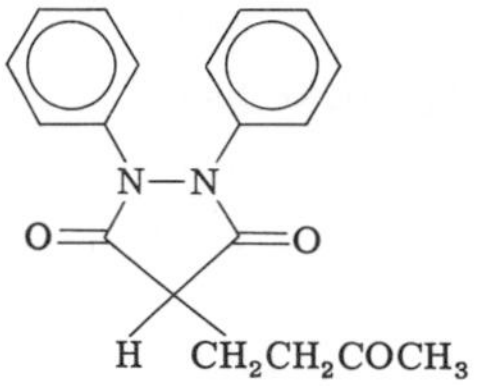

10

Some 1-phenyl-2-styryl analogs (**11**) of phenylbutazone have been made (Yamamoto and Kaneko, 1970) from phenylacetaldehydes and substituted phenylhydrazines, Eq. (5).

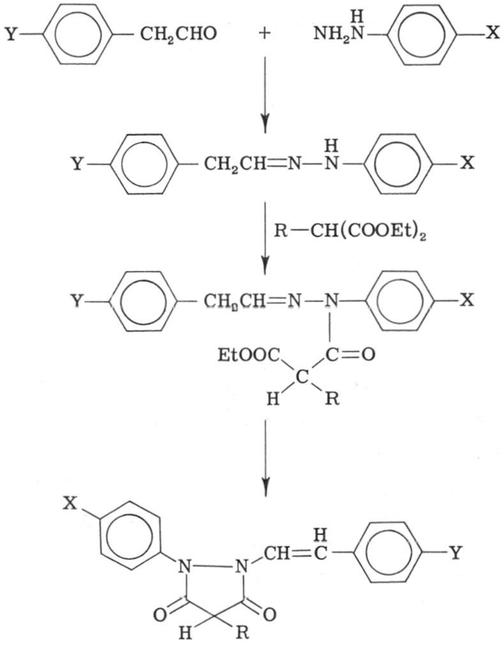

(5)

11

The substituent in (**11**) was maintained as n-butyl for all but one of 31 analogs, while substituents (X, Y) on the phenyl and styryl groups were varied. A 4′-methyl substituent on the phenyl ring appears to improve activity. At the lowest oral dose employed (50 mg/kg), inhibition of carrageenan-induced rat paw edema never exceeds 37% for any of these analogs. These data suggest potency approximately equal to phenylbutazone. However, lack of a dose–response comparison precludes a conclusion on this point.

A 3-keto-4,4-dimethylpentyl group in place of n-butyl at position 4 of phenylbutazone produces compound (**12**), trimethazone, on which only

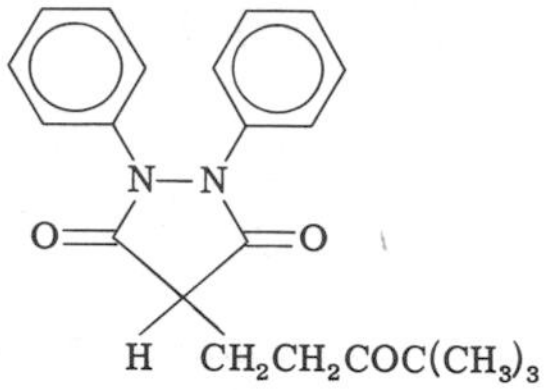

$$O=\underset{\underset{\overset{|}{\text{H}}\quad CH_2CH_2COC(CH_3)_3}{}}{\overset{\overset{\displaystyle\bigcirc\quad\bigcirc}{N-N}}{}}=O$$

12

limited data are published (Muratova and Zahor, 1971). Doses of 50–100 mg/kg in rats produce antiinflammatory activity similar to that of phenylbutazone.

In a special issue of *Arzneimittel-Forschung* [Vol. 22, Issue 1a, pp. 171–232 (1972)], 4-prenylphenylbutazone (prenazone, **13**) is discussed in detail.

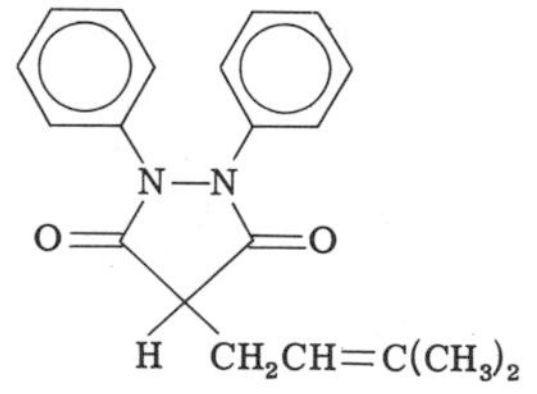

$$O=\underset{\underset{\overset{|}{\text{H}}\quad CH_2CH=C(CH_3)_2}{}}{\overset{\overset{\displaystyle\bigcirc\quad\bigcirc}{N-N}}{}}=O$$

13

The incorporation of an isoprene unit at position 4 is reported (Casadio *et al.*, 1972) to reduce the ulcerating effect of (**13**) in rats and dogs (Marrazi-Uberti *et al.*, 1972). Antiinflammatory activity comparable to that of phenylbutazone is observed in the rat foot edema test (Bianchi *et al.*, 1972; Bianchi, 1972) but the ability to reduce erythema caused by ultraviolet light in guinea pigs is very much less for (**13**) than for phenylbutazone. Structure–activity comparisons of several related terpene-substituted diphenylpyrazolidinediones (Casadio *et al.*, 1972; Pala *et al.*, 1972) reveal (**13**) to possess superior antiinflammatory activity and the lowest ulcerogenicity. A pK_a value of 5.09 (Perego *et al.*, 1972) for (**13**) indicates an acidity quite comparable to that of phenylbutazone. Prenazone exhibits antipyretic properties and inhibits granuloma deposition around a foreign body (Bianchi *et al.*, 1972), even in adrenalectomized animals. The compound also inhibits rat adjuvant arthritis (Lumachi, 1972). Toxicological studies revealed good toleration and no abnormalities in various organs or in hematopoietic systems of the rat or dog when (**13**) is administered for 14–29 weeks (Gaetani *et al.*, 1972a). Comparison with other antiinflammatory agents in rats indicated superior chronic toleration for prenazone (Gaetani *et al.*, 1972b).

The half-life for (**13**) in man of 20–30 hours is considerably shorter than that of phenylbutazone (Buniva *et al.*, 1972). No metabolites of (**13**) have yet been identified and blood levels of (**13**) are considerably lower in both animals and man (Coppi *et al.*, 1972) than levels of phenylbutazone given at comparable doses.

Preliminary indications from early clinical reports on limited numbers of arthritic patients (Passotti *et al.*, 1972; Dotti *et al.*, 1972; Ligniére *et al.*, 1972) are that daily doses of 400–600 mg of prenazone for period of 1–16 weeks are as effective as phenylbutazone (400 mg/day) or indomethacin (75 mg/day). Serum levels of about 30 μg/ml produce satisfactory clinical responses. Prenazone shares the sodium- and water-retentive properties of phenylbutazone (Ghiringhelli *et al.*, 1972) and causes significant decreases in serum (indirect) bilirubin levels.

B. Ring-Fused Pyrazolidinediones

Other approaches to the synthesis of structurally novel antiinflammatory agents containing a pyrazolidinedione ring have been utilized. When a pyrazolidinedione ring was fused to a cinnoline or benzotriazine system, Eqs. (6) and (7), there resulted the antiinflammatory agents cinnopentazone (Scha-306, **14**) and azapropazone (Mi-85, **15**), respectively.

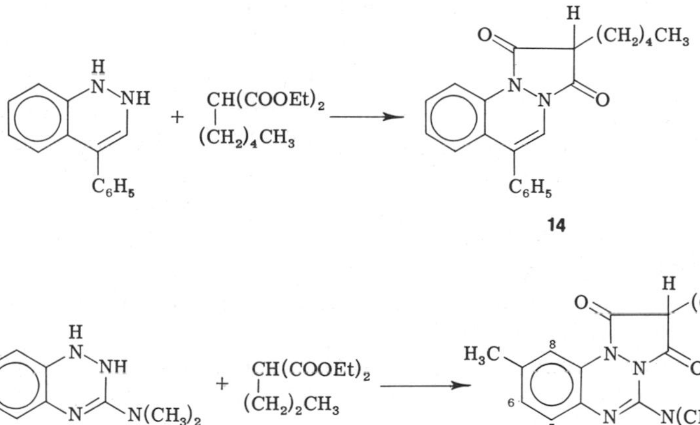

$$(6)$$

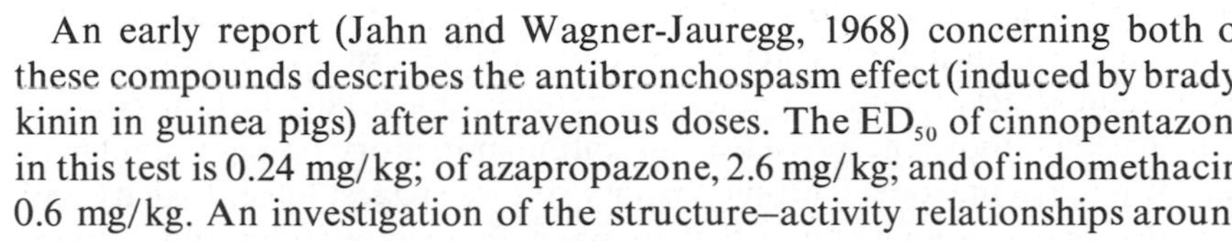

14

$$(7)$$

15

An early report (Jahn and Wagner-Jauregg, 1968) concerning both of these compounds describes the antibronchospasm effect (induced by bradykinin in guinea pigs) after intravenous doses. The ED_{50} of cinnopentazone in this test is 0.24 mg/kg; of azapropazone, 2.6 mg/kg; and of indomethacin, 0.6 mg/kg. An investigation of the structure–activity relationships around cinnopentazone (**14**) (Schatz and Wagner-Jauregg, 1968) reveals that an acidic hydrogen at position 2 is required for activity, that the 2-propyl or 2-butyl analogs are also active, that a 6-*p*-tolyl analog is as active as the

6-phenyl compound, and that the 5-6 double bond is required for antiinflammatory activity.

Cinnopentazone, as well as azapropazone, are capable of stabilizing serum albumin toward heat (Wagner-Jauregg *et al.*, 1969) and a more recent report (Wagner-Jauregg and Burlimann, 1971) corrects an earlier impression that cinnopentazone labilizes rather than stabilizes albumin to heat. Another method employed for classifying antiinflammatory agents involves the measurement of the bacteriostatic activity *in vitro*. Although some standard antiinflammatory agents are active in this test, it is not clear what relationship there is between bacteriostatic activity and antiedema activity. Cinnopentazone and its close analogs are bacteriostatic (Wagner-Jauregg *et al.*, 1970; Wagner-Jauregg and Fisher, 1968), and this has been taken as further evidence of their antiinflammatory usefulness. Despite the antibradykinin and bacteriostatic activity found for cinnopentazone, no clinical reports are available on this drug.

Of the two ring-fused pyrazolidinediones discussed in this section, azapropazone (**15**), more recently assigned the nonproprietary name "apazone," has been most completely described as to its chemical, pharmacological, and clinical properties. A study of the chemical reactivity of (**15**) revealed that a variety of nucleophilic agents either open the pyrazolidine ring or displace the dimethylamino function (Mixich, 1968), perhaps an indication that the compound will not long persist as unchanged drug *in vivo*. The acidity of azapropazone ($pK_a = 6.58$ in 50% aqueous alcohol; personal communication from T. Wagner-Jauregg, 1971) is slightly less than that of phenylbutazone ($pK_a = 544$ in 50% alcohol) when determined in the same solvent system. Although the comparison of pK_a's among different structural types in mixed solvent systems can be misleading, there seem to be only minor effects on the acidity of the pyrazolidinedione ring as a result of fusing it to a benzotriazine system. The structure of azapropazone is best represented as an internal salt (Fehner and Mixich, 1973).

A very complete study has been made of the pharmacological effects of azapropazone (Jahn and Adrian, 1969). In the carrageenan-induced rat paw edema test, azapropazone (ED_{50} of approximately 50 mg/kg, p.o.) and phenylbutazone are found to be equipotent and activity is not reduced in adrenalectomized rats at doses of 100 and 200 mg/kg. Other pharmacological tests, such as guinea pig erythema, the cotton pellet test in rats, and the antibradykinin effects found in guinea pig bronchospasm, support the conclusion that azapropazone possesses an antiinflammatory potency similar to that of phenylbutazone. Chronic toxicity studies suggest lower toxicity and less ulcerogenic activity than that of phenylbutazone (Jahn and Adrian, 1969). It has also been suggested (Lewis *et al.*, 1971) that the lysosome-stabilizing properties of azapropazone may contribute to its antiinflammatory action. Relatively high *in vitro* concentrations of azapropazone will stabilize bovine albumin to heat denaturation (Lewis *et al.*, 1972).

A number of clinical reports on azapropazone have appeared (Kiese-wetter, 1968; Beckschaefer, 1969, 1971; Vokner, 1970; Mennet *et al*., 1971; Schmoekel, 1971; Olbrich *et al*., 1971; Sausgruber, 1971) and some summaries of extensive clinical experience with this drug are also available (Mathies, 1971; Anonymous, 1970). In four double-blind studies, the effectiveness of optimal doses of azapropazone have been equivalent to that of optimal doses of phenylbutazone and indomethacin (Sausgruber, 1971). Open studies in chronic polyarthritis and spondylitis indicate that a daily dose between 600 and 1200 mg can achieve an antiinflammatory effect comparable to that of phenylbutazone (Kiesewetter, 1968; Mennet *et al*., 1971). Azapropazone also reduces inflammation and edema in a variety of traumas when it is administered at a dose of 600–1200 mg/day (Schmoekel, 1971; Ulrych *et al*. 1973). Blood levels of azapropazone increase in a linear manner with increasing oral dose; an 800 mg dose produces approximately 70 μg/ml of drug in plasma 4 hours post dose (Schatz *et al*., 1970). Side effects reported so far include gastric symptoms in 1–10% of patients and exanthema with pruritis (Schmoekel, 1971; Mathies, 1971; Olbrich *et al*., 1971), suggesting fewer toxic effects (Sausgruber, 1971) to date than either phenylbutazone or indomethacin. Azapropazone has an average half-life in man of $8\frac{1}{2}$–12 hours (Schatz *et al*., 1970; Klatt and Koss, 1973a), considerably shorter than that of phenylbutazone, with the 6-hydroxylated metabolite of **15** isolated from human urine (Mixich, 1972a,b). The 6-hydroxylated metabolite is not active in the rat paw edema test and produces a transient hypotensive effect in cats (Jahn, 1973). Metabolic pathways appear to be similar in rat and in man (Klatt and Koss, 1973b; Jahn *et al*., 1973). The uricosuric effect of azapropazone in man has been reported (Frank, 1971) and appears to be caused by enhanced tubular secretion of uric acid.

III. OTHER β-DIKETONES (NON-PYRAZOLIDINEDIONES)

A. 1,3-Indandiones

After demonstrating antiinflammatory activity for 2-phenyl-1,3-indan-dione (**16**), Fontaine *et al*. (1965) concluded that the antiedema (carrageenan-induced rat paw edema) and the antierythema (UV-induced erythema in

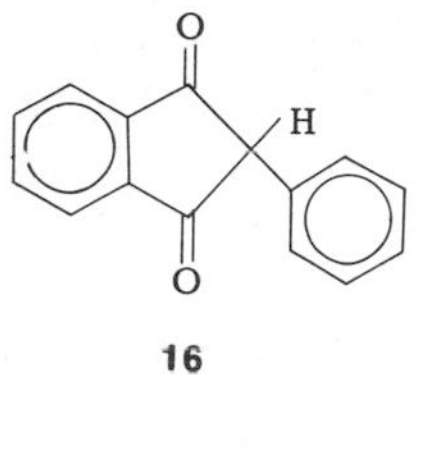

16

guinea pigs) of (16) was probably mediated through the adrenal-stimulating effect of this compound. These same workers (Fontaine *et al.*, 1967) also concluded that the well-known anticoagulant properties of (16) and a few close analogs were not separable from the antiinflammatory activity. However, Lombardino and Wiseman (1968) studied 71 substituted 2-aryl-1,3-indandiones (17) prepared from phthalide and a benzaldehyde or from a phthalic anhydride and a substituted phenylacetic acid, Eq. (8).

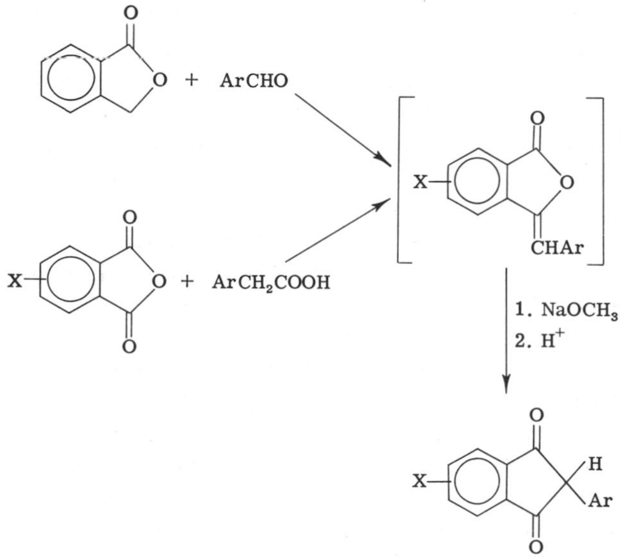

$$\text{(8)}$$

17

They found that several analogs retained antiinflammatory activity when administered orally but were free of anticoagulant effects as measured by inhibition of prothrombin synthesis. For example, in (17), where Ar = 3-$CH_3C_6H_4$ and X = 5-CF_3 or where Ar = 2-naphthyl and X = 5-Br, compounds were obtained that inhibited the carrageenan-induced rat paw edema with a potency approximately equal to phenylbutazone. Furthermore, adrenalectomy was found to have no effect on either the antiedema activity of a number of analogs of (17) or the antiedema activity of (16). The acidity of a majority of the active (antiinflammatory) analogs of (17) was measured in 2:1 dioxane–water and found to be in the range of 4.2–5.9; compounds with higher pK_a's (e.g., 17, X = H, Ar = 2-$CH_3OC_6H_4$, pK_a = 7.6) were probably incapable of achieving a planar enolate anion and were not active antiinflammatory agents.

B. 1,3-Dioxoisoquinoline-4-carboxanilides

The first report of antiinflammatory activity in a class of β-ketoamides was that of Kadin and Wiseman (1969). They found several 1,3-dioxoiso-quinoline-4-carboxanilides (18), prepared from 1,3($2H,4H$)-isoquinoline-dione and arylisocyanates, Eq. (9), to be orally effective inhibitors of

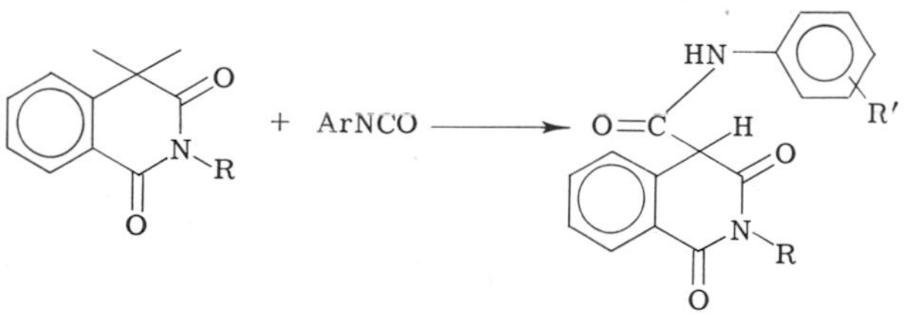

18

carrageenan-induced rat paw edema in either normal or adrenalectom-ized rats. Some analogs of (18), e.g., where R = CH$_3$ and R' = 4'-Cl, were as much as 3 times more potent than phenylbutazone (Wiseman *et al.*, 1970). The compounds were also active in inhibiting the erythemic response to ultraviolet light in guinea pigs, in suppressing cotton string-induced granuloma formation in rats, and in ameliorating the symptoms of adjuvant arthritis in rats. The unexpectedly low pK_a's (in the range of 4–6) found for these compounds were attributed to the ability of the enolate anion, formed on ionization of (18) to form a stable intramolecular hydrogen bond to the amide proton (19). Para substituents (18, R' = 4'-F) prolonged the half-life of (18) in man, probably by blocking the metabolically vulnerable 4'-position. The 4'-unsubstituted compounds were rapidly hydroxylated at

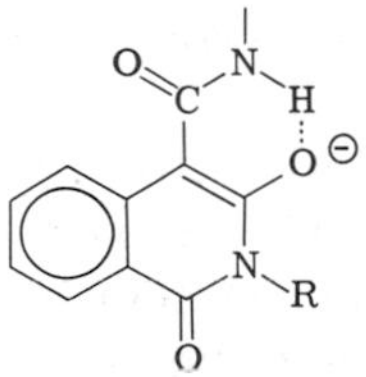

19

the 4'-position to produce an inactive (rat paw edema) compound. The effect of (18), R = H, R' = 4'-Cl, on uric acid clearance, expected from its prolongation of phenol red half-life in rat, was confirmed in man by Wiseman *et al.* (1970).

C. 3-Oxo-1,2-benzothiazine-4-carboxamides

Another example of β-ketoamides with antiinflammatory activity is a series of 3-oxo-1,2-benzothiazine-4-carboxamide 1,1-dioxides (20), Eq. (10)

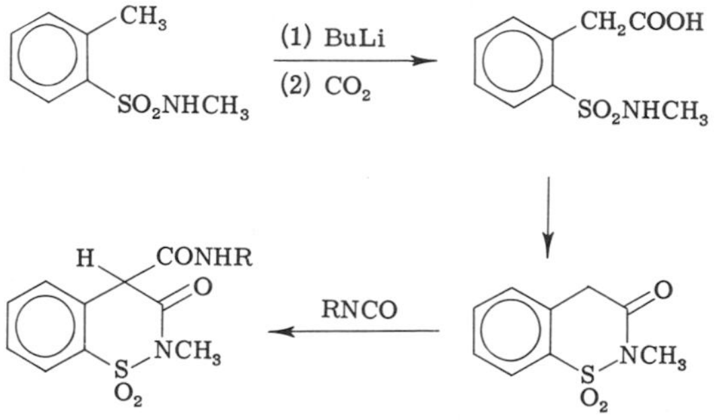

$$ \text{(10)} $$

20

(Lombardino and Wiseman, 1971b). In this class of compounds, 4'-substituted carboxanilides (e.g., $R = 4'\text{-BrC}_6\text{H}_4$ or $4'\text{-NO}_2\text{C}_6\text{H}_4$) are the most potent of 46 analogs of (20) tested in the carrageenan rat paw edema test. Significant inhibition of rat paw edema is observed at oral doses as low as 1 mg/kg and adrenalectomy does not influence the results of this test. A dose–response comparison of the 4'-bromocarboxanilide (20, $R = 4'\text{-BrC}_6\text{H}_4$) with indomethacin indicates the former compound to be 1.5 times more potent (Lombardino and Wiseman, 1971a). Such compounds as 20 are acids of moderate strength with pK_a's in the range of 5–6 when measured in 2:1 dioxane–water. Here again, stabilization of the enolate anion by internal hydrogen bonding seems to explain the enhanced acidity of (20).

D. 4-Hydroxy-1,2-benzothiazine-3-carboxanilides

Certain examples of enolized β-ketoamides derived from 4-oxo-2H-1,2-benzothiazine-3-carboxylic acid 1,1-dioxide (21), Eq. (11), are among the most potent inhibitors of inflammation in animals. Where R = alkyl or aryl (Lombardino et al., 1971), acidity ranging in pK_a's from 6.4 to 8.6 is observed when representatives of 21 are titrated in 2:1 dioxane–water. The unsubstituted carboxanilide (21, $R = C_6H_5$) is twice as potent as phenylbutazone when compared at five dose levels in the rat paw edema test and adrenalectomy does not affect the results of this test. This work was later essentially confirmed by others (DiPasquale et al., 1973) and antipyretic, hypothermic, and adjuvant arthritis activity equivalent to phenylbutazone was reported.

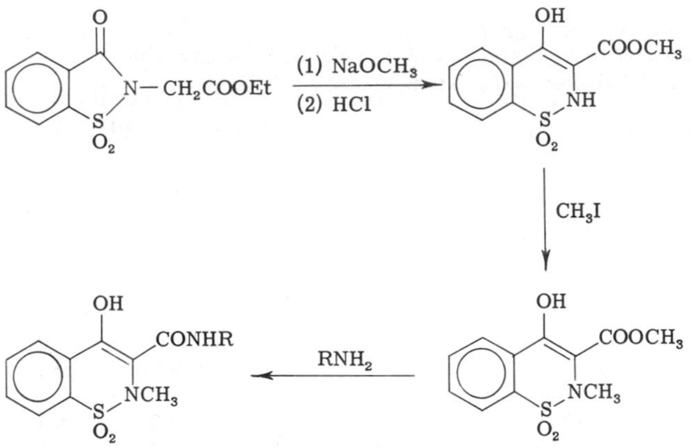

(11)

21

The principle metabolite resulting from administration of the carboxanilide (**21**), R = C_6H_5, to man, monkey, and rat is the 4′-hydroxylated compound (**22**), which is excreted in conjugated form via the urine. The metabolite (**22**) has a longer half-life (37 hours) in man than the parent carboxanilide (21 hours) (Chiaini *et al.*, 1971).

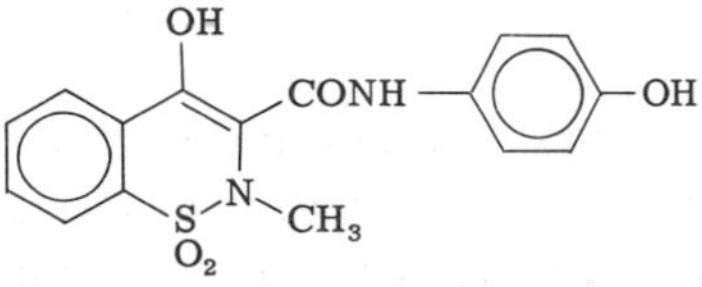

22

Zinnes *et al.* (1973) reported some analogous 1,2-benzothiazines that for the most part displayed only modest or insignificant antiinflammatory activity.

In later reports (Lombardino and Wiseman, 1972; Lombardino *et al.*, 1973), a marked increase in both antiinflammatory potency and in acid strength was described for some N-heterocyclic amides derived from 1,2-benzothiazines (e.g., **23**, sudoxicam). Sudoxicam and related N-heterocyclic analogs (**24–26**) (Table IV) ranged from 0.6 to 2.9 times the potency of

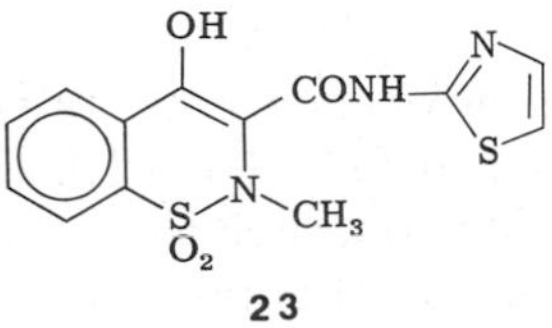

23

TABLE IV

Relative Antiinflammatory Potencies and Acidities of *N*-Heterocyclic
Carboxamides of 4-Hydroxy-2*H*-1,2-benzothiazine 1,1-Dioxides

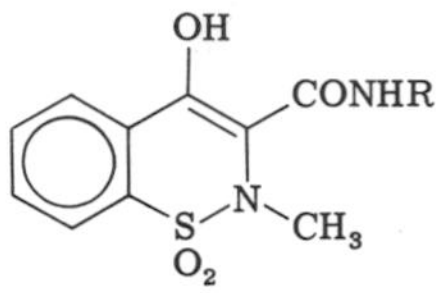

Compound	R	Relative potency[a]	$pK_a{}^b$
23	2-Thiazolyl	2.9	5.3
24	4,5-Dimethyl-2-thiazolyl	1.6	5.8
25	2-Pyridyl	1.6	6.3
26	6-Methyl-2-pyridyl	0.6	6.6
Indomethacin		1.0	7.0

[a] Potency determined by dose–response comparisons at four dose levels in
the carrageenan rat paw edema test. Drugs administered orally 1 hour before
and edema measured 3 hours after injection of carrageenan.

[b] Acidity determinations were carried out potentiometrically in 2:1 dioxane–
water at 25°C using standard sodium hydroxide. pK_a's obtained from the half-
neutralization point in these titrations.

indomethacin when the drugs were compared at four dose levels in the carrageenan rat paw edema test in both normal and adrenalectomized rats.

One explanation for the enhanced acidity of compounds (23)–(26) as compared to such related compounds as (21), R = C_6H_5, involves the possibility
of a dual mode of stabilization of the enolate anion, e.g., tautomeric forms
(25a) and (25b).

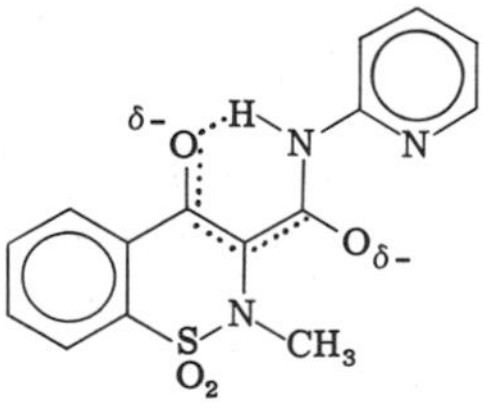

25a 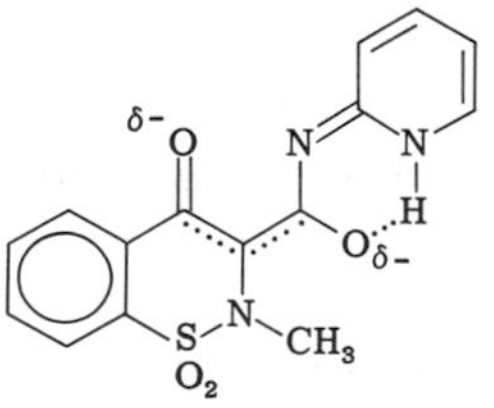   25b

The plasma half-life of sudoxicam is long both in laboratory animals (e.g.,
60 hours in the dog) and in man (24–96 hours), and it exhibits high potency
in animal models of inflammation, such as erythema induced by ultraviolet
light in guinea pigs, suppression of granulation tissue around an implanted

string in rats, and suppression of adjuvant arthritis in rats (Wiseman and Chiaini, 1972). Sudoxicam exhibited superior clinical activity at 20 mg per day when tested in open or in double blind studies against phenylbutazone in rheumatoid arthritis (Rau and Gross, 1973; Roth et al., 1973).

E. 2-Oxobenzofuran-3-carboxanilides

All 19 analogous 2,3-dihydro-2-oxobenzofuran-3-carboxanilides (27) Eq. (12), are antiinflammatory and of a potency at least equivalent to that of

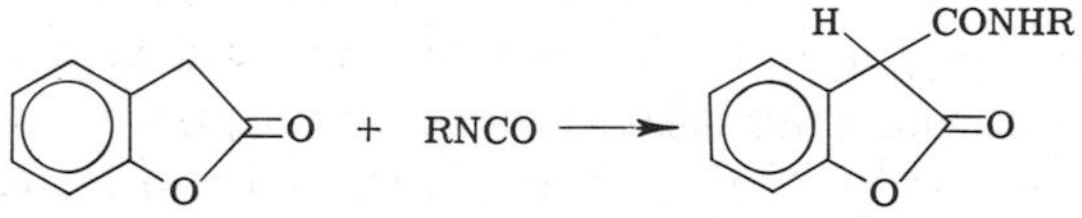

$$\text{(benzofuranone)} + RNCO \longrightarrow \text{(product with } H, CONHR) \tag{12}$$

27

aspirin in the carrageenan-induced rat paw edema assay (Kadin, 1972). Spectral evidence suggests that (27) exists as a diketo rather than an enolized form, and titration of a number of analogs of (27) in 2:1 dioxane–water indicates a pK_a range of 3–4. This markedly enhanced acidity can be attributed to the absence of a stable enol form in the conjugate acid and to stabilization of the enolate anion by hydrogen bonding of the enolate oxygen to the proton on the amide nitrogen atom. Potent analogs in this series include (27), R = 2-CH$_3$C$_6$H$_4$ and (27), R = 2-FC$_6$H$_4$; these two compounds exhibit oral activity at a dose of 10 mg/kg equivalent to that shown by aspirin at a dose of 100 mg/kg.

F. Hexahydropyrimidine-2,4,6-triones

If the two nitrogen atoms in phenylbutazone (1) are separated by a carbonyl group, the substituted barbituric acid, hexahydropyrimidine-2,4,6-trione (28), Eq. (13), is obtained. Senda et al. (1967) describe the antiinflammatory properties of 48 analogs of (28) in the dextran- and ovalbumin-induced rat paw edema test where compounds were administered at a dose

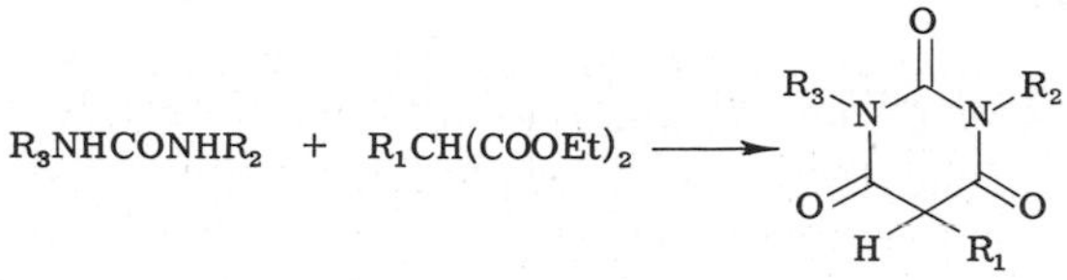

$$R_3NHCONHR_2 + R_1CH(COOEt)_2 \longrightarrow \text{(product)} \tag{13}$$

28

of 100 mg/kg, intraperitoneally. Of 27 of these compounds tested orally in the carrageenan-induced rat paw edema test at 200 mg/kg, (28), $R_1 = C_4H_9$, $R_2 = H$, $R_3 = C_6H_{11}$ (bucolome) is most active (greater than 65% inhibition of edema).

Unfortunately, no dose–response comparison was made of bucolome with standard antiinflammatory drugs. The antiedema activity, combined with a mouse LD_{50} of 550 mg/kg, i.p. (Senda *et al.*, 1967), encouraged several clinical trials of bucolome (Anonymous, 1966). The highest clinical dose (1.2 gm/day) of bucolome produced blood levels of 125–135 μg/ml and an 80–88% improvement in such parameters as erythrocyte sedimentation rate and articular swelling. Gastrointestinal disturbances occurred in 8% of patients and decreased serum urate levels were observed in patients on 0.3–0.6 gm/day of bucolome. Metabolites of bucolome in man included (28), $R_1 =$ butyl, $R_2 = H$, $R_3 = $ 4-hydroxycyclohexyl (Yashiki *et al.*, 1971; Senda *et al.*, 1969a). Toxicological examination of bucolome (Tanabe *et al.*, 1967, 1968) revealed that the lethal effects of the drug in animals were associated with decreased adrenocortical function and atrophy of the lymphoid organs. The acidity constant of bucolome was not reported but might be expected to be in the range of phenylbutazone acidity because the related 5-isopropyl-barbituric acid, for example, has a pK_a of 4.9 (Albert, 1963). Other analogs of (28), e.g., where $R_3 = $ 4'-alkoxycyclohexyl or 4'-hydroxycyclohexyl, were all generally inferior antiinflammatory agents in animals when compared to bucolome (Senda *et al.*, 1969b).

G. Isoxazolidine-3,5-diones

Replacement of one nitrogen atom of phenylbutazone (1) by an oxygen atom produced some antiinflammatory isoxazolidine-3,5-diones (29), Eq. (14)

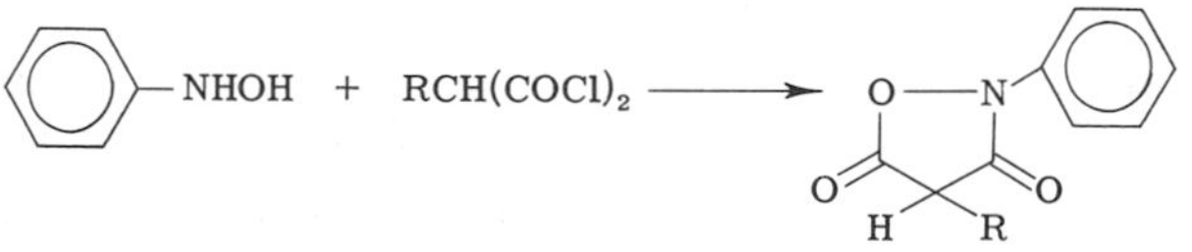

29

(Michel *et al.*, 1965). Titration of several analogs of (29), e.g., $R = C_6H_{11}$ or *t*-butyl, in 80% Methyl Cellosolve solution indicated a pK_a range of 3.2–4.7. Of 44 analogs examined, 16 exhibited antiphlogistic activity in the guinea pig peritonitis test of Bucher (1959) when the compounds were administered subcutaneously. Concurrently run phenylbutazone (15–20 mg/kg) gave a response in this test equivalent to that of either (29), R = C_6H_{11}, or (29), R = t-butyl. Unfortunately, no comparative potency data were presented on these compounds, especially by the oral route, in the more commonly employed animal models of inflammation.

H. 4-Formyl-5-pyrazolones

Formylation of certain 5-pyrazolones produced the 4-formyl-5-pyrazolones (30a), which existed as the internally bonded enol (30b), Eq. (15).

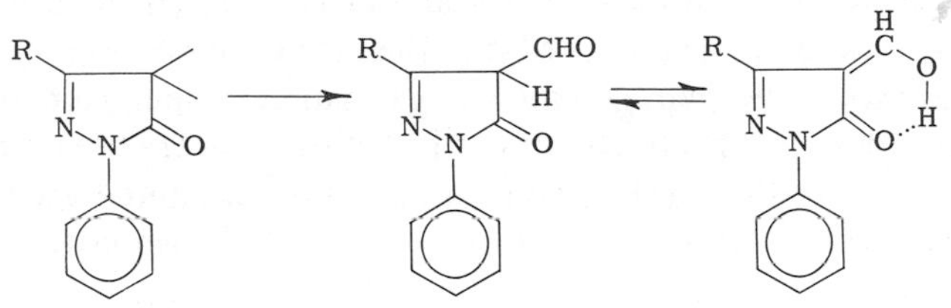

$$(15)$$

30a   30b

Antiinflammatory potency approximately equal to that of phenylbutazone was detected in the carrageenan-induced rat paw edema test when (30b), R = CH_3, was administered by the oral route at doses of 15, 63, and 250 mg/kg (Sinh and Buu-Hoï, 1967; Sinh et al., 1968). This activity could not be detected in the kaolin-induced rat paw edema test but modest anti-granuloma activity (37% inhibition at a dose of 150 mg/kg, p.o.) was observed for (30b) in rats. Surprisingly, two close analogs of (30b), in which R = n-C_3H_7 or C_6H_5, were not active in the carrageenan edema test. The acidity constant for (30b), R = CH_3, was not reported but one might speculate that the stable enol form would tend to decrease the acidity of the compound, perhaps leading to a pK_a of >6.

I. 5-Acetyl-4-hydroxythiophenes

Certain 3-acetyl-5-arylidene-4-hydroxy-2-oxo-2,5-dihydrothiophenes (31), Eq. (16), although not active in the standard acute antiinflammatory

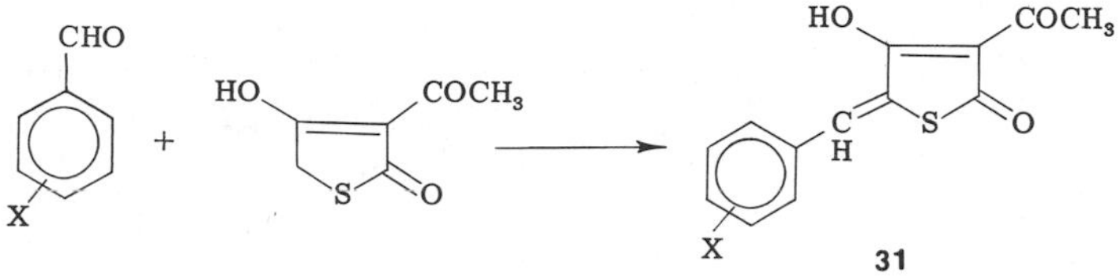

$$(16)$$

31

tests, do inhibit the secondary (immune-mediated) inflammatory lesions of adjuvant arthritis, allergic thyroiditis, and allergic encephalomyelitis in rats (Franklin *et al.*, 1966; O'Mant, 1968). One of the more potent analogs of (31), I.C.I. 47, 776, (X = 4-F), is an inhibitor of nucleic acid synthesis *in vitro* and suppresses the antibody response to either bovine serum albumin or sheep red cells in rats at an oral dose of 5 mg/kg/day. Unfortunately, toxic hematological and histological effects are dose related and parallel the immunosuppressive activity (Franklin *et al.*, 1966). Later work (Davies, 1968) has revealed that the antibody-suppressing activity is species-specific for rats and that no such effect can be demonstrated in guinea pigs or mice.

An acidity constant has not been recorded for I.C.I. 47,776, but the enolic proton is likely to be quite acidic. O'Mant (1968) did not report a value for the acidic proton when he examined the nuclear magnetic spectrum of I.C.I. 47,776; perhaps this acidic proton is not easily distinguished in the spectrum. Although this structurally novel immunosuppressant exhibited the above-mentioned activities in various animal models, no clinical reports on this drug are available.

IV. β-SULFONYLKETONES

Benzo [b] thiophen-3-one 1,1-Dioxides

The successful separation of anticoagulant from antiinflammatory activity in a series of 2-aryl-1, 3-indandiones (see Section III, A), led to the preparation of some 2-arylbenzo [b] thiophen-3(2H)-one 1,1-dioxides (32), using 2-mercaptobenzoic acids as starting materials, Eq. (17) (Lombardino and Wiseman, 1970). The 27 examples of (32) exhibited pK_a's (in 2:1 dioxane–

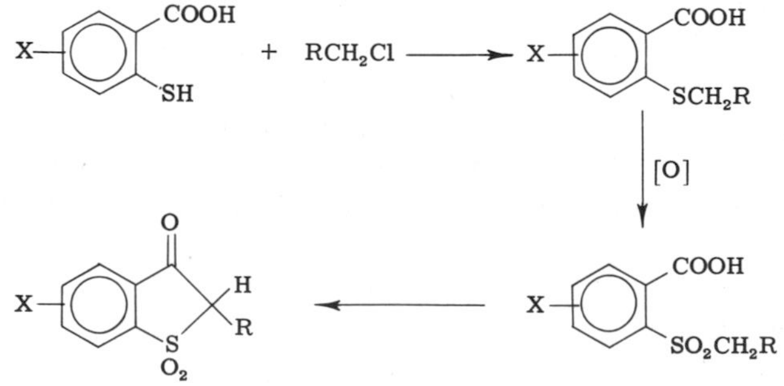

(17)

32

water solvent) in the range of 3.5–7.5. Of these, 16 compounds with pK_a's 4.8–6.2 were effective in suppressing edema resulting from carrageenan injection in the rat paw at oral doses of 10–100 mg/kg. Adrenalectomy had no effect on the results of the rat paw edema test. As in the case of the antiinflammatory 2-aryl-1,3-indandiones (Lombardino and Wiseman, 1968), concurrent anticoagulant properties of (32) could be eliminated in certain analogs by combining fairly large substituents in the benzo ring, e.g., X = 5-Cl, 5-CH$_3$, 5,6-(CH)$_4$, 5,6-(OCH$_3$)$_2$, 5-NO$_2$, or 5-CF$_3$, with meta-substituted aryl groups, e.g., R = 3-CF$_3$C$_6$H$_4$, 3-CH$_3$C$_6$H$_4$, or 3-NO$_2$C$_6$H$_4$. The most active antiinflammatory compound free of anticoagulant effects (32, X = 5-CF$_3$, R = C$_6$H$_5$) was 1.2 times more potent than phenylbutazone when compared at four dose levels in the rat paw edema test.

V. CONCLUDING REMARKS

As a class, acidic organic compounds of diverse structural types have yielded more clinically useful antiinflammatory drugs than either the neutral or the basic classes of compounds. As was first observed for the pyrazolidine dione phenylbutazone, acidic properties can be introduced into antiinflammatory drugs through the use of functionalities other than carboxylic acid groups. Until recently, compounds containing such groups as β-diketones and β-sulfonylketones have received comparatively little attention in the field of antiinflammatory drug research. This is perhaps unfortunate because it is now clear that several types of β-diketones offer an opportunity for manipulating physical and biochemical properties, such as lipophilicity, acid strength (pK_a), and plasma half-life, so as to maximize antiinflammatory effects and minimize undesirable side effects. By extending drug half-life, for example, one may help compensate for a lower intrinsic potency by maintaining higher therapeutic levels of drug for longer periods of time. In man, plasma half-life appears to be generally extended for β-diketones as compared to carboxylic acids (e.g., a 3–4 day half-life for β-diketones, such as phenylbutazone and sudoxicam, versus approximately 2 hours for the carboxylic acids aspirin, ibuprofen, and indomethacin). This extended half-life may be caused by a decreased tendency for β-diketones to undergo O-glucuronide conjugation, a pathway that usually permits rapid excretion of carboxylic acids.

The results reviewed herein suggest that acidic organic molecules other than carboxylic acids may yet yield a drug with the desired combination of high antiinflammatory potency, suitable half-life, and low toxicity that will make it ideally suited for the treatment of inflammation in man.

REFERENCES

Albert, A. (1963). *Phys. Methods Heterocycl. Chem.* **1**, 82.
Anonymous. (1966). *Jap. Med. Gaz.* **3**, 13.
Anonymous. (1970). *Med. Monatsschr.* **24**, 433.
Bavin, E. M., Drain, D. J., Seymore, D. E., and Waterhouse, P. D. (1955). *J. Pharm. Pharmacol.* **7**, 1022.
Beckschaefer, W. (1969). *Arzneim.-Forsch.* **19**, 52.
Beckschaefer, W. (1971). *Praxis* **60**, 447.
Bianchi, C. (1972). *Arzneim.-Forsch.* **22**, 249.
Bianchi, C., Lumachi, B., and Marazzi-Uberti, E. (1972). *Arzneim.-Forsch.* **22**, 183.
Bloch-Michel, H., Gorins, A., and Meyerovitch, A. (1966). *Presse Med.* **74**, 2671.
Bloom, B. M., and Laubach, G. D. (1962). *Annu. Rev. Pharmacol.* **2**, 92.
Brodie, B. B., and Hogben, C. A. M. (1957). *J. Pharm. Pharmacol.* **9**, 345.
Brodie, B. B., Lowman, E. W., Burns, J. J., Lee, P. R., Chenkin, T., Goldman, A., Weiner, M., and Steele, J. M. (1954). *Amer. J. Med.* **16**, 181.
Bucher, K. (1959). *Helv. Physiol. Pharmacol. Acta* **17**, 329.
Buniva, G., Catto, G., Chierichetti, S., Granata, D., and Manieri, G. (1972). *Arzneim.-Forsch.* **22**, 258.
Burns, J. J., Rose, R. K., Chenkin, T., Goldman, A., Schulert, A., and Brodie, B. B. (1953). *J. Pharmacol. Exp. Ther.* **109**, 346.
Burns, J. J., Rose, R. K., Goodwin, S., Reichenthal, J., Horning, B. C., and Brodie, B. B. (1955). *J. Pharmacol. Exp. Ther.* **113**, 481.
Burns, J. J., Yü, T. F., Ritterband, A., Perel, J., Gutman, A. B., and Brodie, B. B. (1957). *J. Pharmacol. Exp. Ther.* **119**, 418.
Burns, J. J., Yü, T. F., Dayton, P., Berger, L., Gutman, A. B., and Brodie, B. B. (1958). *Nature (London)* **182**, 1162.
Burns, J. J., Yü, T. F., Dayton, P. G., Gutman, A. B., and Brodie, B. B. (1960). *Ann. N. Y. Acad. Sci.* **86**, 253.
Casadio, S., Pala, G., Marazzi-Uberti, E., Lumachi, B., Crescenzi, E., Donetti, A., Mantegani, A., and Bianchi, C. (1972). *Arzneim.-Forsch.* **22**, 171.
Chiaini, J., Wiseman, E. H., and Lombardino, J. G. (1971). *J. Med. Chem.* **14**, 1175.
Coppi, G., Bonardi, G., and Perego, R. (1972). *Arzneim.-Forsch.* **22**, 234.
Coyne, W. E. (1970). *In* "Medicinal Chemistry" (A. Burger, ed.), 3rd edition, Part II, p. 953. Wiley (Interscience), New York.
Davies, G. E. (1968). *Immunology* **14**, 393.
Dayton, P. G., Berger, L., Yü, T. F., Sicam, L. E., Landrau, M. A., Gutman, A. B., and Burns, J. J. (1959). *Fed. Proc. Fed. Amer. Soc. Exp. Biol.* **18**, 382.
Dayton, P. G., MacMillan, M., and Chen, W. (1960). *Pharmacologist* **2**, 82.
Di Pasquale, G., Rassaert, C. L., Richter, R. S., and Tripp, L. V. (1973). *Arch. Int. Pharmacodyn.* **203**, 92.
Domenjoz, R. (1960). *Ann. N. Y. Acad. Sci.* **86**, 263.
Domenjoz, R. (1966). *Advan. Pharmacol.* **4**, 143.
Dotti, F., Ongari, R., Carazzi, R., and Chierichetti, S. (1972). *Arzneim.-Forsch.* **22**, 265.
Feeney, G. C., and Carlo, P. (1955). *J. Pharmacol. Exp. Ther.* **114**, 299.
Fehner, H., and Mixich G. (1973). *Arzneim.-Forsch.* **23**, 667.
Fontaine, L., Grand, M., Quentin, Y., and Merle, S. (1965). *Med. Exp.* **13**, 137.
Fontaine, L., Grand, M., Molho, D., and Boschetti, E. (1967). *Med. Pharmacol. Exp.* **17**, 497.
Fowler, P. (1967). *Ann. Rheum. Dis.* **26**, 344.

Frank, O. (1971). Z. Rheumaforsch. **30**, 368.
Franklin, T. J., Newbould, B. B., O'Mant, D. M., Scott, A. I., Stacey, G. J., and Davies, G. E. (1966). Nature (London) **210**, 638.
Fraumeni, J. G. (1967). J. Amer. Med. Ass. **201**, 828.
Gaetani, M., Debeus, R., Bonardi, G., and Coppi, G. (1972a). Arzneim.-Forsch. **22**, 216.
Gaetani, M., Debeus, R., Vidi, A., and Coppi, G. (1972b). Arzneim.-Forsch. **22**, 226.
Ghiringhelli, F., Mazzi, C., and Chierichetti, S. (1972). Arzneim.-Forsch. **22**, 268.
Gibson, T. J., and Burry, H. C. (1971). Clin. Trials J. **8**, 27.
Gutman, A., Dayton, P. G., Yü, T. F., Berger, L., Chen, W., Sicam, L. E., and Burns, J. J. (1960). Amer. J. Med. **29**, 1017.
Hart, F. D. (1953). Lancet **2**, 139.
Horakova, Z., Němeček, O., Pujman, V., Mayer, J., Čtvrtník, J., and Votava, Z. (1958), Arzneim.-Forsch. **8**, 229.
Jahn, U. (1973). Arzneim.-Forsch. **23**, 666.
Jahn, U., and Adrian, R. W. (1969). Arzneim.-Forsch. **19**, 36.
Jahn, U., and Wagner-Jauregg, T. (1968). Arzneim.-Forsch. **18**, 120.
Jahn, U., Reller, J., and Schatz, F. (1973). Arzneim.-Forsch. **23**, 660.
Kadin, S. B. (1972). J. Med. Chem. **15**, 551.
Kadin, S. B., and Wiseman, E. H. (1969). Nature (London) **222**, 275.
Kiesewetter, Von E. (1968). Wien. Med. Wochenschr. **118**, 941.
Klatt, L., and Koss, F. W. (1973a). Arzneim.-Forsch. **23**, 920.
Klatt, L., and Koss, F. W. (1973b). Arzneim.-Forsch. **23**, 913.
Kuhne, H., and Erlenmeyer, H. (1955). Helv. Chim. Acta **38**, 531.
Larsen, V., and Bredahl, E. (1966). Acta Pharmacol. Toxicol. **24**, 443.
Lewis, D. A., Capstick, R. B., and Ancill, R. J. (1971). J. Pharm. Pharmacol. **23**, 931.
Lewis, D. A., Capstick, R. B., and Ancill, R. J. (1972). Biochem. Pharmacol. **21**, 2531.
Ligniére, G. C., Colombo, B., Cárrabba, M., Farrari, P., and Robotti, E. (1972. Arzneim.-Forsch. **22**, 253.
Lombardino, J. G., and Wiseman, E. H. (1968). J. Med. Chem. **11**, 342.
Lombardino, J. G., and Wiseman, E. H. (1970). J. Med. Chem. **13**, 206.
Lombardino, J. G., and Wiseman, E. H. (1971a). Abstr. 161st Nat. Meet., Amer. Chem. Soc. Abstract MEDI 20.
Lombardino, J. G., and Wiseman, E. H. (1971b). J. Med. Chem. **14**, 973.
Lombardino, J. G., and Wiseman, E. H. (1972). J. Med. Chem. **15**, 848.
Lombardino, J. G., Wiseman, E. H., and McLamore, W. M. (1971). J. Med. Chem. **14**, 1171.
Lombardino, J. G., Wiseman, E. H., and Chiaini, J. (1973). J. Med. Chem. **16**, 493.
Lowrie, H. (1962). J. Med. & Pharm. Chem. **5**, 1362.
Lumachi, B. (1972). Arzneim.-Forsch. **22**, 204.
McCarthy, D. D., and Chalmers, T. M. (1964). Can. Med. Ass. J. **90**, 1061.
Marazzi-Uberti, E., Bianchi, C., Gaetani, M., and Pozzi, L. (1972). Arzneim.-Forsch. **22**, 191.
Mathies, H. (1971). Z. Rheumaforsch. **30**, 246.
Mauer, E. F. (1955). N. Engl. J. Med. **253**, 404.
Mennet, P., Olbrich, E., Ulrych, I., Ulrych, J., and Sausgruber, H. (1971). Schweiz. Med. Wochenschr. **101**, 647.
Michel, K., and Matter, M. (1961). Helv. Chim. Acta **44**, 2204.
Michel, K., Gerlach-Gerber, H., Vogel, C., and Matter, M. (1965). Helv. Chim. Acta **48**. 1973.

Mixich, G. (1968). *Helv. Chim. Acta* **51**, 532.

Mixich, G. (1972a). *Helv. Chim. Acta* **55**, 1031.

Mixich, G. (1972b). *Chimia* **26**, 321.

Muratova, J., and Zahor, Z. (1971). *Cesk. Farm.* **20**, 99; *Chem.-Biol. Abstr.* **14**, 4570x (1971).

Nyfos, L., and Lunding, N. C. (1968). *Acta Rheumatol. Scand.* **14**, 148.

Olbrich, E., Ruenzi, J., Sausgruber, H., and Weber, J. (1971). *Med. Welt* p. 1345.

O'Mant, D. M. (1968). *J. Chem. Soc., London* p. 1501.

O'Reilly, R. A., and Aggeler, P. M. (1967a). *Clin. Res.* **15**, 133.

O'Reilly, R. A., and Aggeler, P. M. (1967b). *Ann. Intern. Med.* **66**, 1062.

O'Reilly, R. A., and Levy, G. (1970). *J. Pharm. Sci.* **59**, 1258.

Pala, G., Mantegani, A., Donetti, B., Lumachi, B., Marazzi-Uberti, E., and Casadio, S. (1972). *Arzneim.-Forsch.* **22, 174.**

Passotti, C., Barbieri, C., Buniva, G., and Chierichetti, S. (1972). *Arzneim.-Forsch.* **22**, 262.

Perego, R., Gallazzi, A., Vanoni, P., and Lucarella, I. (1972). *Arzneim.-Forsch.* **22**, 177. **22**, 177.

Perel, J. M., Snell, M. M., Chen, W., and Dayton, P. G. (1964). *Biochem. Pharmacol.* **13**, 1305.

Randall, L. O. (1963). *Physiol. Pharmacol.* **1**, 369–383.

Rau, R., and Gross, D. (1973). *Abstr. 13th Int. Congr. Rheumatology, 1973*. Excerpta Med. Found. Int. Congr. Ser. No. 299, p. 117, Abstract. No. 396.

Rosenthale, M. E. (1973). *Annu. Rep. Med. Chem.* **8**, 214.

Roth, S. H., Englund, D. W., and Harris, B. K. (1973). *Abstr. 13th Int. Congr. Rheumatology, 1973*. Excerpta Med. Found. Int. Congr. Ser. No. 299, p. 117, Abstract No. 397.

Sausgruber, H. (1971). *Arzneim.-Forsch.* **21**, 1230.

Schatz, F., and Wagner-Jauregg, T. (1968). *Helv. Chim. Acta* **51**, 1919.

Schatz, F., Adrian, R., Mixich, G., Molnarova, J., Reller, J., and Jahn, U. (1970). *Therapiewoche* **20**, 2327.

Schmoekel, W. (1971). *Praxis* **60**, 1114.

Seegmiller, J. E., Dayton, P. G., and Burns, J. J. (1960). *Arthritis Rheum.* **3**, 475.

Senda, S., Izumi, H., and Fujimura, H. (1967). *Arzneim.-Forsch.* **17**, 1519.

Senda, S., Izumi, H., Tanimoto, T., and Fujimura, H. (1969a). *J. Pharm. Soc. Jap.* **89**, 254.

Senda, S., Izmui, H., and Fujimura, H. (1969b). *J. Pharm. Soc. Jap.* **89**, 260.

Shen, T. Y. (1967). *In* "Topics in Medicinal Chemistry" (J. L. Rabinowitz and R. M. Meyerson, eds.), Vol. 1, pp. 29–78. Wiley (Interscience), New York.

Shulert, A., Chenkin, T., Goldman, A., and Brodie, B. B. (1952). *J. Pharmacol. Exp. Ther.* **106**, 375.

Siegmeth, W. (1971). *Wien. Med. Wochenschr.* **121**, 784.

Sinh, M. P., and Buu-Hoï, N. P. (1967). *Chim. Ther.* **2**, 106.

Sinh, M. P., Brouilhet, H., Delbarre, F., Buu-Hoï, N. P., and Jouanneau, M. (1968). *Chim. Ther.* **3**, 17.

Solomon, H. M., Schrogie, J. J., and Williams, D. (1968). *Biochem. Pharmacol.* **17**, 143.

Steinbrocker, O., and Argyros, T. G. (1960). *Arthritis Rheum.* **3**, 368.

Stevenson, A. C., Bedford, J., Hill, A. G. S., and Hill, H. F. H. (1971). *Ann. Rheum. Dis.* **30**, 487.

Strandberg, B. (1965). *Acta Rheumatol. Scand., Suppl.* **10**, 5.

Tanabe, K., Takaori, S., and Shimamoto, K. (1967). *Folia Pharmacol. Jap.* **63**, 105.

Tanabe, K., Takaori, S., and Shimamoto, K. (1968). *Excerpta Med.* **21**, 1755.

Thune, S. (1967). *Acta Rheumatol. Scand.* **13**, 63.

Ulrych, J., Olbrich, E. and Sausgruber, H. (1973). *Z. Rheumaforsch.*, **32**, 133.

Unterhalt, B. (1970). *Arch. Pharm.* (*Weinheim*) **303**, 445.

Vokner, J. (1970). *Praxis* **59**, 1756.

von Rechenberg, H. K. (1962). "Phenylbutazone," 2nd ed. Arnold, London.

Wagner-Jauregg, T., and Burlimann, W. (1971). *Arzneim.-Forsch.* **21**, 267.

Wagner-Jauregg, T., and Fischer, J. (1968). *Experientia* **24**, 1029.

Wagner-Jauregg, T., Jahn, U., and Büch, O. (1962). *Arzneim.-Forsch.* **12**, 1160.

Wagner-Jauregg, T., Burlimann, W., and Fischer, J. (1969). *Arzneim.-Forsch.* **19**, 1532.

Wagner-Jauregg, T., Fischer, J., and Jahn, U. (1970). *Arzneim.-Forsch.* **20**, 831.

Weiner, M., and Piliero, S. J. (1970). *Annu. Rev. Pharmacol.* **10**, 171.

Whitehouse, M. W. (1965). *Progr. Drug Res.* **8**, 321–429.

Wilhelmi, G., Herrmann, B., and Tedeschi, G. (1959). *Arzneim.-Forsch.* **9**, 241.

Winter, C. A. (1967). *Progr. Drug Res.* **10**, 139–203.

Wiseman, E. H., and Chiaini, J. (1972). *Biochem. Pharmacol.* **21**, 2323.

Wiseman, E. H., Gralla, E. J., Chiaini, J., Migliardi, J. R., and Chang, Y.-H. (1970). *J. Pharmacol. Exp. Ther.* **172**, 138.

Wissmuller, H. F. (1971). *Arzneim.-Forsch.* **21**, 1738.

Woodbury, J. F. L., Turner, W. A., and Tiongson, R. (1969). *Can. Med. Ass. J.* **101**, 801.

Yamamoto, H., and Kaneko, S. (1970). *J. Med. Chem.* **13**, 292.

Yashiki, T., Matsuzawa, T., Kondo, T., Uda, Y., Shima, T., Mima, H., Senda, S., and Izumi, H. (1971). *Chem. Pharm. Bull.* **19**, 468.

Yü, T. F., Burns, J. J., Paton, D. C., Gutman, A. B., and Brodie, B. B. (1958). *J. Pharmacol. Exp. Ther.* **123**, 63.

Yü, T. F., Burns, J. J., Dayton, P. G., Gutman, A. B., and Brodie, B. B. (1959). *J. Pharmacol. Exp. Ther.* **126**, 185.

Yü, T. F., Dayton, P. G., Gutman, A. B., and Burns, J. J. (1960). *Fed. Proc., Fed. Amer. Soc. Exp. Biol.* **19**, 364.

Zinnes, H., Lindo, N. A., Sircar, J. C., Schwartz, M. L., Shavel, J., Jr., and Di Pasquale, G. (1973). *J. Med. Chem.* **16**, 44.

Chapter 6

Sulfonamides with Antiinflammatory Activity

GEORGE G. I. MOORE

Riker Laboratories, Inc.
3 M Center
St. Paul, Minnesota

I. INTRODUCTION

Relatively few sulfonamide-based chemical systems are reported as acidic, nonsteroidal antiinflammatory agents, in strong contrast to the isosteric carboxylic acid class. In view of the very widespread interest in sulfonamides in other pharmacological areas since 1935, it is logical to assume that many have been routinely screened for antiinflammatory activity and that the dearth of activity reflects a real pharmacological difference between RSO_2NH_2 and RCO_2H, not a lack of synthetic or biological attention. Although these groups are indeed sterically similar, they differ significantly in physical and chemical properties, especially in acidity (pK_a 8–10 versus 3–5) and lipophilicity ($-1.8\,\pi$ versus $-0.3\,\pi$). Furthermore, compounds of the RCO_2H class can act as an acylating agents *in vivo*. Recent reports of antiinflammatory activity in a new class of sulfonamides, the fluoroalkanesulfonanilides, now warrant separate discussion of sulfonamides.

II. FLUOROALKANESULFONANILIDES

A. Background and Chemistry

The fluoroalkanesulfonanilides are a relatively new class of acidic antiinflammatory agents. Their antiedemic activity was discovered and developed during the period 1964–1971 in our laboratories, culminating in the selection of diflumidone (**7**) and triflumidate (**90**) for clinical trials (Harrington *et al.*, 1970). The lead compound, 4-acetyltrifluoromethanesulfonanilide (**3**), was synthesized during a general investigation into the chemical and biological properties of perfluoroalkanesulfonamides. This work also led to potent anticonvulsant agents ($CF_3SO_2NH_2$ and its *N*-acyl and *N*-alkyl derivatives; Moore *et al.*, 1970; Moore and Conway, 1971, 1972; Moore, 1971) and to a variety of herbicides and plant growth regulants (of the fluoroalkanesulfonanilide class) (Trepka *et al.*, 1970).

Our initial interest in these compounds was based on the unique properties of the CF_3SO_2 group as a highly lipophilic ($\pi = 0.95$), powerful electron attractor (Hammett $\sigma = 1.3$). Trifluoromethanesulfonyl fluoride and its higher homologs were synthesized by the Simons electrofluorination of alkanesulfonyl fluorides in liquid HF (Brice and Trott, 1956). Most of the trifluoromethanesulfonanilides were prepared by sulfonylation of the corresponding anilines with $(CF_3SO_2)_2O$ (highly reactive), CF_3SO_2F (less reactive, b.p. $-21°C$, by heating in an autoclave) or CF_3SO_2Cl (relatively unreactive). Homologous perfluoroalkanesulfonanilides were made from the corresponding $C_n F_{2n+1} SO_2 F$ either in an autoclave as above or from the alkali metal salt of the aniline, e.g., ArNHNa, at atmospheric pressure.

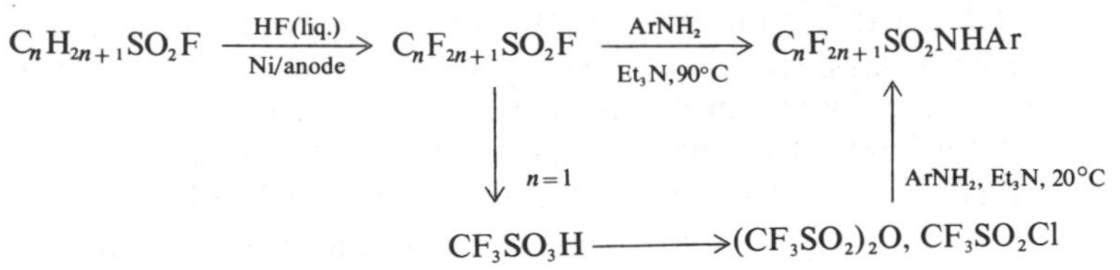

$$C_n H_{2n+1} SO_2 F \xrightarrow[\text{Ni/anode}]{\text{HF(liq.)}} C_n F_{2n+1} SO_2 F \xrightarrow[\text{Et}_3 N, 90^\circ C]{\text{ArNH}_2} C_n F_{2n+1} SO_2 NHAr$$

$$\downarrow n=1 \qquad\qquad\qquad \uparrow \text{ArNH}_2, \text{Et}_3 N, 20^\circ C$$

$$CF_3 SO_3 H \longrightarrow (CF_3 SO_2)_2 O, CF_3 SO_2 Cl$$

The requisite anilines were made by a host of routes that are not discussed here. The $NHSO_2 R_f$* group has proved very stable to acid and base and to conventional functional group interconversions, such as halogenation, oxidation, chemical and catalytic reduction, O-demethylation, Grignard additions, and nucleophilic displacement of aryl halide, allowing convenient synthesis of many more sulfonanilides. Intertwined with this study has been the extensive followup of plant growth regulatory activities. In these combined programs, at least 2500 compounds have been synthesized and most of these screened for antiinflammatory activity. Most of the data in this review are as yet unpublished.

B. Simple Trifluoromethanesulfonanilides

$CF_3 SO_2 NH_2$ and its N-alkyl derivatives were generally inactive at a screening dose of 100 mg/kg (i.e., were less active than aspirin in our assay) for inhibition of the carrageenan-induced edema of the rat's hind paw. The simple (monoaryl) sulfonanilides showed only marginal activity in this assay with few exceptions. Probably the most interesting historically are the acetyl derivatives, (2) and (3), which were very active in our original screen by the subcutaneous route but subsequently proved weaker by the oral route. All screening data reported here were obtained by the latter route of administration. Some higher alkyl homologs of (2) were found inactive at the screening dose but the m-benzoyl derivatives (5) was very potent (Table I). In general, o-acyl derivatives were active but noticeably more toxic than their meta or para isomers. Compound (5) served as a model for subsequent molecular modifications. The main synthetic directions included variations on the acidic group, ring-substituents, linking groups

---

*The term R_f represents an alkyl group substituted with one or more fluorines.

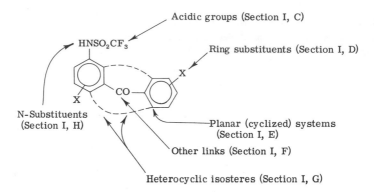

other than carbonyl, cyclization to near-planar systems, heterocyclic isosteres, and *N*-substituents.

C. Acidic Groups

1. PHYSICAL PROPERTIES

Trifluoromethanesulfonanilides are moderately strong organic acids, with ionization constants in the range 2.5–5, roughly similar to those of benzoic acids. The pK_a values of many of these compounds have been determined and representative values are listed in Table II for meta and

TABLE 1

Anticarrageenan Activity[a] of Some
$R - C_6H_4NHSO_2CF_3$

Compound	R	Activity
1	$2-COCH_3$	+, Toxic
2	$3-COCH_3$	+
3	$4-COCH_3$	+
4	$2-COC_6H_5$	±, Toxic
5	$3-COC_6H_5$	+4
6	$4-COC_6H_5$	±

[a] Rating system: $ED_{35} < 5$ mg/kg (p.o.), +5 (e.g., indomethacin); 5–10 mg/kg, +4; 11–25 mg/kg, +3 (e.g., phenylbutazone, flufenamic acid); 26–50 mg/kg, +2; 51–150 mg/kg, + (e.g., aspirin); and no significant activity at 100 mg/kg, ±. Groups of ten rats were used. Phenylbutazone (15 mg/kg) was included as a daily positive control, effecting $40 \pm 5\%$ inhibition of swelling. Maximum inhibition in this screen was 60–70%.

TABLE II

pK_a Values[a] for Some
R—$C_6H_4NHSO_2CF_3$

R	pK_a
H	4.45
3—Cl	3.85
4—Cl	4.00
4—F	4.40
4—CH_2CH_3	4.7
4—OCH_3	4.9
3—CF_3	3.55
4—CF_3	3.4
3—$COCH_3$	3.8
4—$COCH_3$	3.3
3—COC_6H_5	3.7
4—COC_6H_5	3.2
3—SO_2CH_3	3.05
4—SO_2CH_3	2.75

[a] For each solvent system, the half-neutralization potentials (HNP) were determined by titration with tetrabutylammonium hydroxide in 67% dimethylformamide and/or 50% isopropanol and extrapolated to aqueous values. These extrapolations were based on the aqueous pK_a values measured for five water-soluble $RNHSO_2CF_3$ plotted against their HNP values in each solvent system (J. K. Harrington and J. Belisle, unpublished data, 1967).

para monosubstituted derivatives. These pK_a values are linearly related to Hammett's σ constant (the fit to σ^- is poorer) and the slope (ρ value) is 2.15. Therefore, the ionization in its substituent dependence lies between benzoic acids ($\rho = 1.0$) and phenols (2.2).

In the course of an investigation of alternative acidic groups (see Table IV), Harrington discovered a very simple and elegant method to vary the acidity of these agents. He found that stepwise replacement of the α-fluorine by hydrogen gave an incremental decrease in acidity of approximately 1.5 pK_a units per fluorine in two methanesulfonanilide series (Table III). This

TABLE III

Acidity and Lipophilicity of $R-C_6H_4NHSO_2R_f$

R	R_f			
	CF_3	CHF_2	CH_2F	CH_3
	$pK_a{}^a$			
H	4.45	6.0	7.5	8.7
$3-COC_6H_5$	3.7	5.3	6.5	8.2
$4-Cl$	3.9	5.4	6.7	—
	$\log P^b$			
H	3.05	1.95	1.35	0.95
$4-Cl$	3.96	2.84	2.25	1.85
	π of R_fSO_2NH			
	0.92	−0.18	−0.78	−1.13

[a]Extrapolated to water from values determined in 67% dimethylformamide (J. K. Harrington and J. Belisle, unpublished data, 1967).

[b]Log P values derived by partitioning between octanol and 0.1 N perchloric acid (R. D. Trepka, J. K. Harrington, and J. Belisle, unpublished data, 1974).

tool allowed significant changes in the acidity with essentially no alteration of stereochemistry and no change in ring substitution. No other acidic antiinflammatory series possessed such flexibility.

Measurements of lipophilicity are less complete, but it is clear that trifluoromethanesulfonanilides are highly lipophilic. Initially the log D data were determined by partitioning the sulfonanilides between octanol and distilled water (C. D. Green and J. K. Harrington, unpublished data, 1968). These were corrected to log P by dividing by $(1-\alpha)$, α being the degree of ionization. Because α is so large (0.72 for $CF_3SO_2NHC_6H_5$) or because the ionized forms may be significantly soluble in octanol, these values are felt to be less reliable than the log P values obtained by partitioning between octanol and acidic buffer of pH 1, in which α approaches zero (R. D. Trepka, J. K. Harrington, and J. Belisle, unpublished data, 1974). The resulting log P and π data (Table III) show that the changes in pK_a associated with variation of the number of α-fluorines are accompanied by significant changes in lipophilicity. Comparison of parent log P values for various acidic systems emphasizes the unique position of trifluoromethanesulfonanilide (3.05) relative to phenol (1.46), benzoic acid (1.85), phenylacetic acid (1.41), and phenoxyacetic acid (1.28).

2. CHEMISTRY

Known Strecker reaction sequences can be used to prepare the partially fluorinated sulfonyl chlorides, as exemplified below for the important CHF_2SO_2Cl and CH_2FSO_2Cl. [This method, developed by Farrar (1960), works well for small batches but has proven difficult in large scale work.]

$$CH_xF_yCl \xrightarrow{Na_2SO_3} CH_xF_ySO_3Na \xrightarrow{PCl_5} CH_xF_ySO_2Cl$$

$CF_3CH_2SO_2Cl$ was prepared in high yield via the trifluoromethanesulfonate ester, as shown. The corresponding sulfonanilide (17) was readily hydrolyzed in base to the sulfoacetic acid derivative (15).

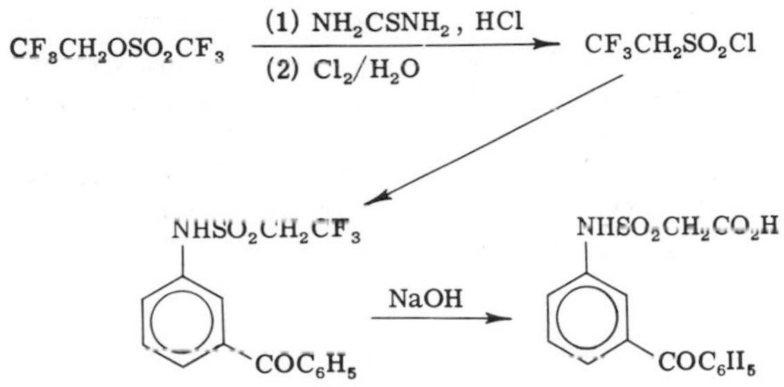

$$CF_3CH_2OSO_2CF_3 \xrightarrow[\text{(2) } Cl_2/H_2O]{\text{(1) } NH_2CSNH_2, \text{ HCl}} CF_3CH_2SO_2Cl$$

17   15

The other acidic and nonacidic alternatives of Table IV were made by conventional routes (Harrington *et al.*, 1971).

3. BIOLOGICAL ACTIVITY

Partially halogenated methanesulfonanilides (7), (8), and (10), were highly potent in the carrageenan assay, whereas the unsubstituted methanesulfonanilide (9) was only marginally active. Generally, sulfonanilides derived from larger alkane/arenesulfonyl groups were less potent (Table IV).

Separation of the aromatic ring and the nitrogen by CH_2 (benzylsulfonamide, 27) substantially reduced activity. Many alternatives to the $NHSO_2R_f$ group were considered as illustrated by (28)–(37). Only the known (Juby, Chapter 4) arylacetic acid (37) had high potency in this test.

Detailed comparison of compounds (5), (7), (8), and (10) in various antiinflammatory–analgetic models is shown in Table V. In the carrageenan test, the relative order of potency is (8) > (5) > (7), (10), but in the guinea pig UV-erythema model, the order becomes (5) > (7) > > (8), (10).

TABLE IV

Anticarrageenan Activity of

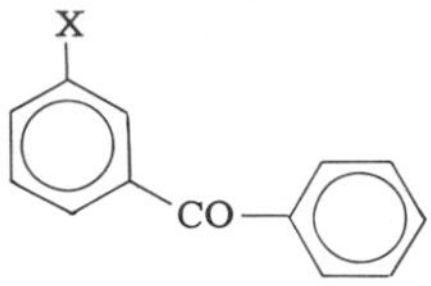

Compound	X	Activity	Compound	X	Activity
5	CF_3SO_2NH	+4	22	$CH_3(CH_2)_3SO_2NH$	$\pm$
7	CHF_2SO_2NH	+3	23	$(CH_3)_2NSO_2NH$	$\pm$
8	CH_2FSO_2NH	+4	24	$4-CH_3-C_6H_4SO_2NH$	$\pm$
9	CH_3SO_2NH	+	25	$4-Cl-C_6H_4SO_2NH$	$\pm$
10	CH_2ClSO_2NH	+3	26	$4-NO_2-C_6H_4SO_2NH$	$\pm$
11	CH_2ISO_2NH	+	27	$CF_3SO_2NH-CH_2$	+
12	$CHCl_2SO_2NH$	+	28	CF_3CONH	+
13	$CH_2=CHSO_2NH$	$\pm$	29	CH_3CONH	+
14	$CH_3COCH_2SO_2NH$	+	30	EtO_2CNH	$\pm$
15	$HO_2CCH_2SO_2NH$	$\pm$	31	$(EtO)_2PONH$	$\pm$
16	$CH_3CH(NO_2)SO_2NH$	$\pm$	32	H_2N	+
17	$CF_3CH_2SO_2NH$	+2	33	HS	+
18	$HCF_2CF_2SO_2NH$	+2	34	HO	+2
19	$C_2F_5SO_2NH$	+3	35	H_2NSO_2	$\pm$
20	$CF_3CHFCF_2SO_2NH$	+	36	HO_2C	+
21	$CF_3(CF_2)_3SO_2NH$	+	37	HO_2CCH_2	+4

Compounds (5) and (7) were compared in a wide variety of laboratory tests and found to be very similar. The pharmacology of (7) (diflumidone sodium) was described in detail by Swingle *et al.* (1971a). Both the dose–response curves in the carrageenan test and the overall profiles paralleled those of indomethacin and phenylbutazone. On the basis of toxicological studies in dogs and rats, (7) was chosen for clinical studies (as the sodium salt).

Ober *et al.* (1971) and Hoogland *et al.* (1969) published preliminary metabolic data gathered with tritiated diflumidone. Marked species differences were seen among rats, dogs, and man in the nature of urinary metabolites, extent of conjugation, and in the plasma half-life (see Chapter 10, by Ober, in Volume II).

D. Ring-Substituted Fluoroalkanesulfonamidobenzophenones

The effects of a variety of substituents and combinations thereof on (5) and (7) were tested. Some of these derivatives showed anticarrageenan potency equal to that of the unsubstituted parent but most were less active.

TABLE V

Pharmacology of

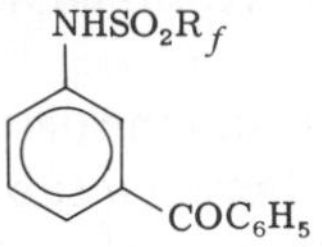

NHSO$_2$R$_f$

(structure: benzene ring with NHSO$_2$R$_f$ and COC$_6$H$_5$ substituents)

Compound	R$_f$	Carrageenan ED$_{35}$ (mg/kg)	UV-erythema[a] ED$_{50}$	Adjuvant[b] arthritis MED	Phenyl-quinone[c] writhing ED$_{50}$	ALD$_{50}$[d]
5	CF$_3$	10	6	18	5	562
7	CHF$_2$	11.5	9.4	16	30	700
8	CH$_2$F	6.7	117	>> 18	>> 25	1750
10	CH$_2$Cl	11	>> 50	—	—	2340
Phenylbutazone		14	—	2	—	—
Indomethacin		1.2	—	< 1	—	—

[a] Guinea pigs, p.o.
[b] Rats, minimum effective dose, p.o., therapeutic assay.
[c] Mice, p.o.
[d] Acute, approximate LD$_{50}$, mice, p.o.

A noteworthy attempt to systematically approach the substituent problem involved preparation of both of the sets of seven possible mono-Cl and mono-CH$_3$ derivatives of (**5**) [Table VI, (**38**)–(**51**) and (**57**)–(**63**) (R. J. Trancik, unpublished data, 1969; Robertson *et al.*, 1971).] The basic premise was that

TABLE VI

Anticarrageenan Activity of Selected

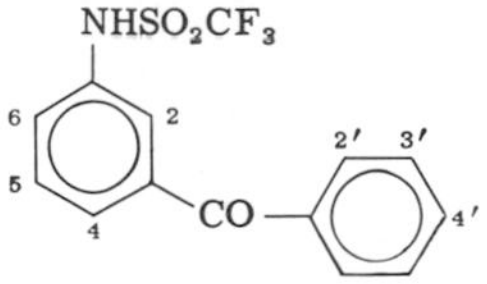

NHSO$_2$CF$_3$

(structure: benzene ring with positions 2, 4, 5, 6 labeled, and CO linked to a second benzene ring with positions 2', 3', 4' labeled)

Compound	Substituent	Activity	Compound	Substituent	Activity
38	2 — Cl	+	**45**	2 — CH$_3$	±
39	4 — Cl	±	**46**	4 — CH$_3$	±
40	5 — Cl	±	**47**	5 — CH$_3$	±
41	6 — Cl	+	**48**	6 — CH$_3$	+
42	2' — Cl	+2	**49**	2' — CH$_3$	+3
43	3' — Cl	+	**50**	3' — CH$_3$	±
44	4' — Cl	+3	**51**	4' — CH$_3$	+2

these groups possessed reasonably similar steric and lipophilic natures with opposite electronic effects. Trancik therefore hoped to identify positions sensitive to stereoelectronic factors. Somewhat disappointingly, no compound in these groups was equivalent or superior to (5).

Related studies of (7), (8), and (10) gave similar results. From the data presently available, no obvious relationship was discernable between substituents (position and steric, electronic, and lipophilic character) and activity.

E. Planar Systems

Continued testing of a large number of monoaryl fluoroalkanesulfonanilides from the herbicide program has emphasized the apparent necessity of a second aryl ring. Several "tied-back" systems have proved active in related carboxylic acid systems (e.g., see Chapter 4 by Juby in this Volume). Some examples of this type are illustrated in Table VII. These coplanar or nearcoplanar systems exhibited considerably reduced activity.

F. Linked Diaryl Systems

A fairly comprehensive examination of linking groups was made (Moore *et al.*, 1971; Moore and Harrington, 1972; Trancik *et al.*, 1972). A broad spectrum of systems had quite good activity in the anticarrageenan assay (Table VIII). Where all three ortho, meta, and para isomers were examined,

TABLE VII

Anticarrageenan Activity of

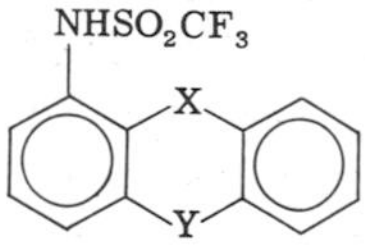

Compound	X	Y	Activity
52	C=O	(σ bond)	$\pm$
53	CH$_2$	(σ bond)	$\pm$
54[a]	C=O	S	$\pm$
55	C=O	O	$\pm$
56	C=O	C=O	$\pm$
57	C=O	CH$_2$—CH$_2$	$+$
58	NH	CH$_2$—CH$_2$	$\pm$

[a]Compound (54) was the CHF$_2$SO$_2$NH derivative.

TABLE VIII

Anticarrageenan Activity of Selected

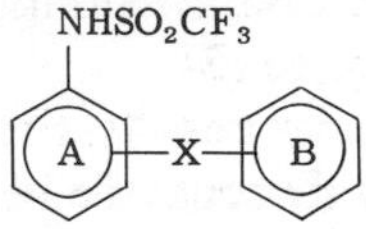

NHSO$_2$CF$_3$

Compound	A — X — B	Meta	Ortho	Para
	C=O	+4	+	±
59	CHOH	+2		
60	CH$_2$	+	+	
61	C=CH$_2$	+3		
62	COCH$_2$	±		
63	CH$_2$CO	+		
64	trans-CH=CH	+3	+3	+3
65	cis-CH=CH	+	+	
66	CH$_2$CH$_2$	±	±	+
67	C≡C	+2	+	+
68	NH	+3	+2	+2
69	O	+3	+2	⊥
70	S	+3	+2	±
71	SO	±	±	±
72	SO$_2$	±	±	±
73	σ bond	+	+	+

activity generally proved best for the meta and lowest for the para isomers, with several ortho isomers proving quite active.

The results suggest that a favorable steric relationship involves a "bent" diaryl system with the second ring ortho or meta to the sulfonamido group. [The term "bent" means here that the center of mass of the B ring can lie below (or above) the plane of the A ring.] The superior activity of *trans*-stilbenes (**64**) is unexpected. Indeed, Dreiding models of the *cis-o*-stilbene (**65**) show that in one noncoplanar configuration it very closely resembles the *m*-benzophenone (**5**); yet this isomer proves less potent than the trans (**64**). Electronic effects of the linking group on the activity do not conform to a pattern, with both active and inactive compounds resulting from electron-donating and electron-attracting linking groups. It may be significant that the more active compounds contain groups that are capable of mesomeric interaction with one or both rings (C=O, **5**; C=CH$_2$, **61**; CH=CH, **64**; NH, **68**; O, **69**; S, **70**. Substituent changes on both rings and on the R$_f$SO$_2$ group have been extensively explored, with results quite similar to those with the benzophenones. The *ortho*-diphenylamine (**68**) is superficially structurally related to the *N*-phenylanthranilic acids, leading to interest in B-ring substituted derivatives, such as (74) and (75). These are less active.

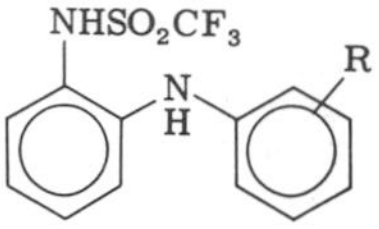

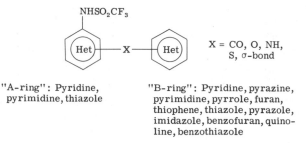

74 R = 3-CF$_3$ (±)

75 R = 2,3-Cl$_2$ (±)

G. Heterocyclic Isosteres

A diverse series of heterocyclic isosteres of (5) and other linked sulfonanilides has been examined (Moore *et al.*, 1972a,b; Moore and Gerster, 1972; Harrington *et al.*, 1972). Some of the more interesting compounds are listed below. Two compounds, (77) and (78), are more potent than (5) in the carra-

X = CO, O, NH, S, σ-bond

"A-ring": Pyridine, pyrimidine, thiazole

"B-ring": Pyridine, pyrazine, pyrimidine, pyrrole, furan, thiophene, thiazole, pyrazole, imidazole, benzofuran, quinoline, benzothiazole

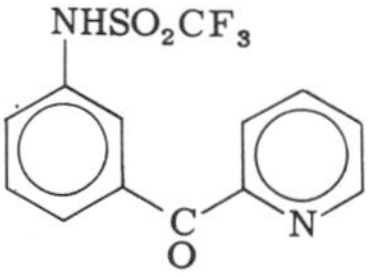

geenan assay. Secondary testing of several of these series has led to the selection of 3-(2-thiazolythio)trifluoromethanesulfonanilide (78) for further studies. The ortho (82) and para (83) isomers are less active (+3, +, respectively). Some other thiazoles and their anticarrageenan activities are illus-

76 (+3)

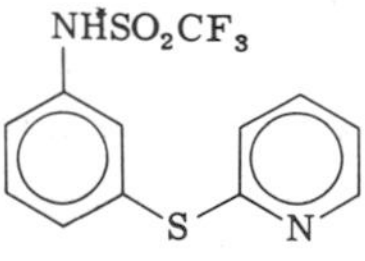

77 (+5)

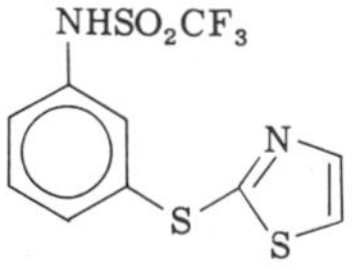

78 (+4)

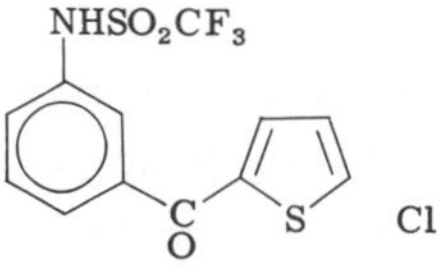

79 (+3)

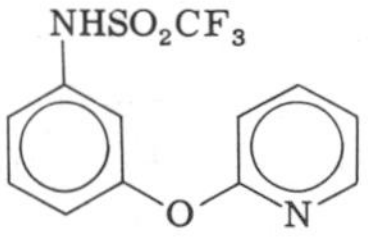

80 (+3)

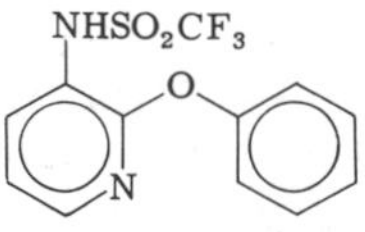

81 (+3)

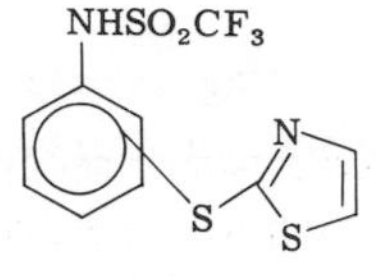

82 ortho (+3)	**84** R = CHF_2 (+3)	**87** X = CO (+2)
83 para (+)	**85** R = CH_2Cl (+3)	**88** X = O (+3)
	86 R = C_2F_5 (+2)	**89** X = SO_2 (+)

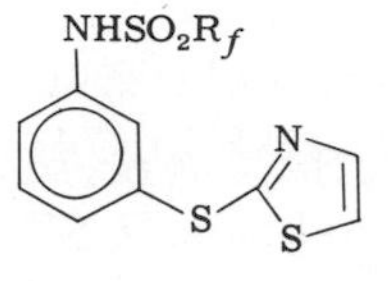

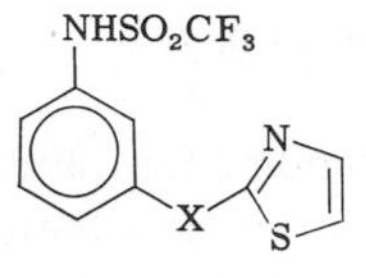

trated by (**84**)–(**89**). Compound (**78**) resembles diflumidone (**7**) in its anti-inflammatory profile. It is highly active in the carrageenan and UV-erythema assays (ED_{35} = 7.5 mg/kg and ED_{40} < 5 mg/kg, respectively) and moderately active against adjuvant arthritis (therapeutic) at 40 mg/kg. An unfavorable subacute toxicity in dogs indicates against further development.

H. N-Substituents

A wide variety of N-substituted derivatives of the fluoroalkanesulfonanilides was prepared in the course of structure–activity relationship (SAR) studies. These derivatives could be active in themselves or in some cases might serve as precursors of the free sulfonanilides. Compounds prepared included R = AlkOCO (Harrington, 1972a), CH_3SO_2 (Harrington, 1972b), NC (Gerster, 1972), and alkyl (Robertson et al., 1971). Generally these compounds were less potent (on a milligram dose per kilogram body weight basis) than the corresponding free acids. A primary advantage of many of these was an improved therapeutic ratio.

The pharmacology of the ethoxycarbonyl derivative of (**5**), triflumidate (**90**), is summarized by Swingle et al. (1971b) and preliminary metabolic data are reported by Chang et al. (1970). It is not currently under active clinical investigation.

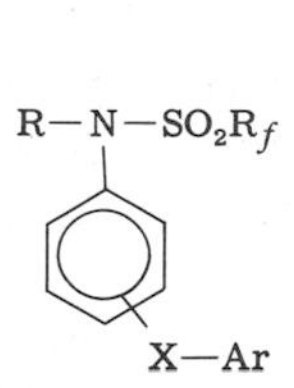

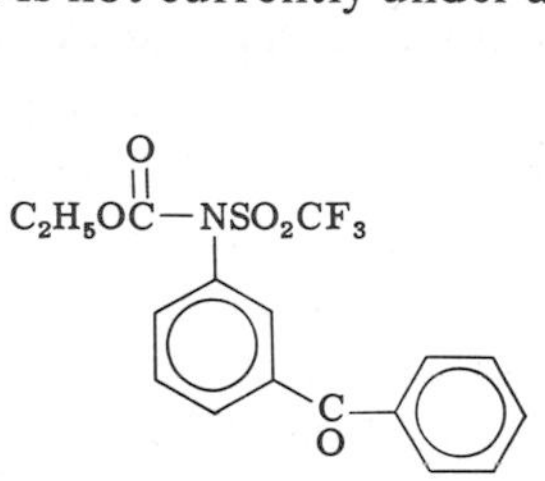

90

We currently feel that the N-substituted derivatives serve as precursors in vivo of the active acidic sulfonanilide. This view is based on the pharmacological similarities between the two classes and on preliminary metabolic data in vitro and in vivo.

I. Summary

Some general aspects of the SAR as presently revealed deserve recapitulation. The key feature seems to be the R_fSO_2NH group, where R_f is preferrably a halomethyl or ethyl group. Nonhalogenated, larger alkyl, and aryl RSO_2NH groups have in general given less active derivatives. High potency is seen with compounds possessing quite different acidities (pK_a 3.2–6.5). There is a potency advantage associated with a second aryl ring meta or ortho to the sulfonamido group. Of the structural links between the two rings that have been tested, the favorable ones have in common high π-electron density. Cyclization of the diaryl system to form near-coplanar molecules lowers the activity, implying a need for either mobility or a "bent" conformation.

Fluoroalkanesulfonanilides differ from their nonfluorinated analogs most obviously in their greater acidity and lipophilicity. However, initial Hansch-type analyses have not revealed any systematic relationship between anti-carrageenan activity and pK_a, π, or π^2. No useful relationships have been discovered between activity and the nature or position of ring substituents in either the A or the B ring, except that most such derivatives were less potent than their parents. Likewise, the isosteric substitution of various heterocyclic rings led to no discernable patterns, although several isosteres were quite competitive in potency with the benzenoid systems. N-Substituents reduced both the activity and, more dramatically, the toxicity. Much circumstantial and some direct evidence favored *in vivo* conversion to the unsubstituted fluoroalkanesulfonanilide.

The haloalkanesulfonanilide class, although chemically distinct, may act pharmacologically in a manner similar to many carboxylic and enolic nonsteroidal antiinflammatory agents and does possess certain structural features in common with the latter, namely an acidic function on a diaryl system. Thus, diflumidone and its congeners can be fitted to the receptor site hypothesized by Scherrer *et al.* (1964) and by Shen (1965). This concept has been applied to acids including $NHSO_2R_f$, CO_2H, $CHRCO_2H$, and OCH_2CO_2H oriented ortho, meta, and para on variously linked diaryl systems, necessitating considerable flexibility in both the macromolecule(s) and the medicinal chemists.

To us, the chief value of the concept lies in the impetus it gives to syntheses designed to test its applicability. Thus, in the link study, this hypothesis induced a broader examination of the ortho and para positions than would be suggested by simple biosteric principles. It also led to a more critical evaluation of the relationship of our series to others. Structurally, the haloalkanesulfonanilides are similar to phenols and enolic compounds, in which the anionic atom is directly bound to the flat (A) ring. However, other comparative data hints that pharmacologically they correspond more closely to the arylacetic acids, although this correspondence is by no means exact.

III. OTHER SULFONAMIDES

Scattered reports of antiinflammatory activity of other sulfonamides do exist, primarily in the patent literature. However, in many of these, the sulfonamide group does not play a key role. Thus, the sulfamoyl and substituted sulfamoyl groups are claimed as substituents on active systems, as in the N-arylanthranilic acid series (Scherrer, Chapter 3 in this volume). Further, the —SO$_2$H— moiety appears as a structural element as in sudoxicam (Lombardino, Chapter 5 in this volume) and in linked analogs (91) of flufenisal (Scherrer, Chapter 3 in this volume) and of phenylacetic acids (92) (Juby, Chapter 4 in this volume).

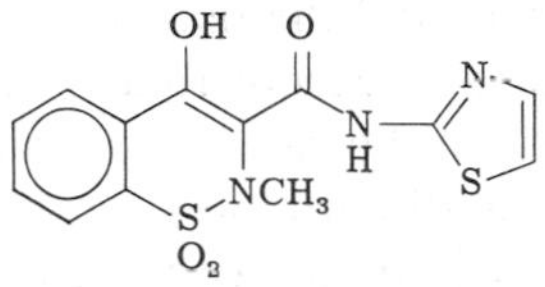

Sudoxicam

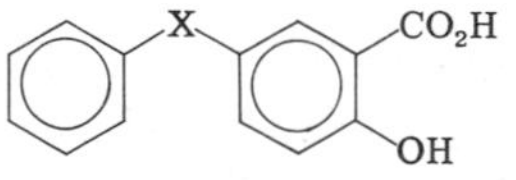

X = SO$_2$NH
NHSO$_2$

91

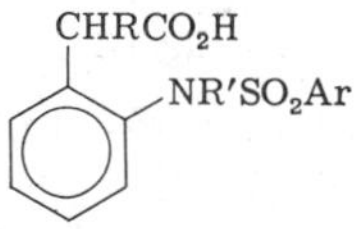

CHRCO$_2$H
NR'SO$_2$Ar

R' = H, alkyl,
acyl

92

The objective in this section is to survey those sulfonamides in which this group seems to be essential for activity and especially those in which it appears to function as the acidic group in the acidic, nonsteroidal antiinflammatory agent.

A. Arenesulfonamides

Pyridinesulfonamides (93) and (94) (Mizzoni and Blatter, 1971) and (95) (Mizzoni and Blatter, 1972) bear an obvious resemblance to the nicotinic acid derivatives niflumic acid (antiinflammatory) and triflocin (diuretic).

All three types are claimed to possess anticarrageenan activity, whereas the sulfonic acids related to (93) and (94) are cited as diuretics.

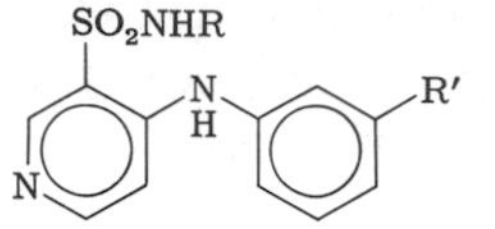

93 R = H
94 R = NH

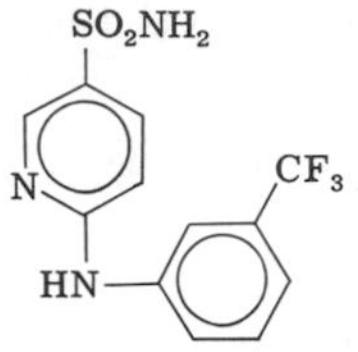

95

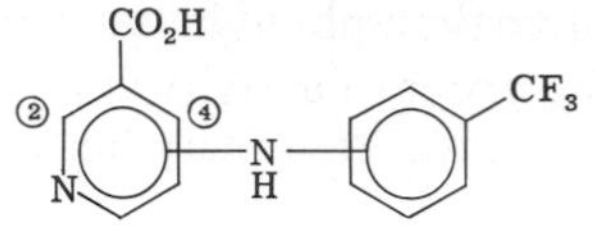

2-Isomer niflumic
acid
4-Isomer triflocin

A sulfonamide isostere (96) of flufenisal has been stated to be active (Sarett, 1969), although the parent sulfonic acid appears to be the primary objective of this patent.

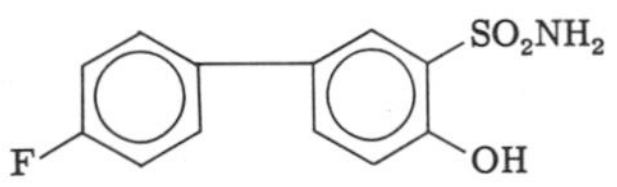

96

B. Sulfonamidoarenes/Alkanes

Tauropyrine (97) has been synthesized from aminopyrine with the hope of favorably altering the metabolism and toxicity of the latter (Naito *et al.*, 1971). In the rat paw carrageenan assay, (97) has weak activity (ED_{35} ca. 300 mg/kg, p.o.). Metabolites in rabbit urine included 4-amino-, 4-acet-amido-, and (traces) 4-hydroxyantipyrine. Compound (98) is claimed active against formalin and dextran edemas, whereas isomer (99) is inactive (Castel-mur, 1972).

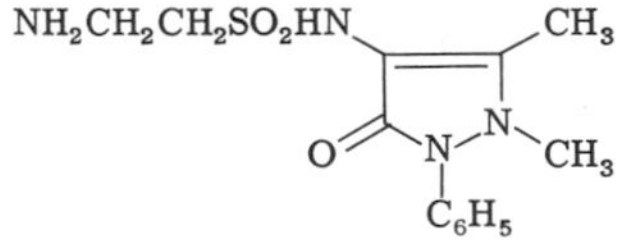

97

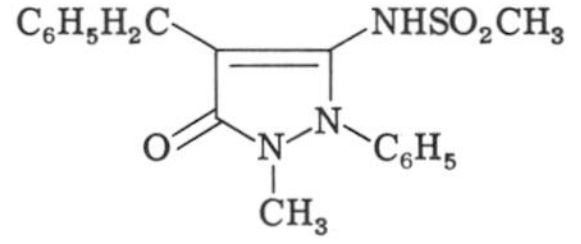

98

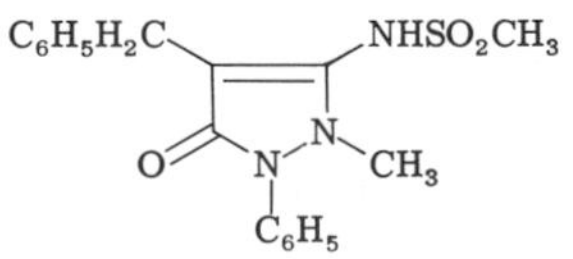

99

Recently, Borne *et al*. (1972) reported a series of *N*-arenesulfonyl derivatives of phenylalanine to be active against carrageenan edema and against heat-induced hemolysis of human red blood cells. Compound (**100**) was more active than phenylbutazone in the edema test and had a similar acute LD_{50}. The order of activity appeared to be DL > L > D, but the significance of the difference in activity between the DL and L forms was questionable.

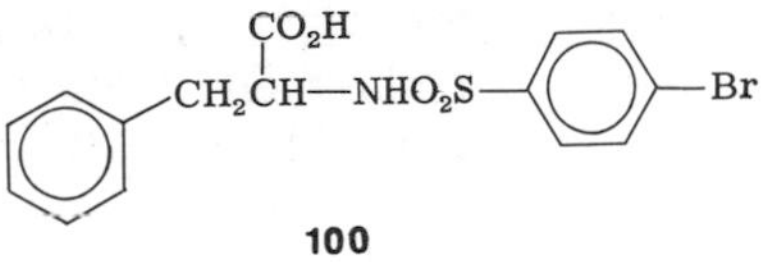

100

C. *N*-Acylsulfonamides

Conversion of active carboxylic acids to the corresponding acylsulfonamides leads to patentably distinct compounds, as typified by (**101**) and (**102**) (Scherrer, 1969) and (**103**) (Childress and Szabo, 1971). The latter compounds are claimed to be approximately as active as their parent acids. Although this class appears to be a latentiated form of the acid (i.e., hydrolyzable *in vivo*), the acidic derivatives (**101**) and (**103**) are isosteric with the carboxylic acids and conceivably can be active in themselves, if sufficiently stable.

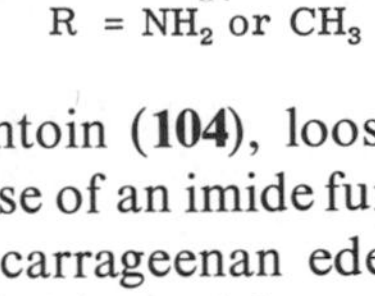

101 R′ = H,
R = NH₂ or CH₃

102 R′ = CH₃,
R = NH₂ or CH₃

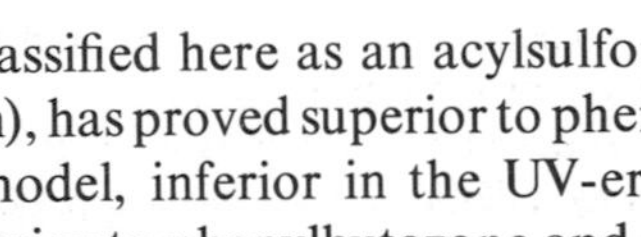

R = CH₃ or Ar
R′ = H or CH₃

103

The hydantoin (**104**), loosely classified here as an acylsulfonamide (but acidic because of an imide function), has proved superior to phenylbutazone in a mouse carrageenan edema model, inferior in the UV-erythema and adjuvant arthritis models, and superior to phenylbutazone and aspirin as an antipyretic (Nakamura *et al*., 1970a). It has modest activity in assays for analgetic activity (phenylquinone writhing, yeast hyperesthesia) and lies between phenylbutazone and aspirin in acute toxicity. Blood level studies in rats, dogs, and monkeys indicate a half-life for (**104**) greater than that of phenylbutazone (Nakamura *et al*., 1970b). Compound (**105**) (inactive against carrageenan-induced edema) has been identified as a metabolite in rat

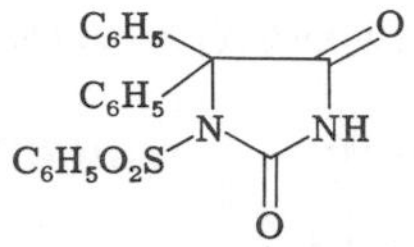

104

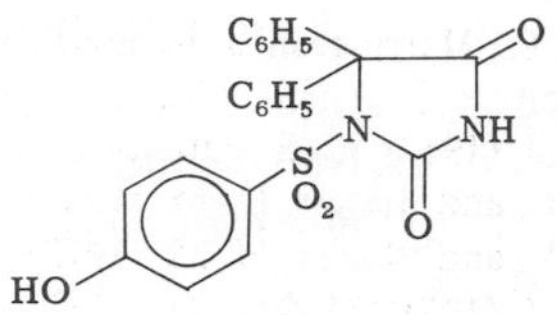

105

plasma; a second, unidentified product has also been found (Nakamura *et al.*, 1970c). Thus, the *N*-benzenesulfonyl derivative of the anticonvulsant diphenylhydantoin has unexpectedly led to (**104**) as an interesting anti-inflammatory agent.

D. Sulfamides

Houlihan (1967) has described two types of sulfamides as active anti-inflammatory agents, as typified by (**105**)–(**107**). These are unlikely to be appreciably ionized at physiological pH.

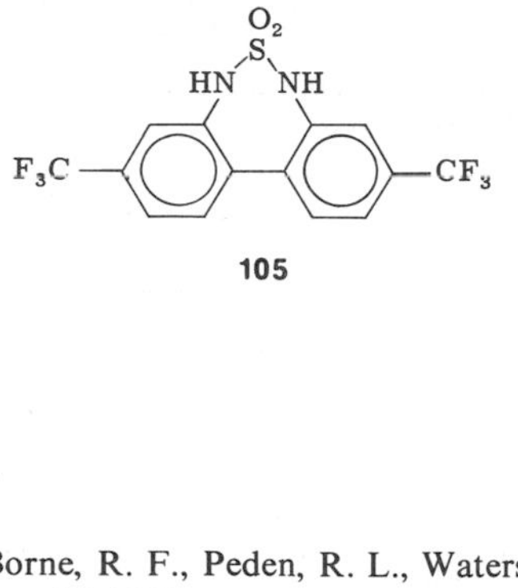

105

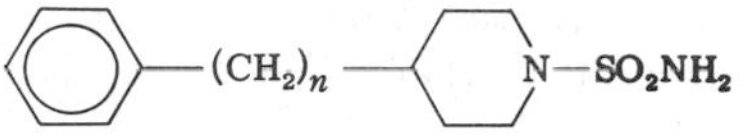

106 $n = 0$
107 $n = 1$

REFERENCES

Borne, R. F., Peden, R. L., Waters, I. W., Weiner, M., and Walz, M. (1972). *J. Med. Chem.* **15**, 1325.

Brice, T. J., and Trott, P. W. (1956). U. S. Patent 2,732,398.

Castelmur, H. V. (1972). U. S. Patent 3,681,383.

Chang, S. F., Hoogland, D. R., Ober, R. E., and Holmes, E. L. (1970). *Fed. Proc., Fed. Amer. Soc. Exp. Biol.* **29**, 678 (abstr.).

Childress, S. J., and Szabo, J. L. (1971). U. S. Patent 3,560,563.

Farrar, W. Y. (1960). *J. Chem. Soc., London.* p. 3058.

Gerster, J. F. (1972). U. S. Patent 3,647,874.

Harrington, J. K. (1972a). U. S. Patent 3,661,990.

Harrington, J. K. (1972b). U. S. Patent 3,663,708.

Harrington, J. K., Robertson, J. E., Kvam, D. C., Hamilton, R. R., McGurran, K. T., Trancik, R. J., Swingle, K. F., Moore, G. G. I., and Gerster, J. F. (1970). *J. Med. Chem.* **13**, 137.

Harrington, J. K., Trancik, R. J., Swingle, K. F., Hamilton, R. R., Robertson, J. E., and Kvam, D. C. (1971). *161st Nat. Meet. Amer. Chem. Soc.* Abstract MEDI 21.

Harrington, J. K., Moore, G. G. I., and Gerster, J. F. (1972). U. S. Patent 3,696,122.

Hoogland, D. R., Harrington, J. K., Funk, M. L., and Kvam, D. C. (1969). *Pharmacologist* 11, 291 (abstr.).

Houlihan, W. J. (1967). U; S. Patents 3,329,687 and 3,334,104.

Mizzoni, R. H., and Blatter, H. M. (1971). German Patent 2,054,142.

Mizzoni, R. H., and Blatter, H. M. (1972). U. S. Patent 3,671,512.

Moore, G. G. I. (1971). U. S. Patent 3,622,626.

Moore, G. G. I., and Conway, A. C. (1971). U. S. Patent 3,609,187.

Moore, G. G. I., and Conway, A. C. (1972). U. S. Patents 3,637,845 and 3,705,185.

Moore, G. G. I., and Gerster, J. F. (1972). U. S. Patent, 3,679,695.

Moore, G. G. I., and Harrington, J. K. (1972). U. S. Patent 3,689,553.

Moore, G. G. I., Lappi, L. R., Bachhuber, J. E., and Conway, A. C. (1970). *160th Nat. Meet. Amer. Chem. Soc.* Abstract MEDI 17.

Moore, G. G. I., Swingle, K. F., and Harrington, J. K. (1971). *Pharmacologist* 13, 524 (abstr.).

Moore, G. G. I., Swingle, K; F., and Gerster, J. F. (1972a). *13th Nat. Meet., Acad. Pharm. Sci., 1972* Abstracts, p. 107.

Moore, G. G. I., Harrington, J. K., and Gerster, J. F. (1972b). U. S. Patent 3,686,192.

Naito, S. I., Ueno, Y., Yamaguchi, H., and Nakai, T. (1971). *J. Pharm. Sci.* 60, 245.

Nakamura, H., Kadokawa, T., Nakatsuji, K., and Nakamura, K. (1970a). *Arzneim.-Forsch.* 20, 1032.

Nakamura, H., Soji, Y., Masuda, Y., and Nakamura, K. (1970b). *Arzneim.-Forsch.* 20, 1579.

Nakamura, H-, Nakatsuji, K., and Nakamura, K. (1970c). *Arzneim-Forsch.* 20, 1729.

Ober, R. E., Chang, S. F., Miller, A. M., Funk, M. L., and Holmes, E. L. (1971). *Pharmacologist* 13, 580 (abstr.).

Robertson, J. E., Harrington, J. K., and Kvam, D. C. (1971). U. S. Patent 3,567,806.

Sarett, L. H., and Hannah, J. (1972). British Patent 1, 263, 220.

Scherrer, R. A. (1969). U. S. Patent 3,471,559.

Scherrer, R. A., Winder, C. V., and Short, F. W. (1964). *Nat. Med. Chem. Symp., Amer. Chem. Soc., 9th, 1964* Abstract p. 11g.

Shen, T. Y. (1965). *Int. Symp. Non-Steroidal Anti-Inflammatory Drugs, Proc., 1964* p. 13.

Swingle, K. F., Hamilton, R. R., Harrington, J. K., and Kvam, D. C. (1971a). *Arch. Int. Pharmacodyn. Ther.* 189, 129.

Swingle, K. F., Harrington, J. K., Hamilton, R. R., and Kvam, D. C. (1971b). *Arch. Int. Pharmacodyn. Ther.* 192, 16.

Trancik, R. J., Moore, G. G. I., and Harrington, J. K. (1972). U. S. Patent 3,689,523.

Trepka, R. D., Harrington, J. K., Robertson, J. E., and Waddington, J. T. (1970). *J. Agr. Food Chem.* 18, 1176.

Chapter 7

Nonacidic Antiarthritic Agents and the Search for New Classes of Agents

T. Y. SHEN

Merck Sharp & Dohme Research Laboratories
Rahway, New Jersey

I. INTRODUCTION

In medicinal chemistry any generalization that associates certain types of biological activity with a specific functional group, such as quaternary ammonium ion or carboxylic acid, is an oversimplification. The word "non-acidic" in the title has been adopted partly to acknowledge the very large number of aryl acids or acid equivalents developed in recent years as anti-inflammatory agents and partly to indicate a natural change of emphasis in many laboratories looking for newer types of antiarthritic compounds.

The development of antiarthritic drugs has been an area of intensive research since the 1940's. Major interest in this prolonged and widespread endeavor seems to evolve in clearly defined stages: the pyrazolones in the early 1940's, a decade of increasingly more potent corticosteroids in the 1950's, and a wide variety of aryl acids in the 1960's. As more substituted arylcarboxylic acids, or acid equivalents, are proceeding steadily into clinical trials, one begins to witness the natural transition of synthetic studies to newer structural types, conveniently designated here as "nonacidic" compounds.

Biologically, efforts are continuing in many laboratories to analyze the classical assays of the early 1960's, the rat paw carrageenan-induced edema assay and the adjuvant arthritis model, and to establish newer ones hopefully bearing closer resemblance to the clinical disease of rheumatoid arthritis. With the advent of modern immunological and histopathological techniques and with the timely coupling of clinical research and molecular pharmacology, a new stage is built for the discovery of superior antiarthritic agents.

II. THE SEARCH FOR NEW STRUCTURAL TYPES

A. Possible Improvement of Efficacy and Tolerance

The search for new types of agents reflects the realization that in spite of the proliferative introduction of many antiinflammatory–analgesic–antipyretic agents in recent years there is still a need for antiarthritic compounds with improved efficacy and tolerance. Many of the new clinical or experimental agents disclosed as far undoubtedly may have some utility in the clinic. However, judging from their pharmacological data in animals, few or none can be expected to be qualitatively superior to such existing drugs as aspirin, indomethacin, or phenylbutazone.

Both the relevance and the predictive value of standard efficacy assays have been continuously under scrutiny. The inadequacy of using the minimal effective dose levels in animal models as a measure for clinical potency has been repeatedly illustrated in this field. The daily clinical dosage of aspirin, phenylbutazone, and indomethacin in rheumatoid arthritis patients is approximately 3 gm, 300 mg, and 100 mg, respectively. Aside from differences in their potential side effects, the observed antiinflammatory effects for all three drugs are generally comparable. These clinical observations are not in accord with expectations based on their potency ratios in several animal assays, which are 1:4:100. [An analysis of these data along pharmacokinetic lines is presented by Wiseman, Chapter 6, Volume II.] Questions have been raised about the clinical correlation of some antiinflammatory assays and the variations of drug bioavailability in different species. The bioavailability of a drug is determined by its pharmacodynamic properties, absorption, distribution, metabolism, and excretion. Antiinflammatory aryl acids, such as indomethacin, have been shown to be well absorbed and distributed mainly in the extracellular fluid. The distribution kinetics of indomethacin between plasma and synovial fluid have been analyzed by Emori and associates (1972). It seems possible, if synovial fluid is considered a representative tissue compartment, to use a two-compartment model to estimate the drug concentration at target sites in this case. Simple formulas, such as

$$\text{Intrinsic potency} \times \text{bioavailability} = \text{drug effect}$$

$$\text{Bioavailability} = \int c \, dt$$

$$c = \text{plasma level of synovial fluid level, } t = \text{duration of drug action}$$

or similar expressions have been used to estimate the potency of a drug.

With nonacidic types of compounds, more complicated tissue distribution and cellular uptake may occur. The predominant metabolic pathway for aryl acids, glucuronide conjugation, and urinary excretion, are also replaced by other modes of drug metabolism. The changes make the correlation of laboratory data and clinical performance of nonacidic agents somewhat less predictable than for aryl acids. However, in a positive manner, these uncertainties have encouraged the initiation of clinical pharmacological studies in the early phase of drug development and put the selection of clinical candidates on a more rational basis.

With respect to patient tolerance or drug safety, the most common side effect of antiinflammatory drugs, gastrointestinal (G.I.) irritation, is routinely checked in all laboratories. The predisposition of rheumatoid patients to G.I. lesions is considered a contributing factor to this widely occurring complaint. In the clinic, hemorrhagic episodes often occur after chronic drug administration but are unpredictable and not always dose related. In contrast, the ulcerogenic data in commonly used laboratory G.I. irritation assays are scored after a single or few daily doses of the test compound at multiples of its antiinflammatory dosage. The predictive value of these assays is further complicated in that the nature of lesions in animals, superficial gastric hemorrhage versus penetrating intestinal erosions, seems to vary according to chemical structure types, e.g., aspirin versus arylacetic acids. A modified ulcerogenic assay employing a 5-day dosing schedule has been shown by Wong (1972) to give better statistical significance and dose–response curves. The therapeutic index, maximum no-lesion dosage/minimum antiinflammatory dosage, for most aryl acids varies within a narrow range of 1–5. For nonacidic agents the therapeutic ratios are generally much better. Indeed, their maximum no-lesion dosage in acute single-dose assays often approaches nonspecific toxic levels of 500–1000 mg/kg. Because therapeutic index is invariably reduced as the duration of daily treatment is increased, the adoption of a 1-week or 2-week ulcerogenic protocol can not only better simulate the chronic administration in man but can also define ulcerogenic potential at nontoxic drug levels. The mechanism of ulcerogenic effect is still not very clear. The influx of hydrogen ion, the inhibition of wound healing, and mucopolysaccharide biosynthesis are possible factors. The biochemical properties of various nonacidic agents have not been thoroughly investigated. The lower degree of ulcerogenicity of certain nonacidic agents in animals remains to be explained.

Renal papillary necrosis and hepatic toxicity are two more common potential side effects of antiinflammatory aryl acids. No substantial data are available to correlate these properties with any chemical structure, acidic or nonacidic.

B. Change of Biological Spectrum

The biological profiles of antiinflammatory aryl acids are generally very similar. Although many nonacidic agents have also been discovered by such standard screening assays, as carrageenan-edema and adjuvant arthritis models, there are considerable variations in their overall biological profiles. The clinical evaluation of these new agents with distinct profiles should help to elucidate the relative importance of various pathological events in arthritis. There is always hope that some new agents may retain the efficacy of aryl acids and show improved patient tolerance.

In the past few years several possible mechanisms of antirheumatic action have been receiving increased attention. The inhibition of prostaglandin biosynthesis by indomethacin, aspirin, and other aryl acids has been publicized by Vane (1971) and others. Newer nonacid structure types have also been found in several laboratories to inhibit prostaglandin synthetase, showing promise as systemic or topical antiinflammatory agents. More effective prostaglandin antagonists or compounds with multiple actions affecting both the function and metabolism of prostaglandins are attractive goals in this field. The dynamic and counterbalancing relationship of prostaglandins and cyclonucleotides (Yin-Yang) have been succinctly generalized by Goldberg (1972) and Kuehl *et al*. (1973) as

$$\downarrow PGE \longrightarrow cAMP \downarrow$$
$$\uparrow PGF \longrightarrow cGMP \uparrow$$

The modulation of intracellular levels of cyclic nucleotides, cAMP and cGMP, by nucleotide analogs or other novel structures is likely to provide a new class of agents. Compounds affecting the prostaglandin–cyclonucleotide pathway may have broad-spectrum activity against many key elements in immunological inflammation, such as lymphocyte transformation, lymphokine production, release of lysosomal contents, and cellular proliferation. The effective inhibition of these processes may interrupt the pathogenesis cycle commonly associated with chronic inflammation. Although no biochemical rationale is available to guide the synthesis of tissue-specific or disease-specific PG–cAMP modulators at the moment, the history of drug development assures that a new chemical entity with adequate selectivity or safety margin is likely to be discovered in the next few years through a combination of semiempirical structure–activity relationship studies and better biochemical understanding of these ubiquitous physiological messengers. The recent identification of the endoperoxide intermediate in PG synthesis and the demonstration of differential inhibition of PG synthetases from different tissues by Flower *et al*. (1973) are encouraging developments.

Other attractive targets not affected by antiinflammatory aryl acids include: the inhibition of the degenerative effect of collagenase, elastase, and possibly cathepsins; complement-mediated immune complex reactions; the production and function of lymphokines (mitogenic factor, cytotoxic factor, macrophage inhibitory factor (MIF); etc.); and the modulation of "angry" macrophages in the amplification of hyperimmunity. Prototypes of selective immunoregulants, some with differential effects on cellular immunity versus humoral responses, have been reported. Other experimental immunological agents will undoubtedly appear in the literature soon.

C. Clinical Experiments

Another potential source of chemical leads for novel antirheumatic agents is the intuitive clinical research by enthusiastic rheumatologists. It may be recalled that three "antirheumatic" drugs, gold, chloroquine, and D-penicillamine, have been discovered more or less in this manner. All three clinical leads are characterized by their slow onset and by their ability to achieve long-term remission of rheumatoid arthritis beyond the scope of conventional antiinflammatory–analgesic drugs. Further improvement of these clinical leads is hampered by the fact that their unusual efficacies have defied explanation by existing acute immunological or inflammatory animal systems. Nevertheless, they remain as valuable tools for characterizing the antiarthritic potential of some new assays. Two recent examples of exploratory antirheumatic experiments are the use of histidine and nitroimidazole. To obtain the valuable clinical feedback in a more systematic manner, human synovial specimens and measurements of patients' immune responses are increasingly employed to guide the development of new drugs. It is hoped that more sophisticated clinical pharmacology will supply the rational basis of laboratory approaches and reduce the high percentage of clinical failures that has plagued this field for so long.

III. NONACIDIC ANTIINFLAMMATORY AGENTS

A. General Discussion

For convenience of organization, nonacidic antiarthritic agents are classified into subgroups mainly on a basis of structural similarities, and this grouping does not necessarily imply any historical or biological relationships. These agents have been selected from a vast amount of scientific and patent literature to illustrate the status of past and current effort to find novel antiarthritic drugs. Without much information on their clinical performance for guidance, the selection is undoubtedly uncomprehensive and unbalanced. Among the examples illustrated in Sections III, B–J are many moderately active antiinflammatory–analgesic compounds with low ulcerogenic properties. A number of natural products has shown antiinflammatory effects in animal assays based on rather different primary biochemical mechanisms. Another group consists of several newly developed immunoregulants that differ from the traditional antimetabolites and cytostatics. These may be considered as prototypes of more effective antirheumatic agents, characterized by their narrow antiinflammatory and immunological profiles. They are probably the forerunners of a variety of new immunoregulants under intensive study in many laboratories at the moment.

B. Indoxole and Diarylpyrroles

1. INDOXOLE ANALOGS

Indoxole (1) is one of the earliest discovered nonacidic antiinflammatory agents (Szmuszkovicz et al., 1966). Its activity is in the range of phenylbutazone but with less ulcerogenic effect.

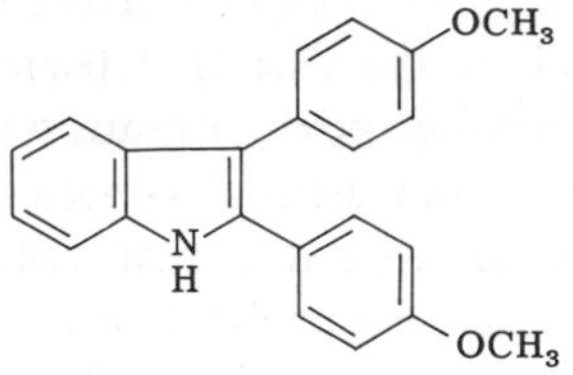

Unfortunately, indoxole showed a tendency to induce photosensitivity during clinical trials in South America and was abandoned. The induced photosensitivity was related to the ultraviolet absorption characteristics of the drug. Several attempts to find a nonsensitizing analog have not been successful (Engel *et al*., 1970). The corresponding indolizines (2) are much less active (Kallay and Doerge, 1972).

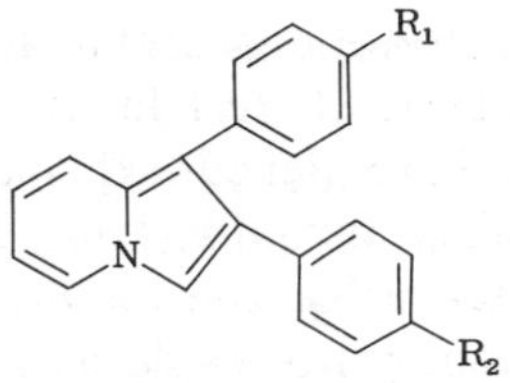

2. DIARYLPYRROLES

Replacing the indole chromophore in indoxole (1) by 2-methylpyrrole was found by the Sankyo group to yield a more potent analog, 2-methyl-4,5-bis(*p*-methoxyphenyl)pyrrole (bimetopyrol) (3) (Tanaka and Iizuka, 1972; Iizuka and Tanaka, 1972; Tanaka *et al*., 1972).

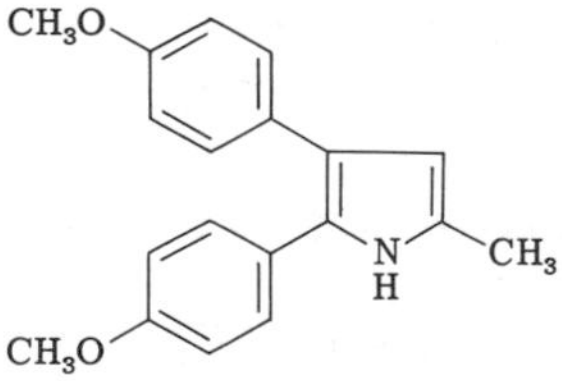

The spectrum of antiinflammatory and other pharmacological activities of bimetopyrol is generally like those of other nonsteroidal antiarthritic agents. Bimetopyrol inhibits carrageenan-induced rat paw edema, UV erythema in guinea pigs, acetic acid-induced writhing in mice, yeast-induced hyperesthesia in rat paw, and yeast-induced fever in rats. It is 2-5 times more potent than phenylbutazone in the carrageenan-edema, cotton pellet granuloma, and adjuvant arthritis assays when given orally at 3–15 mg/kg. It also suppresses leukocyte infiltration *in vivo* and *in vitro*. Like indomethacin and phenylbutazone, bimetopyrol is active against carrageenan edema by subcutaneous administration into the inflamed paw. Its oral activity is not affected by adrenalectomy. Furthermore, the change in bimetopyrol content in the inflamed paw always parallels that in percentage inhibition of paw edema. These findings suggest that bimetopyrol itself is probably the active agent *in vivo*. Bimetopyrol is well tolerated in animals; the acute LD_{50} is 2–3 gm/kg, p.o., in rats. In the chronic toxicity tests no more than 25 mg/kg/day, p.o., is tolerated by rats for 6 months. Higher doses cause gastrointestinal ulceration. In contrast, dogs tolerate daily doses of 150 mg/kg for 3 months without any significant toxicity. No clinical results have been reported.

A brief structure–activity relationship of diarylpyrroles (**4**) is described by Tanaka *et al*. (1972). Antiinflammatory activity is associated with substitution with a chloro or methoxy group in the para position of both the phenyl rings. Among a number of possible alkyl substituents at the 2 position of the pyrrole ring, methyl is distinctly superior to others.

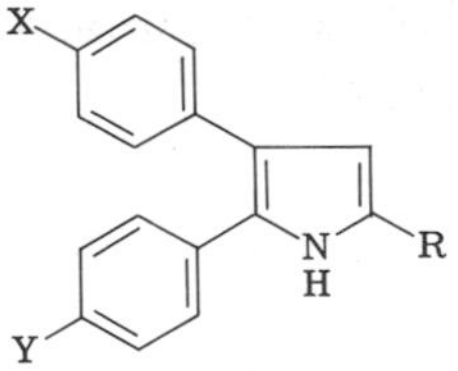

X, Y = CH₃O, Cl > H,

$$\underset{\text{NH\overset{\text{O}}{\overset{\parallel}{C}}CH_3}}{},\ \text{OH}$$

R = CH₃ > C₂H₅ >
    i-Pr, Bu, H

4

3. OTHER DIARYL HETEROARYLS

The promising pharmacological profile of bimetopyrol is reminiscent of the antiinflammatory activities previously observed in several laboratories with other diaryl-substituted heterocyclic compounds, such as 4,5-diphenyl-imidazole and derivatives (**5**). In our own studies both 2-ethyl- and 2-isopropyl-4,5-diphenylimidazoles have inhibited carrageenan-induced rat paw edema about 45% at 30 mg/kg. The 2,4,5-triphenyl analog was less effective. A large number of imidazole analogs were described in a Ciba-

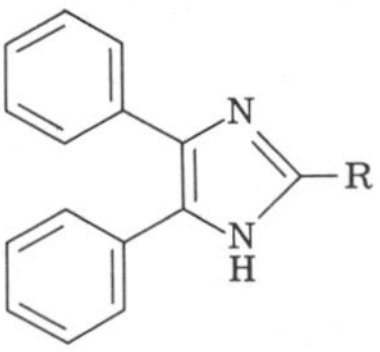

R = C₂H₅ , *i*-C₃H₇ , Ph

5

Geigy patent (1971). Similar to indoxole, these diarylimidazoles inhibited prostaglandin synthesis *in vitro* at 0.5 μg/ml (Shen *et al.*, 1974).

The idea of using a phenyl substituent attached to a ring system to mimic the corresponding benzo analog (having a fused phenyl moiety) has often been explored in medicinal chemistry. Similar analogy apparently exists between diarylheterocycles and arylbenzoheterocycles in this case. Indeed,

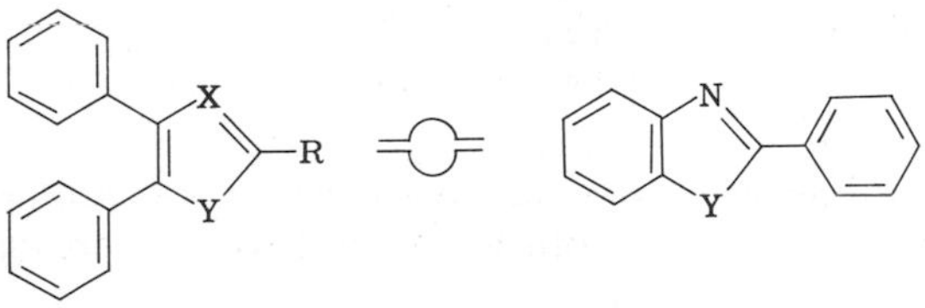

a number of nonacidic 2-arylbenzoheterocycles have already been noted for their antiinflammatory potential.

C. Arylbenzimidazoles and Arylbenzoxazoles

1. THIABENDAZOLE

Thiabendazole (**6**) is a widely used anthelmintic and antifungal agent in animals and in man. Its moderate antiinflammatory and analgesic activities were first noted in the clinic during the treatment of trichinosis at 25–50 mg/kg twice daily (Campbell, 1971).

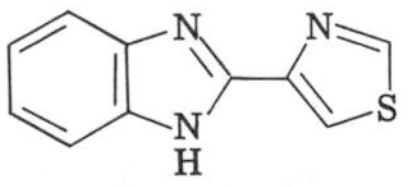

6

In rats, thiabendazole is approximately $\frac{1}{3}$–$\frac{1}{2}$ as potent as aspirin in the antipyretic, carrageenan-edema, yeast-induced hyperesthesia, and adjuvant arthritis assays (C. G. van Arman and W. C. Campbell, unpublished, 1972). It also inhibits the biosynthesis of prostaglandins at 5 μg/ml, being somewhat less potent than aspirin. Numerous thiabendazole analogs have been evaluated for their antiinflammatory effects. There appears to be no correlation of this activity with their antiparasitic and antifungal activities.

2. 2-ARYLBENZOXAZOLES

A series of 2-arylbenzoxazoles (**7**), which may be considered as isosteres of 2-arylbenzimidazoles, was recently investigated by a French group (Rips *et al.*, 1971).

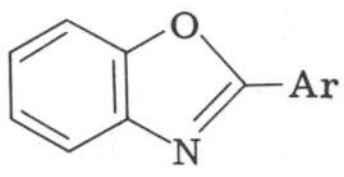

7

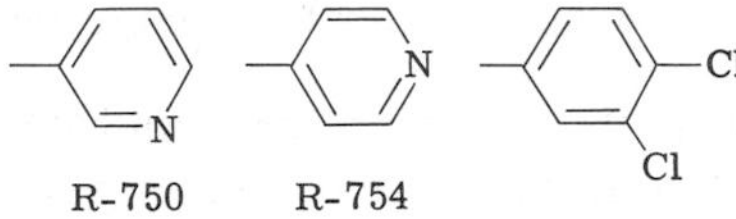

R-750   R-754

In the Kaolin-induced paw edema assay the three compounds of (7) were active at 50–100 mg/kg, i.p. Both R-750 and R-754 were also active in the cotton pellet granuloma assay.

Substituted benzoxazoles have been investigated extensively in medicinal chemistry. In our laboratories, a group of 2-aryloxazolopyridines (8 and 9), i.e., the aza isostere of benzoxazoles, have been found to be relatively potent antiinflammatory–analgesic–antipyretic agents (T. Y. Shen, R. L. Clark, A. A. Pessolano, B. E. Witzel, T. Lanza, C. G. van Arman, E. A. Risley, and G. Nuss, unpublished observations). Several analogs are active at 10–20 mg/kg with a very low degree of gastrointestinal irritation.

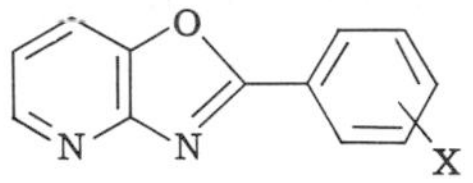

8 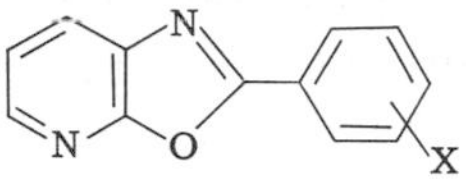   9

Both oxazolo [4,5-b] (8) and oxazolo [5,4-b] pyridines (9) were comparably active, whereas the [4,5-c] isomers were inactive. Some members also inhibited prostaglandin (PG) synthetase at low concentrations *in vitro*. However, no simple correlation between PG synthetase inhibition and carrageenan-edema inhibition was observed in this series. The real antiarthritic potential of this class of 2-aryl bicyclic heteroaryls remains to be ascertained.

D. Thienopyridine and Pyridinothiazinone

1. TETRAHYDROTHIENO [2,3-c] PYRIDINE

A novel series of polyfunctional thiophene derivatives has been reported by the Yoshitomi group (Nakanishi et al., 1970). Their product candidate is 2-amino-3-ethoxycarbonyl-6-benzyl-4,5,6,7-tetrahydrothieno [2,3-c] pyridine (Y-3642, Tinoridine, Nonflamin) (10).

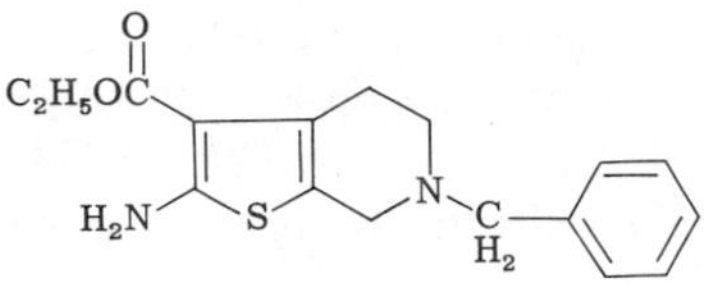

10

Y-3642 is a moderately active analgesic and antipyretic agent comparable to aminopyrine. It nonspecifically inhibits paw edemas induced by carrageenan, dextran, formalin, serotonin, and bradykinin, as well as exudate formation in peritonitis and granuloma pouch in rats at 50–100 mg/kg. However, it is not active in the granuloma pellet and UV-erythema assays. At 50 μM concentration, Y-3642 inhibits platelet aggregation and the histamine release from rat mast cells induced by polymyxin B, dextran, or rabbit lung thromboplastin. It has shown a protective action against polymyxin B shock (death) in rats. These antiphlogistic properties suggest its potential applications in acute allergic responses.

A major metabolic reaction of Y-3642 is the oxidative cleavage of the N-benzyl group to give the debenzyl derivative and various metabolites of benzoic acid (Imamura *et al.*, 1971). Some unchanged drug is found in peripheral fat, whereas only a small amount is in the blood for a short duration. The distribution of this nonacidic agent is obviously rather different from those of aryl acids.

2. PYRIDINO [2,3-b] [1,4]-THIAZIN-2-ONE

Another fused ring structure is Abbott-29590, 2,3-dihydro-1H-pyridino[2,3-b] [1,4]thiazin-2-one (**11**) (Kimura *et al.*, 1972).

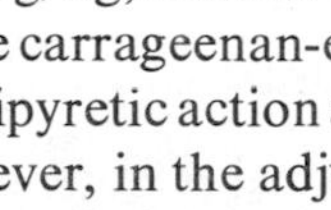

11

At an oral dose of 50–100 mg/kg, Abbott-29590 is approximately half as potent as phenylbutazone in the carrageenan-edema and cotton pellet granuloma assays. It produces an antipyretic action at 20 mg/kg and mild analgesia similar to that of aspirin. However, in the adjuvant arthritis assay its overall effectiveness is less than other antiinflammatory compounds, even at a dose of 200 mg/kg. Abbott-29590 is well tolerated in mice, rats, and guinea pigs in gastrointestinal irritation and acute toxicity studies up to the dose range

of 1–1.5 g/kg, p.o. It seems more toxic to dogs, with side effects induced
at about 300 mg/kg/day after a few days. Abbott-29590 was developed as a
mild, less irritating agent using the ratio of ED_{50}/LD_{50} as a therapeutic index.
An alternate ratio based on chronic toxicity data would seem more relevant
to its intended clinical usage.

Among other biological activities of Abbott-29590 reported are its
weak neuropharmacological actions. In dogs a weak tranquilizing activity.
concomitant with a slight decrease in muscle tone, is observed at 50 mg/kg,
although no central effects are seen in cats and monkeys at less than 400
mg/kg. Its latent central depressant properties are shown in the prolongation of barbiturate sleeping times in mice at 50–200 mg/kg. Whether the
mild tranquilizing action can manifest itself in arthritic patients and produce
an auxiliary beneficial effect remains to be seen.

In a recent multicenter clinical study, Ward, *et al.* (1973) reported that a
daily dose of 1200 mg of A-29590 (q.i.d.) is equivalent to 3900 mg aspirin
(t.i.d.) in rheumatoid arthritis patients. The number of reported side effects
for the two drugs is comparable. Three major side effects were found in
patients receiving A-29590: transient neutropenia (5%), rash (12%), and
exacerbation of the rheumatoid process (12%). The etiology of the last side
effect has not been determined but may reflect a slowly progressive therapeutic effect of A-29590. This kind of exacerbation was also reported to
occur with flazalone (L. Levy, unpublished, 1972).

3. PYRIDONE DERIVATIVES

In our laboratories a group of piperidones (12), pyridones (13) (Merck,
1972), and thienopyridones (14) have been found to have antiinflammatory
activities at 25–50 mg/kg but generally with much less propensity to produce
gastrointestinal lesions. Some also show mild sedative actions at 100 mg/kg
or higher. In spite of their chemical resemblance to Abbott-29590, no correlation of structure–activity relationships is observed.

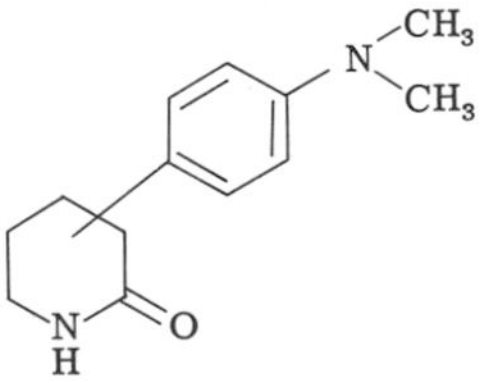

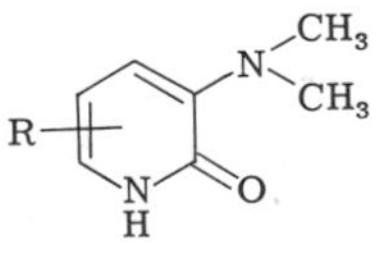

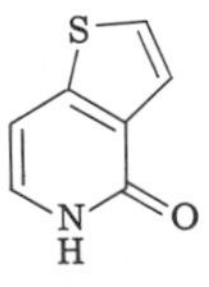

Unlike indoxole and thiabendazole, these aryllactams do not inhibit
prostaglandin synthetase preparations at less than 10 μg/ml. Further delinea-

tion of the biological profile of this class of nonacidic antiinflammatory agents is in progress.

E. Quinazolines

Expansion of the five-membered ring in benzimidazole or benzimidazolone to a six-membered ring gives quinazolines and quinazolinones. These are another class of well-studied nonacidic antiinflammatory agents. Most of these have been disclosed in the patent literature dating back several years. Some of the examples are shown below (**15**, Roussel-UCLAF, 1968; **16**, Glenn *et al.*, 1971; **17**, Sumitomo, 1971).

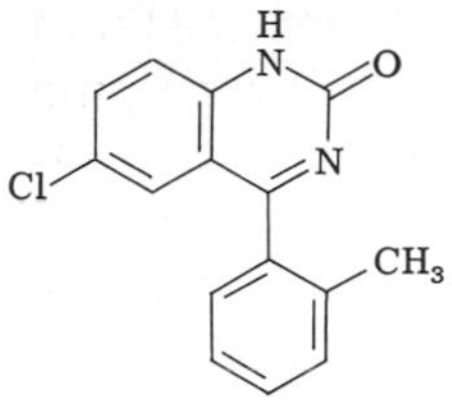

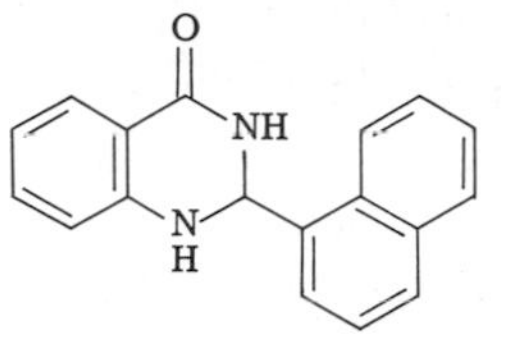

It is of interest that many contain the common feature of a phenyl substituent as in the series discussed above. In most cases their biological properties have not been described in detail. Piroquazone (**18**) (Sandoz-Wander, 1971) is undergoing the late stage of clinical trial. Similar compounds have been investigated by Sumitomo (Komatsu *et al.*, 1972).

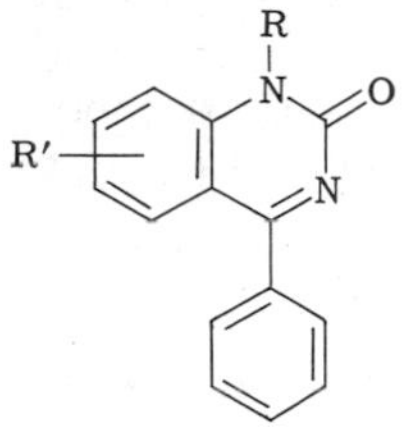

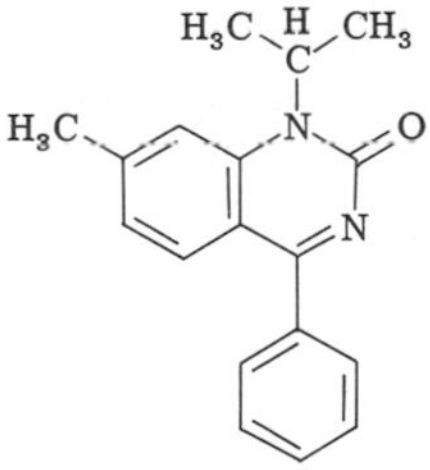

The 2,3-dihydro-4(1*H*)-quinazolinone (**16**) (Upjohn U-29,409) is an antispermatogenic agent that also inhibits the development of adjuvant-induced polyarthritis in rats (at 8 mg/kg, b.i.d.) probably through suppression of circulating leukocytes, particularly the granulocytes.

F. PC-796 and Seclazone

1. PC-796

A hydantoin derivative, 1-phenylsulfonyl-3,5-diphenylhydantoin (PC-796, **19**) was studied by Dainippon Pharmac as a new antiinflammatory agent (Nakamura *et al.*, 1970). PC-796 has a pK_a of 5.0 and forms a stable sodium salt. It inhibits carrageenan edema at 200 mg/kg and croton oil-induced granuloma pouch at 10–7 mg/kg, p.o., but is inactive in the cotton pellet granuloma assay. It has weak activity in the adjuvant arthritis and UV-erythema assays. It exerts strong inhibitory action on the increased vascular permeability induced by bradykinin, serotonin, histamine, and hyaluronidase. It is also more effective than aspirin as an antipyretic and in the inhibition of passive cutaneous anaphylaxis. Clearly, its activity profile is somewhat different from those of other antiinflammatory agents. No clinical data on PC-796 have been noted.

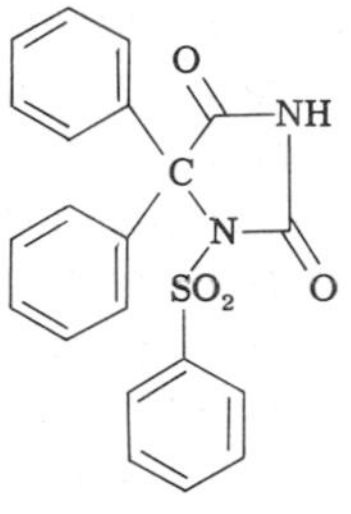

19

2. SECLAZONE (W-2354)

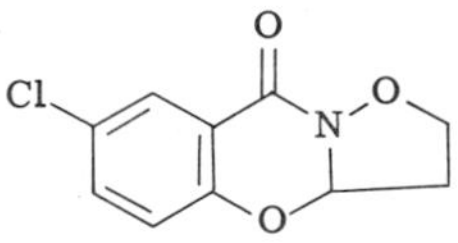

20 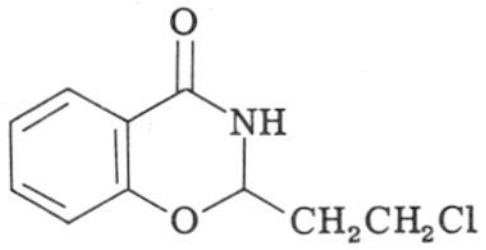   **21**

Formally, seclazone (**20**) is a cyclized salicylamide derivative, reminiscent of chlorthenoxazin (AP 67, **21**) and other related benzoxazinones (Berger *et al.*, 1972). It inhibits adjuvant arthritis when given at 0.1% in the diet (approximately equivalent to 150 mg/kg/day). It produces diuretic action in rats and dogs at 5 mg/kg. In man, seclazone is also a uricosuric agent at its antiinflammatory dose.

Seclazone is hydrolyzable in alkaline solution to 5-chlorosalicylic acid. It is not hydrolyzed in plasma or in the isolated rat stomach but is partially hydrolyzed in isolated intestine segments. In man, the drug is slowly absorbed and no free drug is detected in the plasma. Total [^{14}C] radioactivity reached maximum plasma level at 16 hours with a half-life of 14 hours. The major urinary metabolites in man and in animals are 5-chlorosalicylic acid and its glucuronide (Edelson *et al.* 1973). It seems that 5-chlorosalicylic acid may indeed contribute to the pharmacological action of seclazone. Because salicylic acid itself is more effective than 5-chlorosalicylic acid in many antiinflammatory and analgesic assays, it should be of interest to examine the properties of dechloro seclazone.

G. Cryogenine, Tomatine, and Other Natural Products

1. CRYOGENINE

Cryogenine is an alkaloid isolated from *Heimia salicifolia* Link and Otto and is as effective as phenylbutazone in the carrageenan foot, edema and adjuvant arthritis assays (Nucifora and Malone, 1971; Omaye *et al.*, 1972). In the latter experiment, oral dosing of cryogenine at 100 mg/kg daily for 21 days suppressed the increase of sedimentation rate, reduced foot swelling, and normalized both the leukocyte count and the lymphocyte neutrophil ratio. Cryogenine has very low ulcerogenicity in laboratory animals.

An important property of this alkaloid is its neuroleptic activity. In a comparison psychopharmacologic investigation of cryogenine, indomethacin, phenylbutazone, and lupine alkaloids, it has been found that cryogenine induces a selective CNS depression characterized by pronounced behavioral passivity and a reduction of spontaneous motor activity. No signs of analgesia, hypotension, or decrease in skeletal muscle tone are detected. Cryogenine is also devoid of any ganglionic activity (Kosersky and Malone, 1971). In some tests cryogenine at 25 mg/kg has been more effective than 2 mg/kg of chlorpromazine. It is of interest to note that these CNS effects have been demonstrated at dose levels lower than the antiinflammatory dose. Several neuroleptics, e.g., chlorpromazine and tetrabenazine, have been reported to possess significant oral antiinflammatory activities in animal models. Other central nervous active drugs, e.g., benzoctamine, possessing antihistamine and antiserotonin properties are potent inhibitors of increased vascular permeability occurring in the early phases of inflammatory reaction but are less effective in inhibiting chronic arthritis (Jaques and Riesterer, 1971). Both indomethacin and phenylbutazone show no neuroleptic potential in the above comparison. Clearly, antiinflammatory and neuroleptic actions are not necessarily related. From the therapeutic point of view they are probably not incompatible either. A large-scale trial using a combination of an analgesic and a neuroleptic agent to treat chronic pain, mostly of neoplastic patients, has been claimed a success by Amery *et al.* (1971).

2. TOMATINE

Tomatine (lycopersicin, **26**) is a $C_{50}H_{83}NO_{21}$ alkaloid glycoside that has been investigated for a number of years (Filderman and Kovacs, 1969) and is naturally occurring in certain tomato plants.

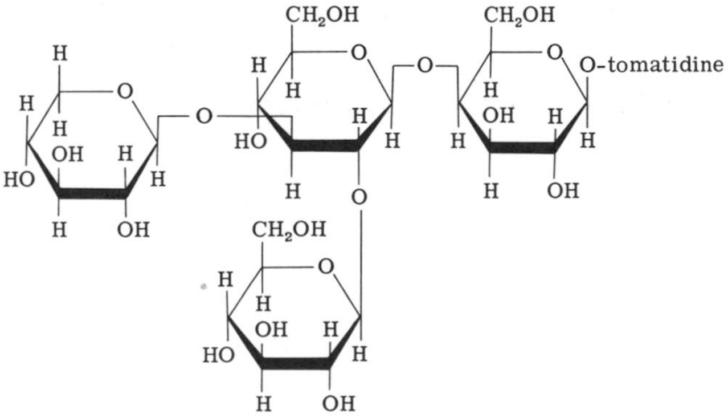

Tomatine

26

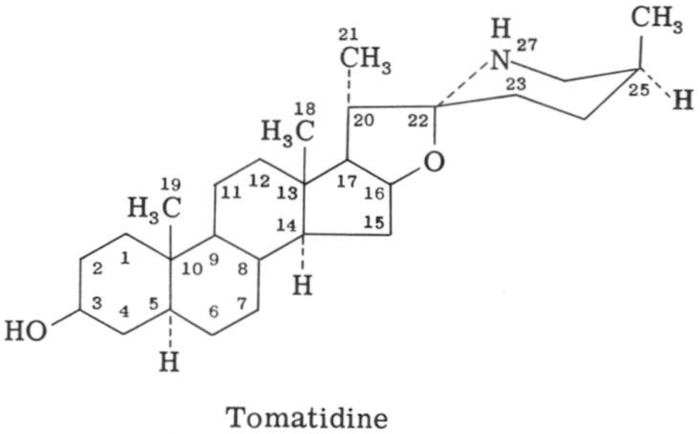

Tomatidine

27

In rats, tomatine exerts a significant inhibition of carrageenan-induced paw edema when administered at 1–10 mg/kg, i.m., or 15–30 mg/kg, p.o. It also inhibits the granuloma tissue formation induced by carrageenan-impregnated cotton pellets. Its antiinflammatory activity is independent of adrenal stimulation but may be related to its antihistamine, antiserotonin, and antibradykinin properties. Tomatine has weak antibacterial and anti-fungal effects. It is not very well absorbed orally. The aglycone, tomatidine **(27)**, has no antihistamine or antiinflammatory activity.

3. CURCUMIN

Curcumin (28), a natural product from *Curcuma longa* (turmeric), is reported as an antiinflammatory agent in India (Arora *et al.*, 1971). Curcuminate, the disodium or dipotassium phenolate, is water soluble and

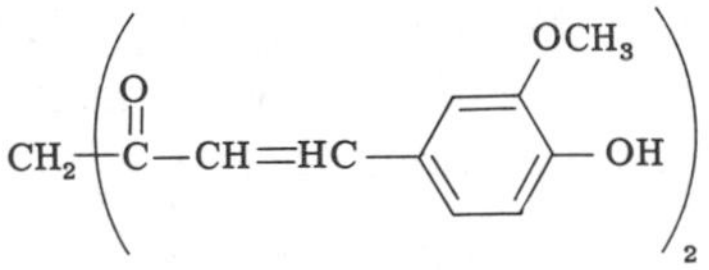

28

orally effective in carrageenan- and formalin-induced edema in rats at 0.1–1.0 mg/kg (Ghatak and Basu, 1972). Sodium curcuminate is well tolerated at 40 mg/kg for 6 weeks in rats. Chronic safety assessment is reported underway for clinical trial. The biological activity of curcumin derivatives may well be associated with the highly conjugated system (29). Its specificity and

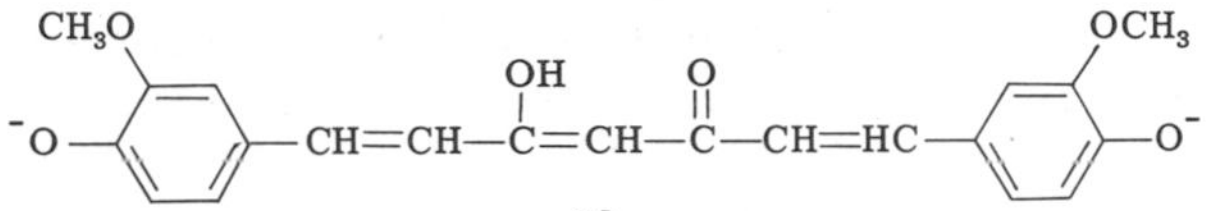

29

other biological effects, including topical actions based on its traditional usage in Indian herb medicine, would be of interest to ascertain.

H. Immunoregulants: Benzothiazines, Flazalone, Methisazone, and Oxisuran

1. BENZOTHIAZINES

An interesting series of antiinflammatory–immunosuppressive agents, the 3-phenyl-2*H*-1,4-benzothiazines (30, 31) was reported by the Squibb Institute (Krapcho and Turk, 1970; Millonig *et al.*, 1971). There was a certain structural resemblance to their earlier immunosuppressant cinanserin (32), but the key intermediate was unexpectedly obtained through a novel chemical rearrangement:

The two most interesting members of this series are SQ 11579 (30) and SQ 11493 (31), the stereochemical configurations of which are assigned on the basis of an X-ray analysis of a methiodide salt. Both compounds are approximately twice as active as phenylbutazone in the carrageenan footedema assay but are moderately active in the adjuvant arthritis model only at nearly toxic levels. SQ 11579 is comparable to indomethacin and phenylbutazone in inhibiting reversed passive Arthus reaction in the rabbit when given intradermally at 200 μg per site and the delayed skin reaction (tuberculin) in the guinea pig at 2 × 50 mg/kg, s.c. Both compounds are also inhibitors of paralysis in experimental allergic encephalomyelitis in rats and the production of hemagglutinin in the mouse. The antiinflammatory activity of these compounds was said to be diminished by adrenalectomy. Their ulcero-

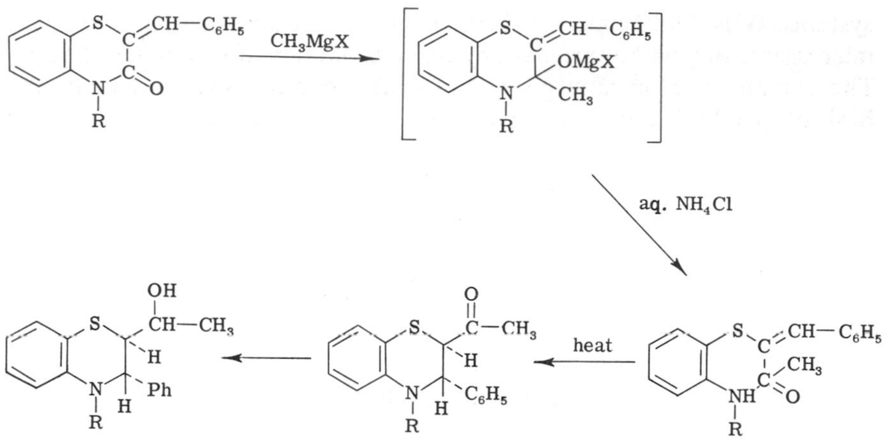

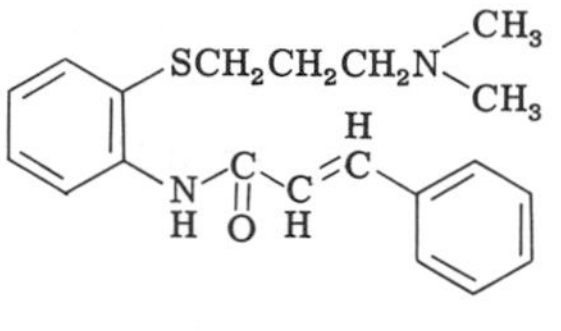

Cinanserin

32

genicity in rats is comparable to that of phenylbutazone. SQ 11579 has been selected for clinical trial. The structure–activity relationship of this series indicates that the inhibition of carrageenan edema is generally reduced when the 3-phenyl group is substituted or replaced by pyridyl or thienyl, and the optimal length of the dialkylamino side chain is propylene.

The metabolism of SQ 11579 has been reported (Lan and Schreiber, 1972). Extensive metabolic conversions, such as N-demethylation, sulfoxidation, N-oxidation, aromatic hydroxylation, and glucuronide conjugation, occur in both the *in vitro* liver microsome system and three animal species, rat, dog, and monkey. Marked species differences have been noted in plasma half-life, major route of excretion, and predominant urinary metabolites. Interestingly, two metabolic inhibitors, SKF-525A and WIN 13099, also show differential inhibition of the oxidative biotransformations in different systems. WIN 13099 blocks N-demethylation and sulfoxidation in rat liver microsomes but inhibits aromatic hydroxylation and sulfoxidation in the dog. The complexity of maximizing bioavailability of a new drug in man on the basis of metabolic data in animals is clearly demonstrated.

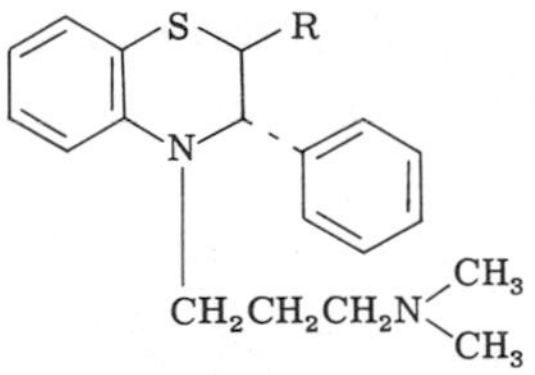

30 R = $\overset{\text{OH}}{\overset{|}{\text{CHCH}_3}}$ (SQ 11579)

31 R = $\overset{\text{O}}{\overset{||}{\text{CCH}_3}}$ (SQ 11493)

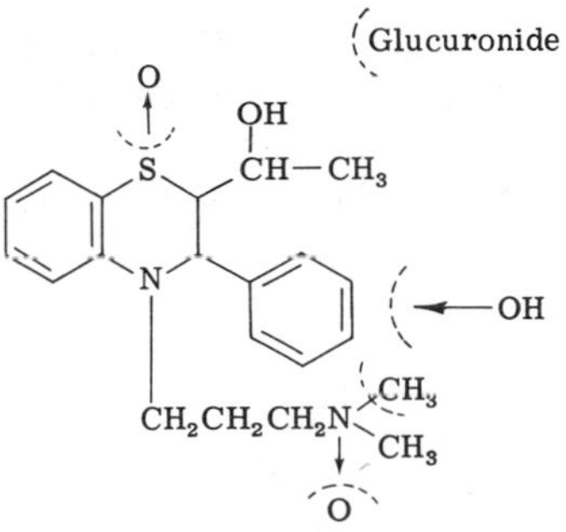

Metabolic transformation of SQ 11,579.

2. FLAZALONE

Flazalone (R-760) is the generic name for *p*-fluorophenyl-4-(*p*-fluoro-phenyl)-4-hydroxy-1-methyl-3-piperidyl ketone (**33**) of 3M-Riker Labora-

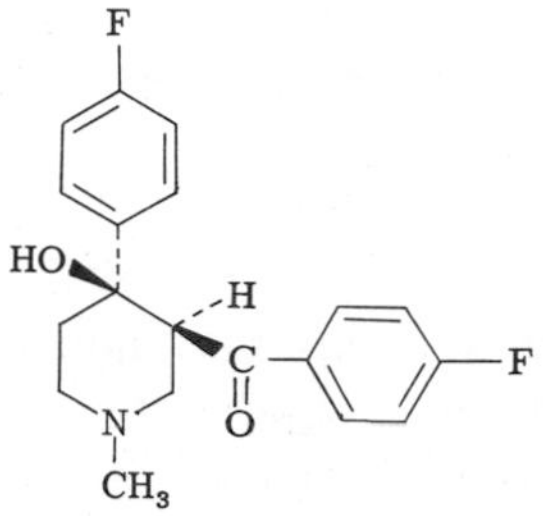

33

tories (Draper *et al.*, 1972; Levy and McClure, 1972). It was prepared by the Mannich reaction of *p*-fluoroacetophenone and methylamine hydrochloride, followed by internal aldolization of the Mannich base with alkali. The stereochemistry of (**33**) was unequivocally established by X-ray analysis. Flazalone inhibits edema induced by a variety of agents, such as carrageenan, serotonin, egg white, dextran, and yeast, at 50–100 mg/kg. It is approximately half as potent as phenylbutazone in the disseminated phase of adjuvant arthritis. It has no effect at 50–200 mg/kg in the UV-erythema assay but inhibits the blueing reaction in hyperimmune passive cutaneous anaphylaxis in the rat. It also inhibits the rejection of goldfish scale homograft and rabbit ear skin homografts. The latter property may be partly related to its antiserotonin activity. Flazalone inhibits the RNA and DNA synthesis of lymphocytes *in vitro* at 0.5 m*M* (Whitehouse, 1971). It has no activity in experimental allergic encephalomyelitis, the Arthus reaction of the rat, or the graft versus host reaction in the mouse.

Flazalone has been evaluated clinically in patients with rheumatoid arthritis. Controlled trials have demonstrated a rather slow onset of activity in some cases that appears to be progressive and sustained. This response is reported to be particularly well defined in some patients who have been refractory to other nonsteroidal antiinflammatory drugs, suggesting a unique mechanism of action. Additional studies are being considered in an effort to determine this mechanism (Riker Laboratories, unpublished, 1972).

3. OXISURAN

Oxisuran, 2-[(methylsulfinyl)acetyl] pyridine (**34**), is a differential inhibitor of cell-mediated hypersensitivity without concomitant suppression of humoral antibody formation (Freedman *et al.*, 1972). The corresponding 3 and 4 positional isomers do not show the selective immunosuppressive effect. Other analogs enhance or inhibit the cellular and humoral immune responses in all possible combinations. The modes of action of this class of compounds are still under investigation (Fox *et al.*, 1973).

34

Oxisuran was developed following the immunological characterization of its congener, which inhibited adjuvant arthritis but not carrageenan edema. Oxisuran prolonged the allograft survival time in mice and rats at 50–100 mg/kg, s.c., but had no effect on the primary and secondary responses to sheep red blood cell (sRBC) in normal mice. It was alleged to be effective against cutaneous delayed reactivity in guinea pigs and rats previously sensitized to ovalbumen or tuberculin. Oxisuran was not cytotoxic or anti-proliferative *in vitro* or *in vivo*. The clinical efficacy of this new immuno-regulant would be of interest to follow.

4. CHLOROPHENESIN

Chlorophenesin (3-*p*-chlorophenoxy-1,2-propanediol, **35**) has been shown to suppress humoral antibody response without affecting antigenic priming of immunocompetent cells (Berger *et al.*, 1967, 1969). It also

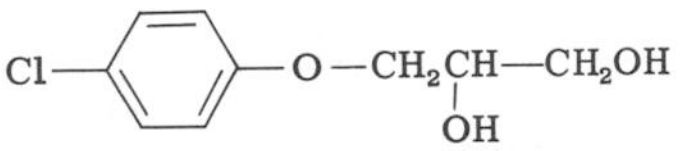

$$Cl-\langle\bigcirc\rangle-O-CH_2CH-CH_2OH$$
$$\underset{OH}{|}$$

35

inhibits the release of both histamine and SRS-A from primate cells and blocks passive cutaneous anaphylaxis. Recently, chlorophenesin has been found to elevate levels of cAMP in treated cells (Malley and Baecher, 1971), an event known to be associated with the action of immunocom-petent lymphocytes and with the inhibition of growth of tumor cells. Chlorophenesin has demonstrated therapeutic activity in a variety of ex-perimental neoplasia (Spencer *et al.*, 1972). It is noncytotoxic but may enhance cell-mediated immune responses of the host, possibly interfer-ing with the synthesis or binding of enhancing antibody to tumor cells. This unusual immunoregulant has no activity in the adjuvant arthritis assay. No information is available on its possible effect on rheumatoid arthritis.

5. METHISAZONE

The antiviral drug methisazone (*N*-methylisatin-β-thiosemicarbazone, Marboran, **36**), was reported by McNeil and co-workers (1972) to be an in-hibitor of the 7S and 19S antibody-forming cell responses to sRBC in mice at daily doses of 23 μg. It reduces the hemolytic antibody titer in the serum. It also suppresses the response of hemopoietic colony-forming cells (granul-ocyte–macrophage progenitor cells) to adjuvant stimulation *in vivo*. It was shown *in vitro* that methisazone at 3 μg/ml inhibits only the earliest stages of the colony development. The drug, in contrast to such nonspecific cytotoxic agents as 6-mercaptopurine and 5-iodo-2'-deoxyuridine, has no effect on subsequent colony development, in terms either of rate of cell division or of morphogenesis. These results indicate the possibility of using drugs to interfere with specific stages of cellular differentiation, thus minimizing the dangerous side effects. Oral methisazone has been used in the clinic for the prophylaxis and treatment of vaccinia infection. Its immunosuppressive effects in man and potential application to immune disorders remain to be elucidated.

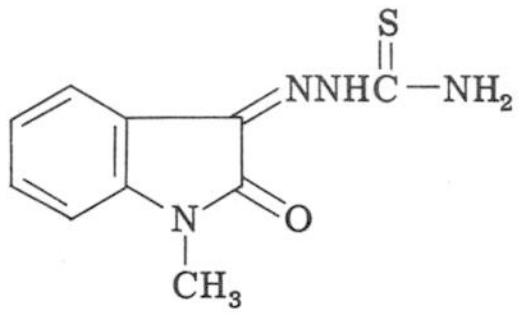

36

I. Antidegenerative Protease Inhibitors

Polymorphonuclear leukocytes (PMN) have been implicated in the pathogenesis of rheumatoid arthritis for a long time. The release of PMN proteases into the extracellular fluid in acute inflammation may overwhelm natural protease inhibitors and cause tissue degeneration. In addition to their direct hydrolytic actions on tissue targets, PMN proteases may play an indirect role in inflammation by activating kinins and cleaving complement factors C_3 and C_5. C_3 and C_5 are chemotactic in nature, thus promoting a vicious cycle of PMN-mediated injury of tissues (Janoff, 1972). In recent years the properties of several proteases (the acid cathepsins, the neutral elastase, and the collagenases) and their relative significance in tissue destruction have been examined in great detail (see Chapter 11 by Fisher).

Many low molecular weight protease inhibitors are known, but most are effective at relatively high concentrations *in vitro*, e.g., 10^{-4} to $10^{-3} M$, only. A naturally occurring peptide, pepstatin (**37**), Isovalyl-L-valyl-L-valyl-4-amino-3-hydroxy-6-methylheptanoyl-L-alanyl-4-amino-3-hydroxy-6-

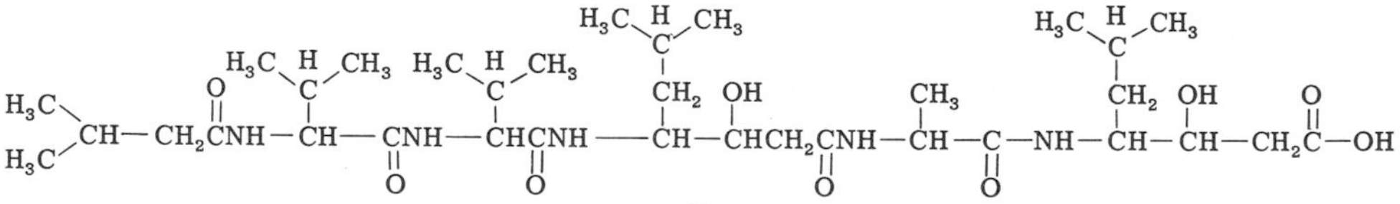

37

methylheptanoic acid, was discovered by Umezawa and co-workers (1970) in their search for enzyme inhibitors from fermentation broths; it is a potent inhibitor of acid proteases, including pepsin and cathepsin D (Dingle *et al.*, 1972). Pepstatin is a noncompetitive inhibitor active at 10^{-9} to $10^{-8} M$ ($\lesssim 0.01$ μg/ml). It is poorly absorbed orally but inhibits carrageenan foot edema in rats at 1.25 mg/kg, i.p. The effects of pepstatin in various acute immunological models, such as Arthus reaction, local Shwartzman, and serum sickness vasculitis, are under investigation in many laboratories. It should be of interest to ascertain whether pepstatin and other cathepsin D inhibitors exert any antidegenerative effect in chronic arthritic models.

For clinical applications protease inhibitors presumably may be used as adjunct therapy in combination with other antiinflammatory–analgesic agents. Aside from the indirect inflammatory effects of proteases mentioned above, the monitoring of long-term antidegenerative effects requires periodic radiography or other measurements. If collagenase, cathepsins, and elastase indeed act in concert or in a broad manner, the ultimate efficacy of any specific protease inhibitor may be very limited. However, the long-term administration of any broad-spectrum protease inhibitor faces the uncertainty of systemic side effects. An alternative to this dilemma is to prevent the release of PMN lysosomal constituents. The current concept of lysosomal leakage from viable PMN involves the "regurgitation" or reverse endocytosis process during phagocytosis. The release of lysosomal enzymes following phagocytosis of immune complexes appears to be modified by changes in intracellular levels of cAMP. Prostaglandin E_1 and theophylline increase cAMP and synergistically suppress leakage of lysosome contents from phagocytizing PMN. The intensive investigation, in many laboratories, of prostaglandin and cyclonucleotide analogs, as well as of agents capable of modulating cAMP or cGMP levels, may well produce new types of antiinflammatory–antidegenerative agents.

J. Carbohydrate Derivatives

1. TRIBENOSIDE

The potential application of Tribenoside (Glyvenol^R), ethyl tri-O-benzyl-D-glucofuranoside (38), as a novel antiarthritic agent (Jaques et al., 1967) excited much curiosity several years ago mainly because of its innocuous chemical structure. Tribenoside has a venotropic effect and inhibits the effects of antigen–antibody reaction. In various in vitro and in vivo test

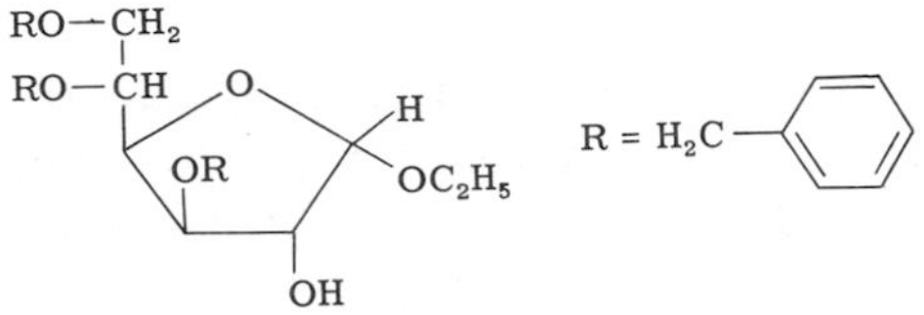

38

systems, it also stimulates fibrinolytic activity (Rüegg *et al.*, 1972). In rats with established adjuvant arthritis it restores the euglobulin clot lysis time to normal but has no positive effect on the secondary lesions. Its anti-rheumatic effect in man is not significant (Dick *et al.*, 1969).

2. SULFATED POLYSACCHARIDES

Various types of polyanionic polysaccharides, such as cellulose sulfate, pentosan polysulfate, dextran sulfate, sulfated amylopectin, and car-rageenan, activate kinin-forming system(s) in the plasma and deplete plasma kininogen(s) after systemic injection (Saeki, 1972; Rocha e Silva *et al.*, 1969). Carrageenan interacts with activated complement C_1'. Its anticomplement-ary action in several species *in vivo* and *in vitro* has been reported. Pretreat-ment of rats with xylan polysulfuric acid or dextrans with molecular weights of 4×10^4 to 200×10^4 produced anticomplementary and antiinflammatory effects. The anticoagulant effect and interaction with the reticuloendothelial system of these polyanions have been noted. Some of these are also known to be weak interferon inducers. The *in vivo* activity profiles of these poly-anions vary according to the polysaccharide backbone, molecular weight, charge density, stereochemistry, and other properties. An oligosaccharide derivative, SP-54, (**39**), is reported (Kalbhen, 1972) to possess a pronounced antiinflammatory effect against all types of experimental edema at 25-100 mg/kg, s.c. or i.p., before or shortly after edema induction. In addition to its suppression of hyaluronidase, histamine, and complement C_1' esterase, SP-54 is considered to have specific vasotropic and stabilizing effects. It is effective in the clinic in treating acute inflammation by i.m. and i.v. ad-ministration. No data on chronic arthritis have been reported.

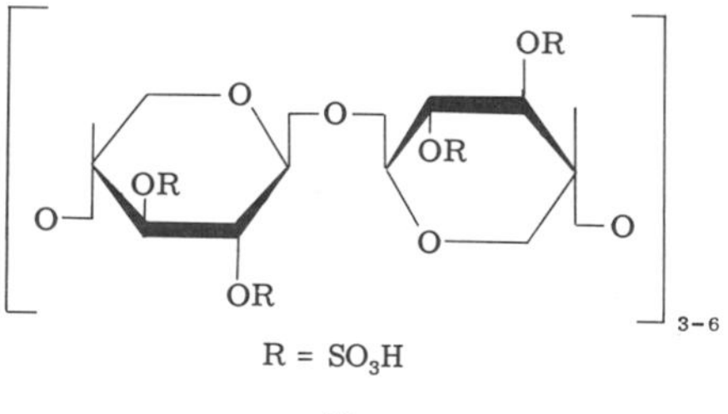

R = SO₃H

39

3. GLYCOPEPTIDE ANALOGS

An experimental biochemical approach to regulate the metabolism and function of immunoglobulins with analogs of the glycopeptide juncture 2-acetamido-1-*N*-(β-L-aspartyl)-2-deoxy-β-glucopyranosylamine (**40**) has been considered (Shen *et al.*, 1972).

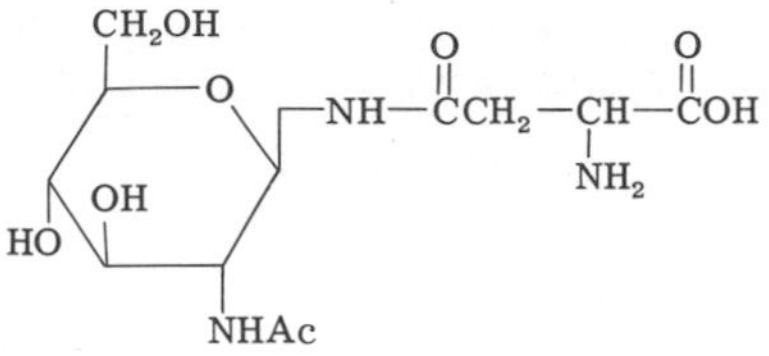

40

A number of analogs have been synthesized as potential inhibitors or acceptors of the glycosyl transfer enzymes. Their effects on the function and catabolism of immunoglobulins possibly involving the participation of the "hinge" region are under study.

IV. CLINICAL ANTIRHEUMATIC STUDIES

A. D-Penicillamine and Other Sulfhydryl Agents

The antirheumatic action of D-penicillamine (**41**), after many years of limited clinical usage, has recently been systematically evaluated in a multi-center cooperative trial in England. Attempts were made to minimize some of its side effects, such as nausea, skin rash, and proteinuria, by a gradually increased dosing schedule. Some individual reports have been released for publication (Huskisson and Hart, 1972 Anonymous, 1973; Jaffe, 1973). A comprehensive official review is awaited.

The mode of action of D-penicillamine is still not clear, although a number of possible mechanisms have been suggested. Among these are pyridoxine antagonism, dermolathyrism, modification of trace metal metabolism, increase in serum sulfhydryl concentration, and a possible effect on immunoglobulin interactions. Closely related compounds, such as cysteine, N-acetylcysteine, and α-mercaptopropionylglycine, have also been considered for clinical experiments.

Attempts to find a better penicillaminelike agent have been hampered by the lack of suitable animal models. Both D-penicillamine and L-cysteine are inactive in the carrageenan edema assay but are weakly active in the adjuvant arthritis model at high doses of 250–500 mg/kg, p.o. Many derivatives, such as S-benzyl- and S-tritylcysteine, are relatively more potent as antiinflammatory agents in laboratory animals, yet their resemblance to D-penicillamine is probably only chemical and not pharmacological in nature. For example, S-trityl-L-cysteine (**42**) is known to exert an acute cytotoxic effect with potential antitumor properties (Coffey et al., 1972). The slow onset (3–6 weeks) of D-penicillamine's clinical efficacy renders the human trials of related analogs with uncertain pharmacological similarity even more difficult.

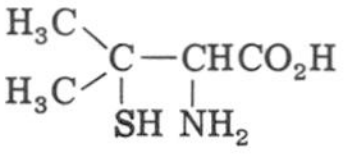

$$
\begin{array}{cc}
\underset{H_3C}{\overset{H_3C}{\diagdown}}C-CHCO_2H & Ph-\overset{Ph}{\underset{Ph}{C}}-S-CH_2-\underset{NH_2}{CHCO_2H} \\
\quad\quad\ \ |\ \ | & \\
\quad\quad\ \ SH\ NH_2 & \\
\end{array}
$$

41 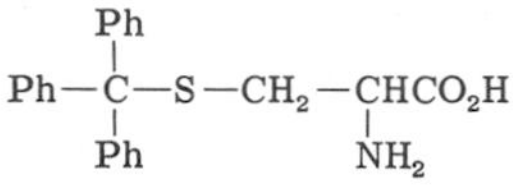   (NSC 83265)

42

B. Histidine

In connection with the investigation of hypohistidinemia in a large number of rheumatoid arthritis patients. Gerber (1969) reported that clinical improvement was observed after oral administration of histidine of 4.5 gm/ day in single-blind studies. The prospect of using a normal amino acid to correct metabolic deviations and to alleviate the pathological syndromes in rheumatoid arthritis (RA) naturally excited many investigators. From the nutritional point of view, excessive histidine loading in ani.nals was known to produce adrenal stimulation. In various arthritis assays, histidine did not show any significant activities. No other pharmacological effect was reported either. The riddle of histidine therapy was partially clarified in a recent disclosure (Pinals et al., 1973). In a double-blind two-center clinical trial of 60 R.A. patients for 30 weeks, no significant differences between histidine- and placebo-treated groups were revealed in such measurements as grip strength, sedimentation rate (ESR), walking time, morning stiffness, or numbers of swollen and tender joints. There was only an indication that patients with long duration of disease, seropositivity, greater impairment of ambulation, and higher ESR improved more often on L-histidine. The therapeutic value of this treatment was obviously very limited.

C. Nitroimidazoles

Nitroimidazoles represent a broad class of antiparasitic agents. Some members also showed weak carcinogenic effects in experimental animals. An amoebicide, BT-985 (E. Merck) has previously been reported to produce clinical remission in acute systemic lupus erythematosus (SLE) patients. Some beneficial effects on 12 rheumatoid arthritis patients at 250 mg/day have been claimed; a controlled trial is suggested by the authors to confirm this observation (Abd-Rabbo et al., 1970, 1972).

V. CONCLUSIONS

For years, the search for new nonsteroidal antiinflammatory agents has been facilitated by the relative abundance of active structures in the screening assays. The discovery of a variety of aryl acids with potencies in the practical range of 1–20 mg/kg enables researchers in this active field to concentrate on safety improvement and to establish the full clinical potential of this class of antiarthritic agents. It is encouraging to see that many novel nonacidic compounds also show potential in the antiinflammatory assays. As a group, they appear to be less irritating to the gastrointestinal tract than aryl acids. On a weight basis, their potency is moderate in comparison, but qualitatively many of them have shown pharmacological profiles distinct from those of aryl acids. It is of special interest to note that a few also possess certain immunoregulatory properties not seen with aryl acids.

With many laboratories intensively pursuing the immunological approach to rheumatoid arthritis, undoubtedly other antiinflammatory compounds with selective immunological activities will soon be discovered. It is generally hoped that these new agents will not have the shortcomings of nonspecific cytotoxic immunosuppressants, particularly with respect to decreased host resistance to infection and enhancement of malignancy. These narrow-spectrum or selective immunoregulants will also be invaluable as experimental tools to delineate the pathogenic mechanisms of rheumatoid arthritis.

Major biomedical advances are often made when the formulation of biological hypotheses coincide with the emergence of active compounds from related investigations. This is attributable in part to the phenomenon of overlapping activities; many drugs have been found to possess broader pharmacological profiles after their initial development. Any clinical feedback, whether positive or negative, further influences the direction of laboratory progress. It seems likely that the treatment of rheumatoid arthritis may soon reach such a fruitful stage.

REFERENCES

Abd-Rabbo, H., Montasir, M., Abaza, H., and El-Gohary, Y. (1970). *J. Trop. Med. Hyg.* **73**, 47.

Abd-Rabbo, H., Abaza, H., Hillal, G., Moghazy, M., and Assur, L. (1972). *J. Trop. Med. Hyg.* **75**, 64.

Amery, W. K. P., Admiraal, P. V., Beck, P. H. M., Bosker, J. T., Crul, J. F., Feikema, J. J., Knape, H., Kuipers Tj., Lampe, C. F. J., van Mansvelt, J., Pearce, C., Pel, J. W. J., van Schaick, D. C. N., Schneider, J. H., van Vark-Berends, J. A., and Zegveld, C. (1971). *Arnzeim-Forsch.* **21**, 868.

Anonymous (1973). *Lancet* **1**, 275.

Arora, R. B., Basu, N., Kapoor, V., and Jain, A. P. (1971). *Indian J. Med. Res.* **59**, 1289.

Berger, F. M., Fukui, G. M., Ludwig, B. J., and Margolin, S. (1967). *Proc. Soc. Exp. Biol. Med.* **124**, 303.

Berger, F. M., Fukui, G. M., DeAngelo, M., and Chandlee, G. C. (1969). *J. Immunol.* **102**, 1024.

Berger, F. M., Kletzkin, M., and Spencer, H. J. (1972). *Fed. Proc., Fed. Amer. Soc. Exp. Biol.* **31**, 578.

Campbell, W. C. (1971). *J. Amer. Med. Ass.* **216**, 2143.

Ciba-Geigy. (1971). German Patent 2,064,520.

Coffey, J. J., Palm, P. E., Denine, E. P., Baranowsky, P. E., and Kensler, C. J. (1972). *Cancer Res.* **31**, 1908.

Dick, W. C., Cunningham, G. M., Nuki, G., Jasani, M. K., and Whaley, K. (1969). *Ann. Rheum. Dis.* **28**, 187.

Dingle, J. T., Barrett, A. J., and Poole, A. R. (1972). *Biochem. J.* **127**, 443.

Draper, M. D., Petracek, F. J., Klohs, M. W., McClure, D. A., Levy, L., and Ré, O. N. (1972). *Arzneim.-Forsch.* **22**, 1803.

Edelson, J., Douglas, J. F., and Ludwig, B. J. (1973). *J. Pharm. Sci.* **62**, 229.

Emori, H. W., Champion, G. D., Paulus, H. E., and Bluestone, R. H. (1972). *Abstr. Pap., Int. Congr. Pharmacol., 5th, 1972* p. 63.

Engel, W., Seeger, E., Teufel, H., and Eckenfels, A. (1970). German Patent 1,922,191; *Chem. Abstr.* **74**, 12995W. (1971).

Filderman, R. B., and Kovacs, B. A. (1969). *Brit. J. Pharmacol.* **37**, 748.

Flower, R. J., Cheung, H. S., and Cushman, D. V. (1973). *Prostaglandins* **4**, 325.

Fox, A. E., Gingold, J. L., and Freedman, H. H., (1973). *Infec. Immun.* **8**, 549.

Freedman, H. H., Fox, A. E., Shavel, J., Jr., and Morrison, G. C. (1972). *Proc. Soc. Exp. Biol. Med.* **139**, 909.

Gerber, D. A. (1969). *Clinical Rev.* **17**, 352.

Ghatak, N., and Basu, N. (1972). *Indian J. Exp. Biol.* **10**, 235.

Glenn, E. M., Lyster, S. C., and Rohloff, N. A. (1971). *Proc. Soc. Exp. Biol. Med.* **138**, 244.

Goldberg, N. D. (1972). *Abstr. Pap. Int. Congr. Pharmacol. 5th; 1972* p. 229.

Huskisson, E. C., and Hart, F. D. (1972). *Ann. Rheum. Dis.* **31**, 402.

Iizuka, Y., and Tanaka, K. (1972). *J. Pharm. Soc. Jap.* **92**, 11.

Imamura, H., Matsui, E., Kato, Y., and Furuta, T. (1971). *Yakugaku Zasshi* **91**, 546.

Jaffe, I. A. (1973). *New England J. Med.* **288**, 630.

Janoff, A. (1972). *Annu. Rev. Med.* **23**, 177.

Jaques, J., Huber, G., Neipp, L., Rossi, A., Schaer, B., and Meier, R. (1967). *Experientia* **23**, 149.

Jaques, R., and Riesterer, L. (1971). *Pharmacology* **6**, 29.

Kalbhen, D. A. (1972). *Abstr. Pap. Int. Congr. Pharmacol., 5th, 1972* p. 118.

Kalley, K. R., and Doerge, R. F. (1972). *J. Pharm. Sci.* **61**, 949.

Kimura, E. T., Young, P, R., Dodge, P. W., and Sweet, L. R. (1972). *Arch. Int. Pharmacodyn. Ther.* **196**, 213.

Komatsu, T., Awata, H., Sakai, Y., Inukai, T., Yamamoto, M., Inaba, S., and Yamamoto, H. (1972). *Arzneim.-Forsch.* **22**, 1958.

Kosersky, D. S., and Malone, M. H. (1971). *J. Pharm. Sci.* **60**, 952.

Krapcho, J., and Turk, C. F. (1970). *Abstr. Pap., 160th Nat. Meet. Amer. Chem. Soc.,* MEDI, 42.

Kuehl, F. A., Jr., Cirillo, V. J., Ham, E. A., and Humes, J. L. (1973). *Advan. Biosci.* **9**, 155.

Lan, S. J., and Schreiber, E. C. (1972). *Abstr., 13th Nat. Meet., Acad. Pharm. Sci., 1972* p. 104.

Levy, L., and McClure, D. A. (1972). *Proc. West. Pharmacol. Soc.* **15**, 22v.

McNeil, T. A. (1972). *Antimicrob. Ag. Chemother.* **1**, 6.

McNeil, T. A., Fleming, W. A., McClure, S. F., and Killen, M. (1972). *Antimicrob. Ag. Chemother.* 1, 1.

Malley, A., and Baecher, L. (1971). *J. Immunol.* 107, 586.

Merck. (1972). U.S. Patent 3,654,291.

Millonig, R. C., Wojnar, R. J., Goldlust, M. B., Turkheimer, A. R., Schreiber, W. F., Brittain, R. J., and Krapcho, J. (1971). *Abstr., 162nd Nat. Meet, Amer. Chem. Soc.* MEDI. 50.

Nakamura, H., Kadokawa, T., Nakatsuji, K., and Nakamura, K. (1970). *Arzneim.-Forsch.* 20, 1032 and 1579.

Nakanishi, M., Imamura, H., and Maruyama, Y. (1970). *Arzneim.-Forsch.* 20, 998–1003.

Nucifora, T. L., and Malone, M. H. (1971). *Arch. Int. Pharmacodyn. Ther.* 191, 345.

Omaye, S. T., Kosersky, D. S., and Malone, M. H. (1972). *Proc. West Pharmacol. Soc.* 15, 205.

Pinals, R. S., Harris, E. D., Frizzel, J., and Gerber, D. A. (1973). *Arthr. Rheum.* 16, 126.

Rips, R., Lachaeize, M., Albert, O., and Dupont, M. (1971). *Chim. Ther.* 6, 126.

Rocha e Silva, M., Cavalcanti, R. Q., and Reis, M. L. (1969). *Biochem. Pharmacol.* 18, 1285.

Roussel-UCLAF. (1968). French Medicament 6,158; *Chem. Abstr.* 72, 066976 (1972).

Rüegg, M., Riesterer, L., and Jaques, R. (1972). *Pharmacology* 7, 51.

Saeki, K. (1972). *Arch. Int. Pharmacodyn. Ther.* 195, 33.

Sandoz-Wander. (1971). U.S. Patent 3,563,990.

Shen, T. Y., Li, J. P., Dorn, C. P., Ebel, D., Bugianesi, R., and Fecher, R. (1972). *Carbohy. Res.* 23, 87.

Shen, T. Y., Ham, E. A., Cirillo, V. J., and Zanetti, M. (1974). "Proceedings of International Symposium on Prostaglandin Synthetase Inhibitors," Nov. 1973, Raven Press, New York (in press).

Spencer, H. J., Runser, R. H., Berger, F. M., Tarnowski, G. S., and Mathé, G. (1972). *Proc. Soc. Exp. Biol. Med.* 140, 1156.

Sumitomo. (1971). South African Patent 70/05270; *Chem. Abstr.* 76, 129828 (1972).

Szmuszkovicz, J., Glenn, E. M., Heinzelman, R. V., Hester, J. B., Jr., and Youngdale, G. A. (1966). *J. Med. Chem.* 9, 527.

Tanaka, K., and Iizuka, Y. (1972). *J. Pharm. Soc. Jap.* 92, 1.

Tanaka, K., Iizuka, Y., Yoshida, N., Tomita, K., and Masuda, H. (1972). *Experientia* 28, 937.

Umezawa, H., Aoyagi, T., Morishima, H., Matsuzaki, M., Hamda, M., and Takeuchi, T. (1970). *J. Antibiot.* 23, 259.

Ward, J. R., Klauber, M., Gleichert, J. E., Willkens, R. F., Rotstein, J., Katz, W. A., and Pierce, W. E. (1973). *J. Clin. Pharmacol.*, p. 218.

Whitehouse, M. W. (1971). *Proc. West. Pharmacol. Soc.* 14, 55.

Wong, S. (1972). *Abstr. Pap. 13th Nat. Meet. Acad. Pharm. Sci., 1972* p. 99.

Vane, J. R. (1971). *Nature (New Biology)* 231, 232.

Vane, J. R. (1973). *Advan. Biosci.* 9, 395.

Chapter 8

Design and Laboratory Evaluation of Gold Compounds as Antiinflammatory Agents

DONALD T. WALZ, MICHAEL J. DIMARTINO,
AND BLAINE M. SUTTON

Smith Kline & French Laboratories
Philadelphia, Pennsylvania

I. INTRODUCTION*

The rationale for chrysotherapy in the treatment of rheumatoid arthritis has its roots deep in empiricism. The use of gold in medicine dates back as far as the eighth century (Smit, 1968; Ellery, 1954; Block and Van Goor, 1959a).

*Editors' note: Nomenclature in this area is vague. The general term "gold" is used in different senses to mean (a) any of the therapeutically effective gold compounds in use, (b) the metal atom in whatever forms or oxidation states it exists after administration to man

The use of gold as a tonic, as an alterative, and as a cure for dipsomania cannot be documented. The basis of the early use of gold probably stems from folklore associated with previous metals, and thus the perpetuation of the adage "gold cures all ills."

The use of gold compounds in the treatment of rheumatoid arthritis was knit to the similarity of the clinical manifestation between tuberculosis and rheumatoid arthritis and was unraveled to a single thread by the observation of Robert Koch (1890), who reported on the ability of gold cyanide compounds to inhibit the growth of tubercle bacilli. The early clinical use of gold was further supported by other investigators for the treatment of lupus vulgaris (Bruck and Glück, 1913) and pulmonary tuberculosis (Junker, 1913). The use of gold in diseases other than tuberculosis was first tried by Landé (1927). His report on the use of gold thioglucose (1) in the treatment

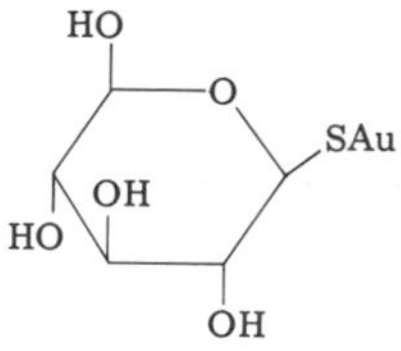

1

of bacterial endocarditis and observation that joint pain was relieved in these patients led him to the conclusion that gold compounds would be beneficial in the treatment of arthritis. Landé's results were not supported by reports by Pick (1927), who could not find any beneficial results in arthritis after the treatment with gold.

The laying of the cornerstone of modern chrysotherapy could be attributed to Forestier (1929, 1932, 1963), who reported positive results in patients with ankylosing spondylitis after treatment with gold compounds. Through the

Editor's note continued

---

or animal, (c) the equivalent metal atom content of a drug or dosage form, or (d) metallic gold, usually qualified as such or as colloidal. There is a practice of referring to the therapeutic gold thio compounds as "gold salts" that we have avoided. This term implies a negligible or fleeting role for the ligand portion of these compounds, which is not the case (Section II,C,3). It also is not consistent with their properties, which include nonconductivity (for compounds without other ionizable groups, Section II,D). The unusual gold–ligand bond strength in Au–S, Au–P, and Au–Cl compounds is attributed to covalent bonding involving d electrons of gold and the p orbitals of the second atom (Dyatkina and Syrkin, 1960). Nuclear quadrupole resonance allows estimation that the Au–Cl bond in $AuCl_4^-$ has 69% covalent character (Sasane et al., 1971). This may be even greater for gold–sulfur and gold–phosphorus bonds.

years conflicting reports on the efficacy of these compounds in the treatment of arthritis stimulated a number of controlled studies that bore out the observations of the early investigators, (Snyder, 1939; Ellman and Lawrence, 1940; Fraser, 1945). Attempts to unequivocally settle the question of efficacy were always plagued by factors that obscured the real assessment of the compounds of their merits as therapeutic agents. It was not until 1958 that the question of gold's efficacy was finally answered, when the Empire Rheumatism Council (E.R.C.) conducted a well-controlled double-blind study with gold sodium thiomalate (2) in a large patient population. The results (Empire

$$\underset{\textstyle 2}{\overset{\textstyle CH_2CO_2Na}{\underset{|}{AuSCHCO_2Na}}}$$

Rheumatism Council, 1961) showed that by practically all criteria improvement was observed, the exception being improvement evidenced by X-ray examination. These beneficial results were even evident after therapy had been stopped and persisted for more than a year. Sigler *et al.* (1972), in a double-blind study, confirmed the results of the E.R.C. study and extended these findings, describing positive radiological evidence that chrysotherapy significantly slowed the progression of the disease in joints of rheumatoid arthritic patients.

The etiology of rheumatoid arthritis is unknown and although a multiplicity of mechanisms are proposed for the disease, to date there is no evidence pointing to a salient one. To further complicate this complex disease the exact mechanism by which clinically used agents alter or palliatively treat the course of disease is unknown, although many hypotheses exist. Because experimentation in man is not possible, we are left with laboratory models to explain and define what we see in man. The laboratory models detect almost all of the clinically used agents, but as in the human counterpart, the mechanisms by which the end effect is achieved are not clearly defined. Gold compounds are probably the one class of agents used to date that successfully alter the course of rheumatoid arthritis and can bring about remission. This activity is also seen in the laboratory models. It is because of this edge that basic laboratory research should be continued and increased to probe the mechanisms by which gold exerts its effects (efficacy and toxicity). Hopefully the fruits of this research will open up new horizons for the future design of new chemical agents and laboratory models, both of which will contribute to curing the disease.

II. LABORATORY EVALUATION OF GOLD COMPOUNDS

A. Efficacy

1. INFECTIOUS ARTHRITIS

Gold compounds were reported to suppress infectious arthritis caused by a number of microorganisms in rodents (Sabin and Warren, 1940; Preston *et al.*, 1942; Findlay *et al.*, 1940; Wiesinger, 1965; Tripi and Kuzell, 1947; Kuzell *et al.*, 1952; Rothbard *et al*, 1941; Jasmin, 1957). This activity of gold compounds was attributed to their bactericidal effects (Findlay *et al.*, 1940; Rothbard *et al.*, 1941), although some investigators could not demonstrate antimicrobial activity of therapeutic gold compounds on the etiological agents (Sabin and Warren, 1940; Wiesinger, 1965). Sabin and Warren (1940) demonstrated that certain gold compounds exerted a dose-related curative effect on an experimental chronic arthritis in mice produced by pleuro-pneumonialike organisms (PPLO). Utilizing this arthritic model, they were able to quantitate the differences in therapeutic effectiveness of various gold compounds that exhibited different physical–chemical properties. The greatest and most rapid therapeutic activity was obtained with soluble inorganic and organic compounds. With insoluble compounds the therapeutic effect was markedly delayed. In the colloidal state, gold had no therapeutic properties. Sabin and Warren (1940) also investigated the toxicity of gold compounds and were able to demonstrate a wide range in the chemotherapeutic index of the different compounds. Apparently, the mode of action of gold in these experiments was not related to antimicrobial activity because neither an effective gold compound (gold sodium thiomalate) nor the blood of treated mice prevented the growth of the etiological agent *in vitro*.

Preston *et al.* (1942) confirmed the chemotherapeutic results of Sabin and Warren (1940) and showed that the therapeutic effects observed in mice were dependent on the presence of gold in the compounds and not results of the sulfur or sulfhydryl components alone.

Findlay *et al.* (1940) reported that organic gold preparations were highly active in preventing arthritis caused by several PPLO types in rats and mice. They attributed this activity to the effect of gold on the microorganisms because the organic gold compounds had a specific action in preventing the growth *in vivo* and *in vitro* of PPLO isolated from rodents.

Kuzell *et al*, (1952) produced PPLO arthritis in rats but were unable to reproduce the mouse arthritis. They reported that the gold compounds, gold thioglucose and gold sodium thiosulfate (**3**) given at the time of infection prevented the development of PPLO-induced arthritis in rats.

Wiesinger (1965) utilized a grip function test to evaluate the effectiveness of various antiphlogistics on *Mycoplasma* arthritis in rats. It was found that Allochrysine (gold sodium 3-thio-2-propanol-1-sulfonate, **4**), given in several doses prophylactically or therapeutically, produced an inhibition of arthritic symptoms that manifested itself in the elimination or diminution of the paw swelling and in improved grip function. It was noted that Allochrysine *in vitro* had no inhibitory effect on the growth of *Mycoplasma*.

$$Na_3Au(S_2O_3)_2 \qquad\qquad \overset{\displaystyle OH}{AuSCH_2CHCH_2SO_3Na}$$

$$\textbf{3} \qquad\qquad\qquad\qquad \textbf{4}$$

Rothbard *et al.* (1941) reported that gold sodium thiomalate was an effective chemotherapeutic agent in the prevention of arthritis produced by a hemolytic streptococcus in rats but noted that the effective dose was close to the lethal dose. They also reported that gold sodium thiomalate did not cure established arthritis and was bactericidal under anaerobic conditions *in vitro*.

Jasmin (1957) showed that gold sodium thiomalate was effective in preventing experimentally induced arthritis produced by Murphy Rat Lymphosarcoma exudate in intact or adrenalectomized rats. This result suggested that the action of gold sodium thiomalate is not mediated by the adrenals.

Although gold compounds have been shown to be effective in infectious arthritis produced by various microorganisms, the lack of antimicrobial activity reported by some investigators (Sabin and Warren, 1940; Wiesinger, 1965) suggests that gold compounds may alter a pathological process of arthritis instead of acting on the infectious microorganisms per se.

2. RAT PAW EDEMA

The inhibitory effects of gold compounds on experimental arthritis induced by various infectious agents (Section II,A,1) suggest that gold may alter the inflammatory process. This possibility is further supported by reports (Vykydal *et al.*, 1956; Gujral and Saxena, 1956) that gold sodium thiomalate exhibited therapeutic activity in experimental formaldehyde arthritis in rats. Sancilio (1969) reported that gold sodium thiomalate reduced Evans blue–carrageenan-induced pleural effusion in rats, and he has been able to determine its relative potency to other nonsteroidal antirheumatic drugs. However, it is apparent from the lack of reports in the literature that the antiinflammatory activity of gold compounds has not been extensively studied in frequently used rat paw edema assays. In several experiments in our laboratories (unpublished data), we have found that a single, high intramuscular dose (44 mg/kg) of gold thiomalate significantly inhibited carrageenan-induced paw edema in intact rats but was inactive in adrenal-ectomized rats.

A lower dose (22 mg/kg, i.m.) of gold sodium thiomalate produced less effective and inconsistent results. In contrast to results obtained in the carrageenan-induced edema assay, gold sodium thiomalate administered intramuscularly at doses of 40, 20, or 10 mg/kg did not significantly inhibit rat paw edema induced by 0.1 ml of 20% brewer's yeast suspension (unpublished data). Because the efficacy of gold compounds in rheumatoid arthritis is delayed (Freyberg, 1966; Freyberg *et al.*, 1972) it may be worthwhile to evaluate the antiinflammatory activity of gold preparations on various rat paw edema assays following extended drug administration.

3. ADJUVANT ARTHRITIS

Adjuvant arthritis in rats has been widely used to evaluate the antiarthritic efficacy of various agents and is considered by some investigators to be one of the best available models of rheumatoid arthritis. This belief is based on the clinical and pathological similarities of adjuvant arthritis to the human disease (Pearson, 1963; Katz and Piliero, 1969; Walz *et al.*, 1971a), the ability of the model to detect most classes of antiarthritic drugs (Newbould, 1963; Graeme *et al.*, 1966; Ward and Cloud, 1966; Winter and Nuss, 1966; Walz *et al.*, 1971b), and its minimal sensitivity to nonspecific biologically active compounds (Walz *et al.*, 1971b). This assay is described in detail in Chapter 2 by Swingle, in Volume II. Briefly, adjuvant arthritis is induced in rats by a single intradermal injection of heat-killed *Mycobacterium butyricum* suspended in oil. The injected site becomes inflamed and represents the primary (non-immune) lesion. Disseminated secondary lesions occur after a delay of approximately 10 days and are believed to be the result of a cellular-type hypersensitivity reaction. Newbould (1963) reported that the development of adjuvant-induced inflammatory lesions were suppressed by gold sodium thiomalate. However, Jessop and Currey (1968) have failed to· confirm these results. In light of these conflicting reports, we (Walz *et al.*, 1971c) have reevaluated the activity of gold sodium thiomalate in adjuvant arthritis. Utilizing highly inbred (Lewis) rats as experimental animals and a volume-displacement apparatus to measure the inflammatory lesions, we have found that gold sodium thiomalate significantly inhibited both the primary and the secondary lesions of adjuvant arthritis in a dose-related manner (Section IV; Figs. 1, 2, and 3). The resulting serum gold levels following daily administration of gold sodium thiomalate were also dose related and were negatively correlated ($P < 0.05$) to the severity of the secondary lesions. The results of these experiments indicate that adjuvant arthritis provides an experimental model by which the antiinflammatory efficacy of gold compounds can be quantitatively compared. We have recently (Walz et al., 1972) used this animal model to compare the anti-arthritic potency of a new orally active gold compound to parenterally administered gold sodium thiomalate (Section IV).

B. Proposed Mechanisms of Action

1. ANTIMICROBIAL

The inception of gold therapy for rheumatoid arthritis was based on the belief that rheumatoid arthritis was a form of tubercular joint disease and the knowledge that gold compounds exhibited bactericidal effects on tubercle bacilli (Section I). Although tubercle bacilli have been ruled out as possible etiologic agents in rheumatoid arthritis, other microorganisms have long been considered as possible causative agents in rheumatoid arthritis. A relationship between PPLO infections and rheumatoid arthritis has been suggested and these organisms have been isolated from the rheumatoid arthritic joint (Bartholomew, 1965; Moore and Redmond, 1965; Thomas, 1970; Jansson et al., 1971). Recently, Jansson et al. (1971) isolated a *Mycoplasma* from every one of 27 patients studied, whereas 24 synovial specimens from cases of traumatic joint lesion were found to be negative for *Mycoplasma*. The possibility that gold compounds may act on an infectious agent was recently suggested (Lewis and Ziff, 1966; Persellin et al., 1967) and was based on evidence that gold therapy reduced the titer of rheumatoid factor in rheumatoid arthritic patients but failed to influence the titer of rheumatoid-like factor in experimental animals. These authors suggested that the decrease in titer observed in man might well be a consequence of the elimination or suppression of an infectious agent ordinarily serving as the underlying antigen for the sustained synthesis of the factor in the rheumatoid patient.

A number of investigators (Robinson et al., 1952; Newsham and Chu, 1965; Davidson and Thomas, 1966; Stewart et al., 1969) have shown that gold sodium thiomalate suppresses the growth of *Mycoplasma in vitro*. However, the results are variable (Robinson et al., 1952; Newsham and Chu, 1965; Stewart et al., 1969) and depend on the gold concentration, *Mycoplasma* species, and inoculum size. Low concentrations of gold have been reported to be more effective in suppressing *Mycoplasma* growth than higher gold concentration (Robinson et al., 1952; Newsham and Chu, 1965; Davidson and Thomas, 1966; Findlay et al., 1940). This "zone phenomenon" has also been noted (Findlay et al., 1940) to occur with the bactericidal action of organic gold compounds on tubercle bacilli *in vitro*. It is interesting that mercaptoethanol and cysteine protected *M. gallisepticum* from gold inhibition (Davidson and Thomas, 1966). This protective effect suggests that the antimicrobial activity of gold compounds may be caused by their reactivity with sulfhydryl groups.

In rodents, gold compounds have been reported to suppress infectious arthritis caused by PPLO (Findlay *et al.*, 1940; Sabin and Warren, 1940; Preston *et al.*, 1942; Wiesinger, 1965; Tripi and Kuzell, 1947; Kuzell *et al.*, 1952), hemolytic streptococcus (Rothbard *et al.*, 1941), and Murphy Rat Lymphosarcoma exudate (Jasmin, 1957). The antiarthritic activity exhibited by gold compounds in certain infectious arthritic models was apparently caused by their bactericidal effects (Findlay *et al.*, 1940; Rothbard *et al.*, 1941), although other investigators (Sabin and Warren, 1940; Wiesinger, 1965) have failed to demonstrate an antimicrobial activity of gold compounds and so could not attribute their antiarthritic activity to an effect on the microorganisms.

Because gold preparations can exhibit antiarthritic activity in experimental arthritis independent of antimicrobial activity, and because no pathogen is as yet identified as the cause of rheumatoid arthritis, the relevance of the antimicrobial activity exhibited by gold compounds remains questionable.

2. IMMUNOLOGICAL RESPONSE

Clinical and experimental evidence suggests that immunologic processes are involved in the pathogenicity of rheumatoid arthritis. It is possible that gold compounds exert their therapeutic effect in rheumatoid arthritis by altering immune responses via inhibition of lysosomal enzymes and/or antigen–antibody reactions. The effect of gold preparations on immune reactions is evidenced by their ability to prolong the survival time of skin homografts in mice and to inhibit lymphocyte proliferative responses and sensitization of rat mast cells. In contrast, antibody titers and delayed hypersensitivity have been found to be unaffected by gold compounds.

It has been reported that the survival time of skin homografts in mice can be prolonged by the injection of aurothiopolypeptide (Scheiffarth *et al.*, 1970). Fikrig and Smithwick (1968) found that peripheral blood lymphocytes from rheumatoid arthritic patients receiving gold treatment did not respond to the blastogenic effects of streptolysin S. Gold thioglucose has been reported to inhibit the Schwartzman phenomenon (Szilágyi *et al.*, 1968). As the blastogenic effects of streptolysin S and the Schwartzman phenomenon are believed to be mediated by lysosomal enzyme release, the inhibitory effects of gold on these reactions may be caused by enzyme inactivation. Persellin *et al.* (1967) reported that gold sodium thiomalate did not affect immune response in animals. Utilizing different antigen systems, they have also found that it did not affect delayed hypersensitivity in guinea pigs or circulating antibody production in rabbits. The level of rheumatoid-factor-like substance in hyperimmunized rabbits was also not affected by gold treatment. Norn (1968) also demonstrated that production of antibodies was not inhibited by gold (gold sodium thiosulfate), although he observed a reduction in histamine release from peritoneal mast cells of gold-treated rats sensitized to horse serum. Norn (1968) postulated that this reduction was caused by inhibition of the antigen-antibody reaction or of the enzymatic processes initiated in the mast cells.

Kuzell and Dreisbach (1948) reported that gold sodium thiosulfate failed to protect guinea pigs against lethal doses of histamine and anaphylactic shock and did not alter the Arthus phenomenon in rabbits. Jessop and Currey (1968) reported that gold sodium thiomalate administered to rats did not suppress the primary antibody response to sheep erythrocytes, delayed skin reaction to tuberculin, or adjuvant-induced arthritis. Other investigators (Newbould, 1963; Walz *et al.*, 1971c), however, demonstrated that gold sodium thiomalate suppressed the development of adjuvant arthritic lesions. We have shown (Walz *et al*, 1971c) that gold sodium thiomalate significantly decreased both the nonimmune (primary lesion) and immune (secondary lesion) inflammation of adjuvant arthritis (Section II,A,3). However, it did not appreciably inhibit antibody production to sheep erythrocytes or cutaneous hypersensitivity to purified protein derivative in adjuvant arthritic rats (unpublished data). In order to determine if gold compounds alter cellular hypersensitivity, we evaluate their effects on experimental allergic encephalomyelitis (EAE) in rats. Gold sodium thiomalate and gold thioglucose significantly delayed the onset of EAE in female Lewis rats but did not inhibit its development (unpublished data). The ability of gold compounds to delay the onset of EAE in rats was also reported by Gerber *et al.* (1972b). These authors suggested that gold preparations might act as antiinjury agents in target tissues through their apparent antiinflammatory properties. In support of this view, we observed a similar delaying effect on EAE in rats following administration of nonsteroidal antiinflammatory drugs, whereas immunosuppressive agents prevented the disease.

It is evident from the above observations that gold compounds do not markedly alter immunological responses of either the immediate or cellular type. The positive results obtained in certain immunological responses appear to be caused by inhibition of (enzymatic) mediators released during the immune response.

3. ENZYME INHIBITION

Evidence obtained from morphological, biochemical, and experimental investigations has strongly implicated lysosomal enzymes in the pathogenesis of rheumatoid arthritis. The role of lysosomes in rheumatoid arthritis has been extensively reviewed by several investigators (Thomas, 1967; Barrett, 1970; Persellin, 1968; Weissman, 1966, 1967, 1972; Chayen and Bitensky, 1971). Because clinically used gold compounds are heavy metal mercaptides, it has been suggested that their mode of action is directed at sulfhydryl groups of enzymes (Ragan and Boots, 1947; Libenson, 1945).

Persellin and Ziff (1966) have shown that gold sodium thiomalate inhibits the lysosomal enzymes acid phosphatase and β-glucuronidase of guinea pig peritoneal macrophage. Their results indicate that the gold derivative was actively transported intracellularly and concentrated in lysosomes. These authors suggested that gold compounds may act by inhibiting lysosomal enzymes of phagocytic cells in the inflamed synovial tissue.

Ennis *et al.* (1968) reported that gold preparations inhibited lysosomal enzymes *in vitro* at concentrations comparable to those found in plasma during gold therapy. The mechanism of gold inhibition appeared to be via the binding of sulfhydryl groups. These investigators reported that gold thiomalate and gold thioglucose produced a marked inhibition of acid phosphatase, β-glucuronidase, and cathepsin from both rabbit liver lysosomes and human synovial fluid. This inhibition was reversible by the addition of a sulfhydryl compound, and other sulfhydryl-binding agents were found to produce similar inhibition when incubated with the free enzymes. Their results also indicated that the enzyme inhibition was not caused by gold competition with other metals required for enzyme activity or by protective effects on the release of the hydrolases from lysosomes.

Enzymes involved in connective tissue metabolism have also been reported to be inhibited by gold compounds (Bollett and Shuster, 1960; Fujihira *et al.*, 1971). Bollett and Shuster (1960) reported that the amount of gold in rheumatoid arthritic patients treated with these agents was sufficient to suppress the synthesis of glucosamine 6-phosphate through enzyme inhibition *in vitro* and that the administration of gold to albino rats resulted in decreased enzyme activity in connective tissue. These observations lend support to the concept that gold may favorably alter enzyme function in patients with rheumatoid arthritis. Fujihira *et al.* (1971) reported that the *in vitro* synthesis of glucosamine 6-phosphate was inhibited by gold thiomalate, as well as nonsteroidal antiinflammatory drugs. They also found a markedly high activity of glucosamine 6-phosphate synthetase in the inflamed hind paws of adjuvant arthritic rats and good correlation was observed between the increase of enzyme activity and the hind paw swelling as the adjuvant disease developed. Because glucosamine 6-phosphate synthesis is a limiting step in the biosynthesis of mucopolysaccharides, the inhibition of this enzyme by antiarthritic drugs may have clinical significance in view of the altered connective tissue metabolism observed in inflammation. The activity of many enzymes that are required for biosynthesis of mucopolysaccharides depends on the presence of certain trace metals. The observation that the concentrations of these trace metals were abnormal in blood serum and synovial fluid in rheumatoid arthritis (Niedermeier and Griggs, (1971) has suggested to Niedermeier et al. (1971) that the therapeutic action of gold may be mediated through an effect on trace metal metabolism. These investigators found that the concentrations of certain trace metals in blood serum shifted toward the concentrations observed in normal blood serum in response to chrysotherapy and postulated that gold may displace certain essential trace metals from their abnormal binding sites, thus modifying a series of disease-producing events.

Gold compounds were also shown to uncouple oxidation phosphorylation. Whitehouse (1965) noted that gold sodium thiosulfate was a potent uncoupling agent that was effective at 0.3 mM in vitro; whereas, gold sodium thiomalate uncoupled oxidation phosphorylation of isolated liver mitochondria at a relatively higher level (2.5 mM). Whitehouse further noted that the more water-soluble gold preparations, such as gold thioglucose and sodium aurothiopropanol sulfonate, failed to uncouple oxidative phosphorylation, and he suggested that their activity in vivo might be caused by their transformation within the body to less hydrophilic compounds or complexes.

4. PROTEIN INTERACTION

Rheumatic diseases, arthritis, and secondary inflammation in general are characterized by a disturbance of the plasma colloids that is caused not only by a relative increase in the less hydrophilic protein fractions but also by the appearance of abnormal fractions (Silvestrini, 1968). Sera from certain patients with rheumatoid arthritis have been reported to be abnormal in electrophoretic, ultracentrifugal, and serologic patterns (Franklin et al., 1958). It has been suggested that biochemical abnormalities found in connective tissue diseases reflect in vivo denaturation of proteins and formation of macroglobulins that may render the proteins antigenic and play a role in inflammation associated with rheumatoid arthritis (Lorber et al., 1964; Gerber, 1965). Furthermore, several reports suggest that denaturation of protein may cause certain types of allergic and nonspecific inflammation (Ishizaka and Campbell, 1959; Ishizaka and Ishizaka, 1960; Opie, 1962, 1963). The above observations suggest that protein denaturation may be involved in the initiation and perpetuation of rheumatoid arthritis instead of in the secondary effects of inflammation. Silvestrini (1968) proposed a working hypothesis in an attempt to link antirheumatic action with the ability to stabilize proteins. He suggested that the ability to protect proteins from denaturation is a particular property of nonsteroidal, antirheumatic drugs and that drugs that combat inflammation of the primary type (normal systemic reactivity) are only slightly active in arthritis and are devoid of antidenaturant effects. Gerber (1964) reported that heat and urea denaturation of bovine serum albumin was altered in the presence of gold thiomalate. The denatured albumin formed in the presence of this compound resembled that formed in the presence of reagents that prevent the sulfhydryl–disulfide interchange reaction.

Gerber (1971) also reported that gold sodium thiomalate inhibited heat-induced aggregation of human γ-globulin. He postulated that the rather specific antiinflammatory effects of gold sodium thiomalate in rheumatoid arthritis may be caused by its effect on the formation of aggregated γ-globulin, which is believed to be inflammatory, antigenic, and a stimulus for the formation of rheumatoid factors.

Lorber et al. (1972) suggested that the distribution of gold binding to various serum proteins may relate to its therapeutic action. These authors compared the serum protein distribution of gold at high serum gold levels, attained by adjusting gold dosage, with the lower levels characterizing the regimen in current use. They found that with conventional chrysotherapy the majority of gold was bound to albumin, whereas with attainment of higher serum gold levels there was progressively increased and significant binding to other serum protein fractions, including those proteins (immunoglobulin and complement) thought to be instrumental in the pathogenesis of rheumatic disorders. These authors considered it possible that the increased binding of gold (observed at higher gold levels) to immune complexes may enhance the access of gold to cells involved in phagocytosis of such complexes.

Gold has also been reported to react with collagen (Adam et al., 1964, 1965a,b, 1968; Adam and Kühn, 1968). Adam et al. (1964, 1965a,b) have shown that gold reacts with rat tail collagen when administered as the thiosulfate complex resulting in increased number of crosslinkages in collagen and higher structural stability. In further studies to elucidate the mechanics of the reaction, Adam and Kühn (1968) reported that the administration of gold sodium thiosulfate to rats produced a hardening of the collagen that was attributed to crosslinkage of the fibrils by the gold ion. The gold complex was apparently first taken up into the fibril by virtue of electrostatic forces and, in a second slower reaction, the thiosulfate groups were displaced by the side chain groups resulting in the crosslinkage. Adam *et al*. (1968) have also investigated biochemical changes in the collagen of rat skin following administration of gold sodium thiosulfate to normal and lathyritic rats. They demonstrated that the insoluble collagen content was increased and that the lathyritic effect was partly reversed. The gold sodium thiosulfate thus reacted with the insoluble collagen introducing additional crosslinks. Adam and Kühn (1968) have assumed that stabilization of the collagen fibrils causes reduced reactivity of the collagen, which may have an important effect on the pathological process in connective tissue. Adam *et al*. (1968) noted that the increase in the crosslinking of collagen decreased its liability to denaturation and to subsequent enzymatic degradation with the formation of products that may act as antigens. These authors speculated that the higher degree of collagen crosslinking induced by gold may affect the genesis and course of the disease because of a possible decrease in the rate of autoantigen formation. Furthermore, the decreased capacity of gold-treated collagen for swelling and increased resistance to enzymatic attack may be of relevance to other pathological processes in connective tissue.

5. SULFHYDRYL GROUP REACTIVITY

Serum protein sulfhydryl–disulfide interchange reactions are believed to play important roles in various biological phenomena, including protein denaturation, blood clotting, and cell division (Jensen, 1959). Subnormal levels of serum sulfhydryl groups have been observed in various connective tissue diseases, including rheumatoid arthritis (Lorber *et al*., 1964, 1971; Kosaka, 1970), and some researchers have suggested that this abnormality is a reflection of biochemical defects that may be involved in the initiation and perpetuation of this disease.

Gerber *et al*. (1965) reported an inability of N-ethylmaleimide or cysteine to alter the viscosity of heated serum of patients with rheumatoid arthritis and suggested that rheumatoid serum protein might be characterized by increased disulfide interchange.

Lorber *et al*. (1964) also postulated that impaired sulfhydryl group reactivity in rheumatoid arthritis might be caused by accelerated formation of disulfide bonds, which could result in macroglobulin formation, protein denaturation, and autoimmunity.

Because currently used gold drugs are heavy metal mercaptides, it has been frequently suggested that their biological activity is caused by reactivity with sulfhydryl groups. Various investigators have demonstrated that the sulfhydryl reactivity of gold compounds plays a role in their inhibition of lysosomal enzyme activity (Ennis *et al*., 1968), protein denaturation (Gerber, 1964), and *Mycoplasma* growth (Davidson and Thomas, 1966). In order to measure directly the sulfhydryl group reactivity of standard gold compounds, we have evaluated the effects of gold sodium thiomalate and gold thioglucose on a sulfhydryl–disulfide interchange reaction between rat serum sulfhydryl groups and dithiobisnitrobenzoic acid (Walz and DiMartino, 1972). The clinically used golds were found to produce a potent, dose-related inhibition of the interchange reaction rate following their *in vitro* administration. Gold sodium thiomalate inhibited the interchange reaction rate by 50% at an estimated concentration of 13 μg gold per milliliter and was calculated to be 2.9 (2.6–3.2) times more potent than gold thioglucose in this procedure. In *in vivo* experiments, the administration of gold sodium thiomalate at a single intramuscular dose of 20 mg gold per kilogram produced a marked decrease in rat serum reactivity with dithiobisnitrobenzoic acid. These results suggest that the sulfhydryl–disulfide interchange reaction utilizing rat serum sulfhydryl groups is a sensitive and quantitative procedure to measure sulfhydryl group reactivity of gold compounds following their *in vitro* or *in vivo* administration.

C. Metabolism

The metabolism of gold compounds has been extensively investigated in attempts to gain insight into the therapeutic and toxicological mechanisms of these agents and to determine the optimal combination of gold preparations, route of administration, and dosing regimen that can provide improvement in drug efficacy with minimal toxicity.

Although this section is divided into separate topics of absorption, transport, distribution and retention and excretion for convenience of presentation, it is important to bear in mind that these topics are significantly interrelated.

1. ABSORPTION

Most investigators have utilized blood levels of gold as an indicator of drug absorption. It is obvious, however, that blood concentration of gold also depends on other factors, such as dosing schedule, excretion rates, and tissue retention. Freyberg *et al.* (1941) have shown that the soluble gold compounds, gold sodium thiomalate and gold sodium thiosulfate were rapidly absorbed from intramuscular sites in humans. These compounds produced maximum plasma gold levels within 1 hour after injection and remained at high levels for at least 24 hours. Although the plasma gold levels were related to the amount of gold injected, they were not proportional to the weekly intake of gold. Freyberg *et al.* (1942) have further substantiated the rapid absorption of soluble gold compounds by demonstrating that plasma gold levels following intravenous and intramuscular injections were essentially the same. When soluble gold thioglucose was suspended in oil, however, a slower rate of absorption was observed.

Similar findings concerning gold absorption were obtained in recent studies utilizing atomic absorption spectrophotometric methods (Mascarenhas *et al.*, 1972). Gold sodium thiomalate and gold thioglucose were rapidly absorbed from injection sites and reached peak blood levels between 4 and 6 hours. Although the absorption of gold sodium thioglucose suspended in oil was slightly slower than that of an aqueous solution of gold sodium thiomalate, there were no apparent differences in absorption or excretion between these compounds after the first day of treatment.

In contrast to soluble gold compounds, the administration of insoluble or colloidal gold compounds to humans produced much lower plasma gold levels (Freyberg *et al.*, 1941, 1942). Following administration of insoluble gold calcium thiomalate, practically no gold was absorbed from intramuscular deposits. The plasma gold levels were found to be small and unpredictable. In addition, toxic manifestations were frequently observed.

The injection of colloidal gold sulfide also produced variable results and even when relatively large doses were administered, only small amounts of gold appeared in plasma. Freyberg *et al.* (1942) administered colloidal gold and colloidal gold sulfide intravenously and found that no gold was present in plasma or urine 30 minutes after injection; whereas large amounts of colloidal gold were found phagocytized in the reitculoendothelial cells. Because colloidal particles were found to be quickly phagocytized and held inert in the tissues, colloidal preparations of gold have not been recommended for treatment of rheumatoid arthritis (Freyberg, 1966; Freyberg *et al.*, 1972).

It is apparent from these investigations that in order to be therapeutically effective, injectable gold must be in a form that is readily absorbed. Therefore, current chrysotherapy utilizes the intramuscular injections of soluble gold compounds. Because these are readily absorbed from muscle deposits and because their therapeutic effect is delayed, there appears to be no advantage to intravenous administration (Freyberg, 1966; Freyberg *et al.*, 1972).

The absorption of gold compounds in animals was found to be generally similar to human studies. Block *et al.* (1941, 1942, 1944) studied the absorption of gold in rats following intramuscular administration of various gold compounds by measuring gold levels in both the injected site and in plasma. The soluble crystalline preparations (gold sodium thiosulfate, gold sodium thiomalate, sodium succinimidoaurate (**5**) and gold thioglucose) were rapidly absorbed, whereas the insoluble crystalline preparation (gold calcium thiomalate) was intermediate in rate of absorption and the colloidal preparations (colloidal gold sulfide and colloidal gold) were slowly absorbed. These invest-igators also found that the plasma levels were similar for compounds with similar rates of absorption.

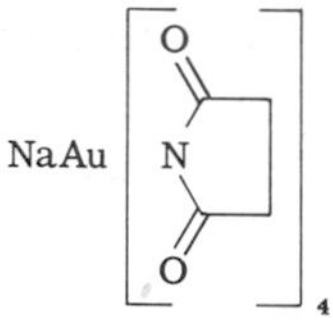

5

Gold thioglucose was also found to be rapidly absorbed in mice following intramuscular or intraperitoneal injections. Peak blood levels of gold were attained in 30–60 minutes. The use of an oil vehicle produced retarded absorption and lower plasma levels (Deter and Liebelt, 1964).

Although gold levels in blood of humans and experimental animals have been a useful indicator of drug absorption, gold blood levels do not appear to correlate with either the therapeutic or toxic effects in man (Freyberg, 1966; Freyberg et al., 1972; Gerber et al., 1972a; Mascarenhas et al., 1972).

In view of their negligible absorption from the gastrointestinal tract, currently used gold preparations must be administered parenterally. How-ever, gold compounds have been developed recently that exhibit signi-ficant absorption and therapeutic activity following oral administration to experimental animals (Sections III and IV). Their therapeutic potential in man awaits further study.

2. TRANSPORT

Freyberg et al. (1941) found that when gold sodium thiomalate and gold sodium thiosulfate were administered intramuscularly to humans, all the gold in the blood appeared in the plasma fraction. There have been disagree-ments, however, on the mechanism by which the gold was transported in the blood. Lawrence (1961) reported that following administration of gold sodium thiomalate to humans, the gold in the plasma appeared to be mostly bound to fibrinogen. However, other investigators found that administration of gold sodium thiomalate to humans (Mascarenhas et al., 1972; Sliwinski, 1968) or rabbits (McQueen and Dykes, 1969) resulted in most of the gold binding to the albumin fraction, whereas no gold was bound to fibrinogen.

As McQueen and Dykes (1969) indicated, however, metabolites of gold sodium thiomalate formed after prolonged treatment, or other gold prepara-tions, may exhibit different binding characteristics.

Lorber *et al.* (1972) confirmed the observation that albumin contained most of the gold in the circulation system, but these investigators found that with higher serum gold levels, attained by adjusting gold dosage, there was a progressive and significant increase in the binding of gold to other serum protein fractions, including proteins (immunoglobulins and complement) thought to be involved in the pathogenesis of rheumatoid arthritis. These authors therefore speculated that the manner by which gold was bound to serum protein fractions might determine its mechanism of action.

3. DISTRIBUTION

Lawrence (1961) found that when radioactive gold sodium thiomalate was injected in rheumatoid patients more gold was present in painful joints than in symptomless joints. Kantor *et al.* (1970), using radioactive gold thioglucose intravenously, also found a high initial accumulation of gold in inflamed joints, which he attributed to increased blood supply. In Lawrence's studies, however, the high levels of radioactive gold remained in painful joints at least 20 days after injection and were not related to plasma levels. This persistence of high levels of gold in painful joints was thought to be caused by gold deposition in articular cartilage and/or gold combination with fibrin deposits.

Gold levels in the synovial fluid of arthritic patients who received gold sodium thiomalate (Freyberg *et al.*, 1941; Lawrence, 1961) or gold thioglucose (Gottlieb *et al.*, 1972) were generally found to be less than or equal to plasma levels. These results suggest that gold does not concentrate in synovial fluid but may diffuse from the plasma.

Gottlieb *et al.* (1972) reported postmortem findings from a patient who had received chrysotherapy which demonstrated that articular and paraarticular tissues exhibited significantly less affinity for gold than the organs of the reticuloendothelial system. Of the articular structures, the synovium had the highest gold concentration and cartilage had the least. Bertrand *et al.* (1948) also demonstrated the great affinity of gold for the synovial membrane compared to other articular tissues. However, Lawrence (1961) found low gold concentration in synovial membrane and attributed this discrepancy to the difference in sampling time postinjection. The tendency of gold to accumulate in areas of inflammation was also observed in animal studies. In rabbits with chemical synovitis, inflamed tissues took up more gold than similar tissues of normal joints (Bertrand *et al.*, 1948). The uptake of gold by these tissues, however, was regarded as nonspecific. Szporny and Ezer (1962; Ezer and Szporny, 1962) found that colloidal gold accumulated in inflamed tissues in rats, but the degree of accumulation decreased with increasing time interval between administration of inflammatory substance and colloidal gold. The accumulation of colloidal gold was thought to be caused by increased capillary permeability.

Gottlieb et al. (1972) observed that although the tissue distribution of gold had been adequately studied in animals, the concentrations of gold in human tissues had not been systematically measured. According to these authors, before their study of one patient no information was available on gold concentration in internal organs or the musculoskeletal system from rheumatoid arthritic patients on long-term chrysotherapy. Gottlieb et al. (1972) examined postmortem specimens from a patient who had received gold thioglucose therapy and found that the highest concentration of gold occurred in the lymph nodes, followed by the adrenal gland, renal cortex, and other organs of the reticuloendothelial system, comparatively low concentrations were found in tissues comprising the joint structure.

Lawrence (1961), utilizing whole body scintillation of patients who received radioactive gold sodium thiomalate, found that within 5 minutes counts were detected in all parts of the trunk and in the proximal parts of the limbs. The highest counts during the first 2 weeks were over the injection site. At the twentieth day, however, levels over the liver, spleen, and kidneys were highest. In renal tissues obtained by biopsy from patients receiving gold sodium thiomalate, gold was found in the glomerular tuft and in macrophages of the interstitial space. Shortly after injection, gold was found in the proximal tubules, but after 1–4 years, more was localized in the distant tubules (Brun et al., 1964).

Root et al. (1954) found that radioactive colloidal gold localized primarily in the reticuloendothelial system following intravenous administration. Most of the gold was present in the liver but did not alter liver function. Sheppard et al. (1947) also found radioactive gold colloid to concentrate in liver and spleen with moderate to low amounts in kidney.

Subepithelial deposits of crystalline gold compounds have also been demonstrated (Rodenhäuser and Behrend, 1969) and corneal and conjunctival deposits are frequently found (Henkind, 1964).

Distribution studies following parenteral administration of various soluble and insoluble gold compounds to rats, rabbits, and guinea pigs have shown that gold accumulates in high concentrations in kidneys, liver, and spleen (Block et al., 1941, 1942, 1944; Jeffrey et al., 1958; Elftman et al., 1946; Bertrand et al., 1948; Rubin et al., 1967).

Gold thioglucose differs from other soluble gold compounds in that it is selectively deposited in the hypothalamus of mice (Debons et al., 1962) and produces hyperphagia and obesity in these animals (Brecher and Waxler, 1949). This specificity of gold thioglucose is believed to be related to structural similarities with the glucoreceptors located in the satiety region of the hypothalamus. Tissue selectivity of other gold compounds has been demonstrated by Rubin *et al.* (1967). In their evaluation of chelation on gold meta-bolism in rats, they have found that the gold carrier was an important determinant in the distribution and excretion of the metal. These authors also suggested that amelioration of gold toxicity by chelation therapy is caused partly by gold redistribution as well as by excretion. The evidence that gold compounds exhibit different distribution patterns suggests the possibility that improved chrysotherapy with decreased toxicity may be achieved by developing gold carriers that provide controlled and selective gold deposition.

4. RETENTION AND EXCRETION

Freyberg *et al.* (1941, 1942) found that following administration of soluble gold compounds to patients with rheumatoid arthritis, gold was excreted chiefly in the urine. The largest amounts of gold were eliminated on the first day and the amount of gold in urine increased with increased dosage. Ap-parently, the larger amounts of gold in urine on injection days did not result from significantly higher plasma levels. The sharp decrease in urinary excretion of gold after the injection day suggested that soon after injection, gold circulated through the kidneys in a state that could be readily elimin-ated. After several hours, however, less gold circulated in this readily excretable form. Fecal excretion of gold was found to be small and irregular. Although slightly larger amounts of gold were excreted in the feces when larger doses were injected, the increased fecal excretion of gold following increased gold dosage was not as consistent as that found with urinary excretion.

Recent results obtained utilizing atomic absorption spectroscopy (Mas-carenhas *et al.*, 1972) were generally similar to results obtained by Freyberg *et al.* (1941, 1942). However, the recent studies found that the amount of gold excreted in feces constituted a considerable portion of the total excre-tion. Although fecal excretion varied considerably among patients, the weekly fecal excretion ranged from about 25 to 64% of the total excretion, and in one patient fecal excretion of gold was consistently greater than that of urine.

It is apparent from excretion data that the bulk of the injected gold is retained in the body during the period of its administration (Freyberg *et al.*, 1941, 1942). Because the excretion of gold does not increase significantly following constant weekly gold doses, the magnitude of gold retention during chrysotherapy becomes great.

After gold therapy is terminated, gold is found in the blood and excreta for long periods of time, the duration of which depends on the size of the weekly dose. The gradual buildup and subsequent prolonged excretion of gold are believed to be responsible for the delayed and long-term benefits and toxicity observed in chrysotherapy.

Block et al. (1941, 1942, 1944) studied the retention and excretion of gold in rats following administration of various gold preparations. The water-soluble compounds were found to be excreted mostly in urine, whereas colloidal gold and insoluble gold calcium thiomalate were excreted more in feces than urine. The rate of excretion of all compounds studied was comparatively rapid during the first 8 days postinjection, followed by a rapid decrease in rate. In general, gold compounds that were most rapidly absorbed were most rapidly excreted. Gold was found to be retained in the liver, spleen, and kidney and to be present in plasma for as long as 85 days after intramuscular injections in rats.

Jeffrey et al. (1958) studied the excretion of radioactive gold calcium thiomalate following single intramuscular injections to rabbits and rats. The rate of excretion reached its maximum about 6 days after injection, when up to 3% of the dose was excreted daily, and then declined. The rates of excretion were similar in both species and after 4 weeks, 40% of the dose had been excreted.

Rubin et al. (1967) studied the effects of various gold-chelating compounds on excretion of gold in rats. The administration of 2,3-dimercapto-propanol (BAL), thiomalic acid, 1,8-diamino-3,6-dimercaptooctane-N, N-tetraacetic acid (BATA), or D,L-penicillamine increased the urinary excretion of gold thioglucose but also caused a concomitant increase in gold concentration in the kidney. Penicillamine and BATA appeared to be the most effective agents because the ratio of urine gold to kidney gold was highest for these compounds. As penicillamine mobilized the most gold, it was thought to be superior to BATA. Rubin et al. (1967) suggested that the most useful compounds for treating gold toxicity were those that induced urinary gold excretion with least deposition in the kidney. Careful attention to renal function is mandatory in the chelate therapy of gold toxicity.

D. Toxicity

Toxic effects produced by gold compounds are usually manifest at areas of penetration into the body, in the organ or tissue of elimination and excretion, and at points where an active cellular turnover is occurring.

The toxicity in man of gold compounds has been reported to involve skin, mucus membranes, liver, hematopoietic organs, kidney, central nervous system, and ocular tissues.

The most frequently encountered toxic effects, clinically, are dermatological (Anonymous, 1961; Forestier, 1963; Freyberg, 1966; Freyberg et al., 1942, 1972). These, as well as other forms of toxicity, usually do not appear until a cumulative dose of 300–400 mg of gold has been injected; these reactions are almost always preceded by pruritis (Freyberg, 1966; Freyberg et al., 1972). The forms of dermatitis include nonspecific dermatitis (Anonymous, 1960, 1961; Freyberg et al., 1942; Bayles and Fremont-Smith, 1956; McCarty et al., 1963; Ragan and Boots, 1947; Saiyanen and Laaksonen, 1962; Smith et al., 1958; Sorensen, 1963) exfoliative dermatitis (Hill, 1968), lichenoid eruptions (Reed and Becker, 1962), photosensitivity (Lewis and Ziff, 1966), and local rash (Lewis and Ziff, 1966). Skin biopsies show that gold dermatitis is not caused by parenchymatous poisoning in the skin because of the accumulation of gold (Freyberg et al., 1942).

The more serious effects seem to be less frequent (Forestier, 1963); included in these are such reactions as blood dyscrasias, which may be fatal (McCarty et al., 1963). The types of dyscrasias include eosinophilia (Saiyanen and Laaksonen, 1962; Sievers et al., 1963; Garrel, 1960), leukopenia (Bayles and Fremont-Smith, 1956; Saiyanen and Laaksonen, 1962; Smith et al., 1958; Sorensen, 1963; Goodwin, 1964), aplastic anemia (McCarty et al., 1963), granulocytosis (Forestier, 1963; Sorensen, 1963), granulocytopenia (Saiyanen and Laaksonen, 1962), and thrombocytopenia (Forestier, 1963; Saiyanen and Laaksonen, 1962; Lockie et al., 1947; Saphir and Ney, 1966). Gold is thought to produce the latter effect by depressing platelet production and by increasing platelet destruction (Crosby and Kaufman, 1964). Bone marrow depression per se appears not to be induced by gold, but the irregular rise in reticulocyte count in arthritic patients disappears with gold therapy (Denman et al., 1965).

Toxic effects on internal organs (kidney and liver) are also rare and usually disappear after gold therapy is stopped (Forestier, 1963; Lee et al., 1965). Hepatitis has been reported infrequently (Anonymous, 1960; Sorensen, 1963). There have been reports of nephrotic syndrome, nephritis, and nephrosis associated with gold therapy (Sorensen, 1963; Lee et al., 1965; vanden Broek and Han, 1966; Wilkinson and Eccleston, 1970). Reversible proteinuria, primarily in female patients (Freyberg et al., 1942; Lewis and Ziff, 1966; Saiyanen and Laaksonen, 1962; Sievers et al., 1963; Sorensen, 1963), and hematuria (Bayles and Fremont-Smith, 1956; Saiyanen and Laaksonen, 1962) have also been reported to occur with chrysotherapy. However, findings of gold in proximal tubules early in therapy and in distal tubules after several years of therapy fail to account for proteinuria nor does gold found in macrophages of interstitial tissues after several years of therapy (Brun et al., 1964). Creatinine clearance studies show that gold compounds do not reduce kidney function (Lee et al., 1965; Sorensen, 1963).

There are other isolated reports of toxic reactions to gold. Mucous membrane lesions, such as stomatitis (Anonymous, 1965; Smith, 1963; Sievers *et al.*, 1963; McCarty *et al.*, 1963), ulcer (Anonymous, 1960), and colitis (Anonymous, 1965), have occurred. Other reactions include anaphylactic shock (Sievers *et al.*, 1963), articular pain (Saiyanen and Laaksonen, 1962), fever (Anonymous, 1960; Sievers *et al.*, 1963), tachycardia and chest pain (Saiyanen and Laaksonen, 1962), optic atrophy (Bayles and Fremont-Smith, 1956), keratitis (Anonymous, 1960), and edema (Goodwin, 1964). EEG changes in rheumatoid arthritis patients receiving gold therapy are associated with the total amount of gold received (Dale and Patterson, 1967). Ocular toxicity is also seen in rheumatoid patients treated with parenteral gold preparations. These toxicities are of two types: (a) subepithelial deposits of gold in the cornea (chrysiasis) and (b) an allergic manifestation causing marked corneal ulceration (Behrend and Rodenhäuser, 1969). Reactions that are not considered significant or limiting to continuing gold treatment are often seen on the initial regimen of therapy. These include hyperthermia, which may or may not be associated with the exacerbations of the symptoms; headache; flushing; dizziness; syncope; and mild euphoria (Dawson *et al.*, 1941; Kuzell, 1949; Price and Leichentritt, 1943).

The exact mechanism by which gold compounds induce toxicity in man and animals is not known (Lee *et al.*, 1965). A number of theories have been proposed to explain gold pathogenesis, but to date none has been unequivocally substantiated either experimentally or clinically. Some of these theories include: nonspecific metal toxicity (Feldt, 1917, 1924), vitamin deficiency (Secher, 1938), liver dysfunction (Umber, 1929; Heuck, 1937; Mann, 1938), activation of latent diseases (Milian, 1926), liberation of toxins (Møllgaard, 1924), allergic phenomena (Heinild, 1937), and binding to sulfhydryl-containing substances in the body (Libenson, 1945).

Although no unequivocal evidence supports any of the above theories, allergic phenomena appear to explain some of the pathogenetic properties of gold (Block and Van Goor, 1959b; Freyberg, 1966; Freyberg *et al.*, 1972). The evidence is based on the following observations. The most prevalent toxic manifestation of gold therapy involves the skin. Dermatological reactions can occur after a single dose of gold, where there is hardly any gold concentrated in the skin. The mechanism for these reactions is postulated (Freyberg, 1966) to involve a gold–protein haptenelike linkage to form an allergen, which now becomes a neoantigen that immunologically induces the dermatitis and blood dyscrasias. The eosinophilia seen with gold administration, which also occurs in allergic manifestations, tends to support this concept. It should be noted that exact allergens, in spite of the research efforts of many, have not been identified (Bayles and Fremont-Smith, 1956;

Forestier, 1963; Freyberg, 1966; Freyberg *et al.*, 1944, 1972; Lee *et al.*, 1965; Ragan and Boots, 1947; Garrel, 1960; Stavem *et al.*, 1968; Denman *et al.*, 1965; Key *et al.*, 1939; Svanberg, 1952; Denman and Denman, 1968).

Common forms of clinical toxicity are not often seen in laboratory animals. Kidney damage is one of the few consistently reproducible toxic effects in the laboratory (Freyberg, 1966; Freyberg *et al.*, 1972). Nephritis has occurred after the administration of the soluble gold derivatives, gold sodium thiomalate and gold sodium thiosulfate (Freyberg *et al.*, 1942; Jasmin, 1957; Wagner and DeGroot, 1963). This observation has also been reported for gold thioglucose and gold chloride (Deter and Liebelt, 1962) but not for colloidal gold preparations. The latter, however, do cause damage to the liver and spleen (Freyberg *et al.*, 1944). A single injection of gold thioglucose in rats, 0.1–0.5 mg/gm body weight, causes pyknosis and cloudy swelling in the cells of the proximal and distal convoluted tubules 2 hours postinjection, necrosis at 6 hours post-injection, and casts and hemorrhagic foci at 8 hours postinjection (Deter and Liebelt, 1962). Albuminuria occurs in proportion to dose (Freyberg *et al.*, 1944). The parenteral administration of gold sodium thiomalate at doses from 2.5 to 20 mg of gold per kilogram in the adjuvant-induced arthritic rat produces marked gold retention in the kidneys (Walz *et al.*, 1972). At autopsy, all kidneys from these animals exhibit an abnormal pale colored appearance with a concomitant increase in kidney weight that is dose dependent.

The skin toxicity produced in man has not been observed in animals except in isolated cases. Reactions ranging from subjective symptoms to a breakdown of epithelial tissue with multiple hemorrhages have been observed in dogs and horses (Fennel, 1969). In our laboratory, gold sodium thiomalate given intramuscularly to rats and dogs has not produced any skin lesions. Eosinophilia seen in man on gold therapy and in allergic manifestations can also be detected in the peripheral blood of rabbits receiving gold sodium thiomalate injections over a long period of time (Nineham, 1963).

Gastric mucosal lesions have been reported to be induced by gold thioglucose in mice (Liebelt and Perry, 1957) and rats (Deter and Liebelt, 1962; Wagner and DeGroot, 1963) and are associated with hypothalamic lesions. In contrast, a lethal dose of gold sodium thiomalate or gold chloride did not produce either gastric or hypothalamic lesions.

In mice injected with gold sodium thiosulfate an experimental pathoclisis was established by gold poisoning of the nerve cells of the central nervous system (Querido, 1947). Furthermore, gold thioglucose was reported to enhance the experimental allergic encephalomyelitis (EAE) response in mice (Bochme *et al.*, 1970), whereas in rats we found delaying effects on the

EAE response with the parenteral administration of gold sodium thiomalate and oral administration of SK&F 36914 (**6**) (Walz *et al.*, unpublished observations, 1972). These observations were also reported by Gerber *et al.* (1972b).

$$(C_2H_5)_3P \rightarrow AuCl$$

SK & F 36914

6

Voluminous reports of the toxicological effects associated with gold thioglucose have accumulated. Some toxicity is associated with hypothalamic lesions, which are postulated as caused by a specific affinity of the ventro-medial nucleus for the glucose moiety of the gold that accumulates there (Brecher *et al.*, 1965; Chang and Persellin, 1968). Other toxic effects observed include: weight gain (Friedman *et al.*, 1962, 1963), hyperglycemia and reduced response to insulin (Edelman *et al.*, 1965; Hazama, 1965; Katsuki *et al.*, 1962), glycosuria (Goodwin, 1964), degenerative pathology and physiology of the liver (Larsson, 1959; Meyer *et al.*, 1961; Peterson and Hellman, 1962), thyroid hypofunction (Hazama, 1965; Schindler and Liebelt, 1967), and alteration of reproductive tissue and function (Liebelt *et al.*, 1966; Rudali and Silberman, 1966; Browning and Kwan, 1964; Browning *et al.*, 1965/1966). Teratogenic effects were produced in rats by gold sodium thiomalate injected at various times between $7\frac{1}{2}$ and $11\frac{1}{2}$ days of gestation. The doses of gold sodium thiomalate used produced gold levels in these animals comparable to those seen in rheumatoid arthritis patients treated with this compound (Kidston *et al.*, 1970).

The interaction of gold mercapto derivatives with sulfhydryl groups has been postulated as a mechanism of toxicity (Libenson, 1945). This interaction has also been proposed as a mechanism by which gold mercapto derivatives may exert a therapeutic effect (Lorber *et al.*, 1971; Gerber, 1964; Ennis *et al.*, 1968; Persellin and Ziff, 1966). In rat serum nonsteroidal antiinflammatory agents accelerate the SH-SS interchange reaction (Walz and DiMartino, 1972), whereas gold sodium thiomalate and gold thioglucose inhibit this reaction (Section II,B,5). The importance of this observation is that one can experimentally distinguish the nonsteroidal antiinflammatory agents from the gold compounds.

Whether either mechanism (inhibition or acceleration of SH–SS interchange) prevents protein denaturation or operates to inhibit inflammatory conditions in man is equivocal at this point. It is conceivable that both efficacy and toxicity may operate through similar mechanisms, the degree and/or location of which should determine the therapeutic *vis à vis* toxic effects.

In our laboratory both gold sodium thiomalate and gold thioglucose, administered orally and intramuscularly, were investigated for their ulcerogenic effects on the rat's gastric mucosa 4 hours postdrug. Gold sodium thiomalate administered orally produced erosions, mucus depletion, vascular congestion, hemorrhage, and diarrhea, whereas when it was given intramuscularly only vascular congestion was produced. Gold thioglucose given both orally and intramuscularly produced erosions. In the nonfasted rat, gold sodium thiomalate at 44 and 22 mg/kg intramuscularly produced marked food retention in the stomach. This latter observation bears further investigation.

SK&F 36914 (**6**), an orally acting gold compound (see Section IV) administered orally to the rats, did not produce gastric erosions but vascular congestion and diarrhea were noted.

The acute lethal dose (LD_{50}) in the rat receiving gold sodium thiomalate intramuscularly could not be calculated because of the minimal lethality (two out of ten animals) up to 200 mg gold per kilogram. For SK&F 36914, the oral acute LD_{50} was calculated to be 63 mg of gold per kilogram.

In a 5-day toxicity study in ten rats, gold sodium thiomalate produced 100% deaths at 10 mg of gold per kilogram per day, i.m., whereas at doses of 5 and 20 mg of gold per kilogram per day there were no deaths and two deaths, respectively. Investigations to elucidate this interesting phenomenon were without success, and we concluded that it was associated with erratic absorption. Marked weight loss was seen in all animals receiving the drug.

In a 5-day toxicity study, SK&F 36914 produced death in only two out of ten rats at 20 mg of gold per kilogram per day, p.o.

It is evident from data in both man and animal that gold compounds exhibit delayed rather than acute toxicity. One must design extended (rather than acute) studies for the investigation of gold toxicity with this salient fact in mind. Acute toxicity studies do not give an accurate profile of a compound's toxicity, because multiple dosing over a reasonable period of time is mandatory in these tests. Furthermore, the need for baseline data on gold sodium thiomalate in chronic toxicity studies in various species is needed for preclinical assessment of any new gold or nongold compounds with similar profiles of activity.

III. DESIGN OF CHRYSOTHERAPEUTIC AGENTS

All valence states of gold have been evaluated for the treatment of rheumatoid arthritis. The monovalent form has proved superior to either the colloidal or the trivalent state. Although the aurous ion (Au^+) has only fleeting existence in solution, being rapidly converted to metallic gold or the auric (Au³⁺) species (Cotton and Wilkinson, 1967), ligand complexation results in compounds with varying degrees of stability. Gold compounds in use today are complexes of aurous gold with different sulfur-containing ligands, such as thiomalic acid (Myochrysine, **2**), thioglucose (Solganal **1**), sodium thiosulfate (Sanochrysine, Crisalbine **3**), and thioacetanilide (gold thioglycanide, **7**). The first three complexes are freely soluble in water, but

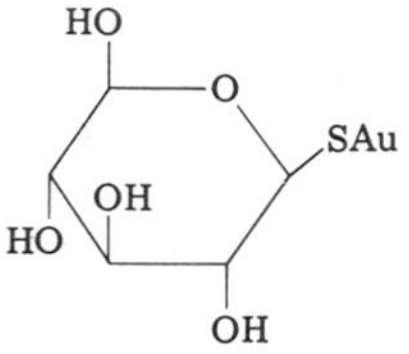

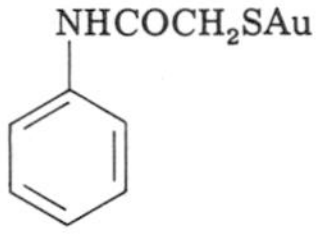

Gold thioglucose	Gold sodium thiomalate	Gold sodium thiosulfate	Gold thioglycanide
1	**2**	**3**	**7**

their solutions slowly decompose on standing. Because they are not absorbed orally, they are administered by the intramuscular route for therapeutic effect. In the blood, gold is bound strongly to protein. Recent reports indicate that this binding is limited mainly to the albumin fraction (Mascarenhas *et al.*, 1972; Sliwinski, 1968; McQueen and Dykes, 1969).

Attempts to improve upon the effectiveness of soluble gold preparations by chemical manipulation have not been rewarding (Nineham, 1963); however, the nature of the ligand carrier has been shown to modify both the tissue distribution properties of gold and its excretion rate (Rubin *et al.*, 1967).

Recently we (Sutton *et al.*, 1972) expanded on the chemistry of Mann *et al.* (1937) and prepared a series of compounds (**8, 9a, 9b**) in which aurous gold was complexed with trialkylphosphines. Coordination of monovalent gold with ligands of the phosphine type is known to stabilize the reduced

R₃PAuCl

Chloro(trialkyl-
phosphine)gold

R = Me, Et, *i*-Pr, Bu

8

R₃PAuSR′

9

R = Me, Et, *i*-Pr, Bu

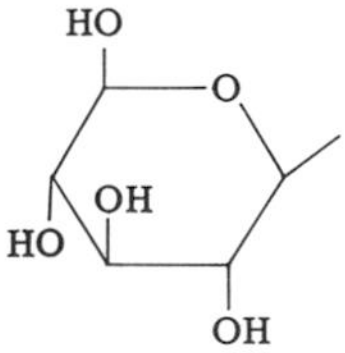

(Trialkylphosphine)-
[(β-D-glucopyranosyl)-
thio]gold

9a

R = Et, Bu

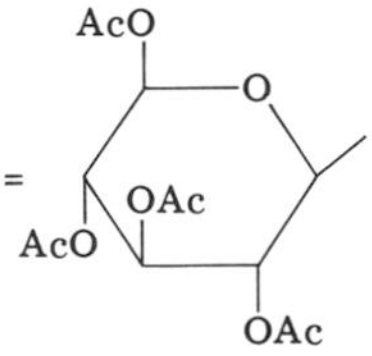

[Tetra-*O*-acetyl-β-D-
glucopyranosyl)thio]-
(trialkylphosphine)gold

9b

valence state and to result in nonionic complexes soluble in organic solvents (Booth, 1964). In compounds of this type, gold has a coordination number of 2. The molecules are monomers in solution and nonconducting.

Unlike water-soluble gold preparations, the new compounds were absorbed after oral administration and protected rats from the development of adjuvant arthritis when administered by this route. The nongold phosphine compounds studied gave no protection against adjuvant arthritis. All compounds in which gold was in the form of a phosphine complex gave demonstrable serum gold levels after oral administration to rats, and the degree of arthritis prevention paralleled the magnitude of the serum gold concentration. Comparative studies of **8**, **9a**, and **9b** in adjuvant arthritic rats indicated that the nature of the phosphine ligand in the gold coordination complexes played a greater role in bringing about changes in antiarthritic activity than did the other group bonded to gold. Such diverse ligand groups as chloro, thioglucosyl, acetylated thioglucosyl, thiohydroxyethyl, or thiocyano did not markedly modify the protective activity of coordinated gold when the other ligand was triethylphosphine. In any homologous series (**8**, **9a**, **9b**), the greatest activity resided in the triethylphosphine gold derivative.

IV. PHARMACOLOGY OF ORALLY ABSORBED GOLD COMPOUNDS

We recently reported (Walz *et al.*, 1972) on a new gold compound, chloro-(triethylphosphine)gold (SK&F 36914, **6**; **8**, R = Et), that produced antiarthritic activity and serum gold levels after oral administration to adjuvant arthritic rats. In contrast, a clinically used gold compound, gold sodium thiomalate, did not produce a therapeutic effect or significant serum gold levels after oral administration. The oral activity of SK&F 36914 was recently confirmed by Gerber *et al.* (1972b). These investigators found that SK&F 36914, given either i.m. or p.o., was approximately as effective as equal doses of gold sodium thiomalate in delaying the onset and decreasing the severity of experimental allergic encephalomyelitis in rats. SK&F 36914 administered orally to rats was equipotent with parenterally administered gold sodium thiomalate in suppressing the development of adjuvant-induced inflammatory lesions. It produced lower gold levels in both serum and kidneys than equivalent therapeutic doses of parenteral gold sodium thiomalate.

Adjuvant arthritis was produced and assessed as previously described (Section II,A,3). Drugs were administered once daily, beginning on the day of adjuvant injection (day 0), for 17 days with the exception of weekend days (days 4, 5, 11, and 12 postadjuvant).

Administration of SK&F 36914 orally or gold sodium thiomalate intramuscularly produced significant suppression of the injected hind leg inflammation (primary lesion) on day 3 (Fig. 1). Although the flat dose response of SK&F 36914 precluded the calculation of relative potencies, it is evident that at 5 mg gold per kilogram per day, SK&F 36914 (p.o.) was more effective than the same dose of gold sodium thiomalate (i.m.) in suppressing the primary lesion.

Administration of SK&F 36914, p.o., and gold sodium thiomalate, i.m., produced parallel dose–response suppression of both the injected and uninjected (secondary lesion) hind leg volumes measured on day 16 (Figs. 2 and 3). The calculated dose–responses on these parameters were not significantly different.

On day 17, kidneys and/or serum were obtained from the adjuvant arthritic rats. Both SK&F 36914, p.o., and gold sodium thiomalate, i.m., produced measurable serum gold levels at all doses tested (Fig. 4). However, SK&F

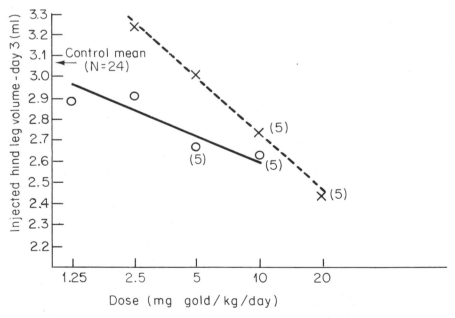

Fig. 1 Relative potency of SK&F 36914, p.o. (——), and gold sodium thiomalate, i.m. (– – –), in suppressing the primary lesion (injected hind leg volume on day 3) of adjuvant arthritis. Each datum represents a mean of six rats per dose level. Control mean represents pooled hind leg volumes of p.o. and i.m. control groups. (S), Significant difference from control ($P \leq .01$). Data from Walz *et al.* (1972).

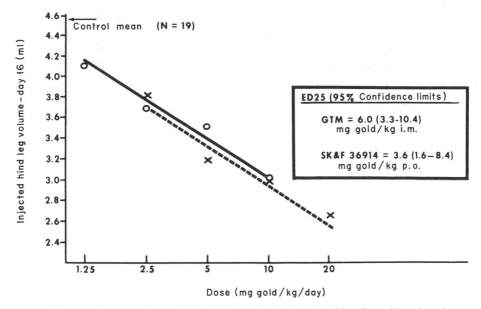

Fig. 2 Relative potency of SK&F 36914, p.o. (——), and gold sodium thiomalate, i.m. (– – –), in suppressing the injected hind leg volume on day 16 of adjuvant arthritis. Control mean represents pooled hind leg volumes of p.o. and i.m. control groups. Each datum is a mean of three to six rats per dose level. Data from Walz *et al.* (1972).

36914 differed from gold sodium thiomalate in that it produced lower serum gold levels at equal therapeutic doses. In this study, SK&F 36914 administered orally at therapeutic doses produced little or no gold retention in the kidney, whereas the parenteral administration of gold sodium thiomalate at either equivalent therapeutic doses or doses producing equivalent serum gold levels led to marked gold retention in the kidneys. At autopsy, kidneys obtained from rats treated with gold sodium thiomalate exhibited an abnormal (pale colored) appearance and increased weight, whereas no such abnormalities were noted in rats treated with SK&F 36914.

These results suggest that the tissue distribution and gold retention characteristics of SK&F 36914 may differ from those properties of the gold preparations currently in use.

V. SUMMARY

The empirical rationale for the use of gold preparations in rheumatoid arthritis, a disease in which the mechanisms of etiology and chronicity are ill defined, is a challenging enigma for the researcher.

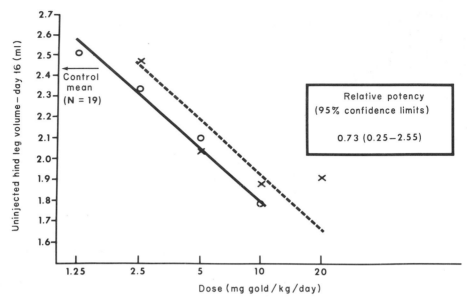

Fig. 3 Related potency of SK&F 36914, p.o. (——), and gold sodium thiomalate, i.m. (– – –), in suppressing the secondary lesion (uninjected hind leg volume on day 16) of adjuvant arthritis. Each datum is a mean of three to six rats per dose level. Control mean represents pooled hind leg volumes of p.o. and i.m. control groups. Data from Walz *et al.* (1972).

That gold compounds are effective in rheumatoid arthritis is well documented. The laboratory evaluation of the efficacy of these compounds, however, is based empirically on their effectiveness in experimental models of arthritis that appear to reflect the human disease. Chrysotherapy has been found to suppress experimental arthritis in animals induced by various infectious, chemical, or immunological methods. This suggests that the therapeutic activity of gold is caused by its effect on common sites in the inflammatory process.

The mechanism of action of gold compounds has been postulated to involve interaction with proteins. They may act by (a) preventing denaturation and formation of macroglobulins, (b) increasing the stability of collagen, (c) uncoupling oxidative phosphorylation, (d) inhibiting lysosomal enzymes, or (e) inhibiting antigen–antibody reactions.

The metabolism of gold derivatives in both man and animals has been studied. This fertile field of research is contributing to our understanding of the mechanisms by which they produce their efficacy and toxicity. In the past, the design of new gold drugs has not contributed significant improvements to chrysotherapy. The newly developed, orally absorbed gold compounds that have been described here may contribute to the fields of chemical, experimental, and clinical research in chrysotherapy.

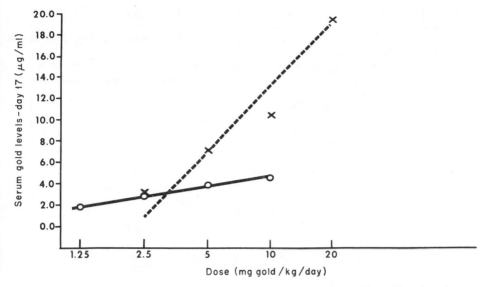

Fig. 4 Relative potency of SK&F 36914, p.o. (———), and gold sodium thiomalate, i.m. (– –), in producing serum gold levels after administration to adjuvant arthritic rats. Each datum is a mean of three to six samples per dose. Data from Walz *et al.* (1972).

Future advances in chrysotherapy will depend on a multidiscipline approach in both clinical and laboratory investigations.

REFERENCES

Adam, M., and Kühn, K. (1968). *Eur. J. Biochem.* **3**, 407.
Adam, M., Bartl, P., Deyl, Z., and Rosmus, J. (1964). *Experientia* **20**, 203.
Adam, M., Bartl, P., Deyl, Z., and Rosmus, J. (1965a). *Ann. Rheum. Dis.* **24**, 378.
Adam, M., Deyl, Z., and Rosmus, J. (1965b). *Int. Symp. Non-Steroidal Anti-Inflammatory Drugs, Proc., 1964* pp. 73–77.
Adam, M., Fietzek, P., and Kühn, K. (1968). *Eur. J. Biochem.* **3**, 411.
Anonymous. (1960). *Ann. Rheum. Dis.* **19**, 95.
Anonymous. (1961). *Ann. Rheum. Dis.* **20**, 315.
Anonymous. (1965). *Med. Lett. Drugs Ther.* **7**, 109.
Barrett, A. J. (1970). *Advan. Sci.* **27**, 140.
Bartholomew, L. E. (1965). *Arthritis Rheum.* **8**, 376.
Bayles, T. B., and Fremont-Smith, P. (1956). *Ann. Rheum. Dis.* **15**, 394.
Behrend, T., and Rodenhäuser, J. H. (1969). *Z. Rheumaforsch.* **28**, 441.
Bertrand, J. J., Waine, H., and Tobias, C. A. (1948). *J. Lab. Clin. Med.* **33**, 1133.
Block, W. D., and Van Goor, K. (1959a). *In* "Metabolism, Pharmacology and Therapeutic Use of Gold Compounds" (A. C. Curtis, ed.), p. 3. Thomas, Springfield, Illinois.
Block, W. D., and Van Goor, K. (1959b). *In* "Metabolism, Pharmacology and Therapeutic Uses of Gold Compounds" (A. C. Curtis, ed.), p. 39. Thomas, Springfield, Illinois.

Block, W. D., Buchanan, O. H., and Freyberg, R. H. (1941). *J. Pharmacol. Exp. Ther.* **73**, 200.

Block, W. D., Buchanan, O. H., and Freyberg, R. H. (1942). *J. Pharmacol. Exp. Ther.* **76**, 355.

Block, W. D., Buchanan, O. H., and Freyberg, R. H. (1944). *J. Pharmacol. Exp. Ther.* **82**, 391.

Boehme, D. H., Wardelin, O., Cottrell, J. C., and Bernardis, L. L. (1970). *J. Reticuloendothel. Soc.* **8**, 522.

Bollett, A. J., and Shuster, A. (1960). *J. Clin. Invest.* **39**, 1114.

Booth, G. (1964). *Advan. Inorg. Chem. Radiochem.* **6**, 1–69.

Brecher, G., and Waxler, S. H., (1949). *Proc. Soc. Exp. Biol. Med.* **70**, 498.

Brecher, G., Laqueur, G. L., Cronkite, E. P., Edelman, P. M., and Schwartz, I. L. (1965). *J. Exp. Med.* **121**, 395.

Browning, H. C., and Kwan, L. P. (1964). *Tex. Rep. Biol. Med.* **22**, 678.

Browning, H. C., Larke, G. A., and Gibbs, W. E. (1965/1966). *Neuroendocrinology* **1**, 93.

Bruck, C., and Glück, A. (1913). *Muenchen. Med. Wochenschr.* **60**, 57.

Brun, C., Olsen, S., Raaschou, F., and Sorensen, A. W. S. (1964). *Nephron* **1**, 265.

Chang, R. J., and Persellin, R. H. (1968). *Proc. Soc. Exp. Biol. Med.* **129**, 598.

Chayen, J., and Bitensky, L. (1971). *Ann. Rheum. Dis.* **30**, 522.

Cotton, F. A., and Wilkinson, G. (1967). *In* "Advanced Inorganic Chemistry" (F. A. Cotton and G. Wilkinson, eds.), p. 1047. Wiley (Interscience), New York.

Crosby, W. H., and Kaufman, M. C. (1964). *Med. Ann. D. C.* **33**, 194.

Dale, P. W., and Patterson, M. B. (1967). *Electroencephalogr. Clin. Neurophysiol.* **23**, 493.

Davidson, M., and Thomas, L. (1966). *Antimicrob. Ag. Chemother.* **6**, 312.

Dawson, M. H., Boots, R. H., and Tyson, T. L. (1941). *Trans. Ass. Amer. Physicians* **56**, 330.

Debons, A. F., Silver, L., Cronkite, E. P., Johnson, H. A., Brecher, G., Tenzer, D., and Schwartz, I. L. (1962). *Amer. J. Physiol.* **202**, 743.

Denman, A. M., Huber, H., Wood, P. H. N., and Scott, J. T. (1965). *Ann. Rheum. Dis.* **24**, 278.

Denman, E. J., and Denman, A. M. (1968). *Ann. Rheum. Dis.* **27**, 582.

Deter, R. L., and Liebelt, R. A. (1962). *Gastroenterology* **43**, 575.

Deter, R. L., and Liebelt, R. A. (1964). *Tex. Rep. Biol. Med.* **22**, 229.

Dyatkina, M. E., and Syrkin, Y. K. (1960). *Zh. Neorg, Khim.* **5**, 1663–1668. *Chem. Abstr.* **56**, 13555c.

Edelman, P. M., Schwartz, I. L., Cronkite, E. P., Brecher, G., and Livingston, L. (1965). *J. Exp. Med.* **121**, 403.

Elftman, H., Elftman, A. G., and Zwemer, R. L. (1946). *Anat. Rec.* **96**, 341.

Ellery, R. S. (1954). *Med. J. Aust.* **41**, 762.

Ellman, P., and Lawrence, J. S. (1940). *Brit. Med. J.* **2**, 314.

Empire Rheumatism Council. (1961). *Ann. Rheum. Dis.* **20**, 315.

Ennis, R. S., Granda, J. L., and Posner, A. S. (1968). *Arthritis Rheum.* **11**, 756.

Ezer, E., and Szporny, L. (1962). *Arch. Int. Pharmacodyn. Ther.* **138**, 263.

Feldt, A. (1917). *Klin. Wochenschr.* **54**, 1111.

Feldt, A. (1924). *Klin. Wochenschr.* **6**, 1136.

Fennel, C. (1969). *Vet. Rec.* **84**, 259.

Fikrig, S. M., and Smithwick, E. M. (1968). *Arthritis Rheum.* **11**, 478.

Findlay, G. M., Mackenzie, R. D., and MacCallum, F. O. (1940). *Brit. J. Exp. Pathol.* **21**, 13.

Forestier, J. (1929). *Bull. Soc. Med. Hop. Paris* **53**, 323.

Forestier, J. (1932). *Lancet* **1**, 441.

Forestier, J. (1963). *Arch. Interamer. Rheumatol.* **6**, 15.

Franklin, E. C., Kunkel, H. G., and Ward, J. R. (1958). *Arthritis Rheum.* **1**, 400.

Fraser, T. N. (1945). *Ann. Rheum. Dis.* **4**, 71.
Freyberg, R. H., Block, W. D., and Levey, S. (1941). *J. Clin. Invest.* **20**, 401.
Freyberg, R. H., Block, W. D., and Wells, G. S. (1942). *Clinics* **1**, 537.
Freyberg, R. H., Block, W. D., and Preston, W. S. (1944). *J. Amer. Med. Ass.* **124**, 800.
Freyberg, R. H. (1966). *In* "Arthritis and Allied Conditions" (J. L. Hollander, ed.), pp. 302–332. Lea & Febiger, Philadelphia, Pennsylvania.
Freyberg, R. H., Ziff, M., and Baum, J. (1972). *In* "Arthritis and Allied Conditions" (J. L. Hollander, ed.), pp. 455–482. Lea & Febiger, Philadelphia, Pennsylvania.
Friedman, G., Waye, J. D., and Janowitz, H. D. (1962). *Amer. J. Physiol.* **203**, 631.
Friedman, G., Waye, J. D., and Janowitz, H. D. (1963). *Amer. J. Physiol.* **205**, 919.
Fujihira, E., Tsubota, N., and Nakazawa, M. (1971). *Chem. Pharm. Bull.* **19**, 190.
Garrel, M. (1960). *Arch. Intern. Med.* **106**, 874.
Gerber, D. A. (1964). *J. Pharmacol. Exp. Ther.* **143**, 137.
Gerber, D. A. (1965). *Proc. Soc. Exp. Biol. Med.* **119**, 100.
Gerber, D. A. (1971). *Arthritis Rheum.* **14**, 383.
Gerber, D. A., Shapiro, M. M., and Follows, J. W., Jr. (1965). *In* "Proceedings of the Eleventh Interim Scientific Session" (R. W. Lamont-Havers, ed.), Vol. XV, p. 373. Arthritis Found., New York.
Gerber, R. C., Paulus, H. E., Bluestone, R., and Pearson, C. M. (1972a). *Ann. Rheum. Dis.* **31**, 308.
Gerber, R. C., Whitehouse, M. W., and Orr, K. J. (1972b). *Proc. Soc. Exp. Biol. Med.* **140**, 1379.
Goodwin, J. F. (1964). *Mich. Med.* **63**, 437.
Gottlieb, N. L., Smith, P. M., and Smith, E. M. (1972). *Arthritis Rheum.* **15**, 16.
Graeme, M. L., Fabry, E., and Segg, E. B. (1966). *J. Pharmacol. Exp. Ther.* **153**, 373.
Gujral, M. L., and Saxena, P. N. (1956). *Indian J. Med. Res.* **44**, 657.
Hazama, F. (1965). *Folia Endocrinol. Jap.* **40**, 385.
Heinild, S. (1937). *Acta Med. Scand.* **92**, 308.
Henkind, P. (1964). *Ann. Phys. Med.* **7**, 258.
Heuck, W. (1937). *Beitr. Klin. Tuberk. Spezifischen Tuberk. Forsch.* **89**, 646.
Hill, D. F. (1968). *Med. Clin. N. Amer.* **52**, 733.
Ishizaka, K., and Campbell, D. H. (1959). *J. Immunol.* **83**, 318.
Ishizaka, K., and Ishizaka, T. (1960). *J. Immunol.* **85**, 163.
Jasmin, G. (1957). *J. Pharmacol. Exp. Ther.* **120**, 349.
Jansson, E., Mäkisara, P., Vainio, K., Vainio, U., Snellman, O., and Tuuri, S. (1971). *Ann. Rheum. Dis.* **30**, 506.
Jeffrey, M. R., Freundlich, H. F., and Bailey, D. M. (1958). *Ann. Rheum. Dis.* **17**, 52.
Jensen, E. V. (1959). *Science* **130**, 1319.
Jessop, J. D. and Currey, H. L. F. (1968). *Ann. Rheum. Dis.* **27**, 577.
Junker, (F.) (1913). *Muenchen. Med. Wochenschr.* **60**, 1376.
Kantor, T. G., Bishko, F., Meltzer, M., and Harley, N. (1970). *Arthritis Rheum.* **13**, 326.
Katsuki, S., Hirata, Y., Horino, M., Ito, M. Ishimoto, M., Makino, N., and Hososako, A. (1962). *Diabetes* **11**, 209.
Katz, L., and Piliero, S. J. (1969). *Ann. N.Y. Acad. Sci.* **147**, 515
Key, J. A., Rosenfeld, H., Tjoflat, O. E. (1939). *J. Bone Joint Surg.* **21**, 339.
Kidston, M. E., Beck, F., and Lloyd, J. B. (1970). *Proc. Anato. Soc. G. Brit. Ireland* **108**, 590.
Koch, R. (1890). *Deut. Med. Wochenschr.* **16**, 756.
Kosaka, S. (1970). *Tohoku J. Exp. Med.* **100**, 349.
Kuzell, W. C. (1949). *Calif. Med.* **71**, 140.
Kuzell, W. C., and Dreisbach, R. H. (1948). *Proc. Soc. Exp. Biol. Med.* **67**, 157.

Kuzell, W. C., Gardner, G. M., Fairley, De L. M., and Tripi, H. B. (1952). *In* "Rheumatic Diseases: Based on the Proceedings of the VII International Congress on Rheumatic Diseases, 1949", *Amer. Rheum. Ass.*, p. 409. Saunders, Philadelphia, Pennsylvania.

Landé, K. (1927). *Muenchen. Med. Wochenschr.* **74**, 1132.

Larsson, S. (1959). *Acta Physiol. Scand.* **46**, 159.

Lawrence, J. S. (1961). *Ann. Rheum. Dis.* **20**, 341.

Lee, J. C., Dushkin, M., Eyring, E. J., Engleman, E. P., and Hopper, J., Jr. (1965). *Arthritis Rheum.* **8**, 1.

Lewis, D. C., and Ziff, M. (1966). *Arthritis Rheum.* **9**, 682.

Libenson, L. (1945). *Exp. Med. Surg.* **3**, 146.

Liebelt, R. A., and Perry, J. H. (1957). *Proc. Soc. Exp. Biol. Med.* **95**, 774.

Liebelt, R. A., Sekiba, K., Ichinoe, S., and Liebelt, A. G. (1966). *Endocrinology* **78**, 845.

Lockie, L. M., Norcross, B. M., and George, C. W. (1947). *J. Amer. Med. Ass.* **133**, 754.

Lorber, A., Pearson, C. M., Meredith, W. L., and Gantz-Mandell, L. E. (1964). *Ann. Intern. Med.* **61**, 423.

Lorber, A., Bovy, R. A., and Chang, C. C. (1971). *Metab. Clin. Exp.* **20**, 446.

Lorber, A., Bovy, R. A., and Chang, C. C. (1972). *Nature (London) New Biol.* **236**, 250.

McCarty, D. J., Brill, J. M., and Harrop, D. (1962). *J. Amer. Med. Ass.* **179**, 655.

McQueen, E. G., and Dykes, P. W. (1969). *Ann. Rheum. Dis.* **28**, 437.

Mann, E. (1938). *Z. Tuberk.* **81**, 23.

Mann, F. G., Wells, A. F., and Purdie, D. (1937). *J. Chem. Soc. London.* p. 1828.

Mascarenhas, B. R., Granda, J. L., and Freyberg, R. H. (1972). *Arthritis Rheum.* **15**, 391.

Meyer, J. S., Hideshige, I., and Scott, H. W. (1961). *Yale J. Biol. Med.* **33**, 308.

Milian, G. (1926). *Presse Med.* **34**. 1575.

Møllgaard, H. (1924). *Ugeskr. Laeger* **86**, 1035.

Moore, R. W., and Redmond, H. E. (1965). *Arthritis Rheum.* **8**, 458.

Newbould, B. B. (1963). *Brit. J. Pharmacol. Chemother.* **21**, 127.

Newsham, A. G., and Chu, H. P. (1965). *J. Hyg.* **63**, 1.

Niedermeier, W., and Griggs, J. H. (1971). *J. Chronic Dis.* **23**, 527.

Niedermeier, W., Prillaman, W. W., and Griggs, J. H. (1971). *Arthritis Rheum.* **14**, 533.

Nineham, A. W. (1963). *Arch. Interamer. Rheumatol.* **6**, 113.

Norn, S. (1968). *Acta Pharmacol. Toxicol.* **26**, 470.

Opie, E. L. (1962). *J. Exp. Med.* **115**, 597.

Opie, E. L. (1963). *J. Exp. Med.* **117**, 425.

Pearson, C. M. (1963). *J. Chronic Dis.* **16**, 863.

Persellin, R. H. (1968). *Med. Clin. N. Amer.* **52**, 635.

Persellin, R. H., and Ziff, M. (1966). *Arthritis Rheum.* **9**, 57.

Persellin, R. H., Hess, E. V., and Ziff, M. (1967). *Arthritis Rheum.* **10**, 99.

Peterson, B., and Hellman, B. (1962). *Acta Pathol. Microbiol. Scand.* **55**, 401.

Pick, E. (1927). *Wien. Klin. Wochenschr.* **40**, 1175.

Preston, W. S., Block, W. D., and Freyberg, R. H. (1942). *Proc. Soc. Exp. Biol. Med.* **50**, 253.

Price, A. E., and Leichentritt, B. (1943). *Ann. Intern. Med.* **19**, 70.

Querido, A. (1947). *Acta Psychiat. Neurol.* **22**, 97.

Ragan, C., and Boots, R. H. (1947). *J. Amer. Med. Ass.* **133**, 752.

Reed, W. B., and Becker, S. W. (1962). *C. R. Soc. Biol.* **160**, 546.

Robinson, L. B., Wichelhausen, R. H., and Brown, T. McP. (1952). *J. Lab. Clin. Med.* **39**, 290.

Rodenhäuser, J. H., and Behrend, T. (1969). *Deut. Med. Wochenschr.* **94**, 2389.

Root, S. W., Andrews, G. A., Kniseley, R. M., and Tyor, M. P. (1954). *Cancer* **7**, 856.

Rothbard, S., Angevine, D. M., and Cecil, R. L. (1941). *J. Pharmacol. Exp. Ther.* **72**, 164.

Rubin, M., Sliwinski, A., Photias, M., Feldman, M., and Zvaifler, N. (1967). *Proc. Soc. Exp. Biol. Med.* **124**, 290.

Rudali, G., and Silberman, C. (1966). *C. R. Soc. Biol.* **160**, 546.

Sabin, A. B., and Warren, J. (1940). *J. Bacteriol.* **40**, 823.

Saiyanen, E., and Laaksonen, A. L. (1962). *Ann. Paediat. Fenn.* **8**, 105.

Sancilio, L. F. (1969). *J. Pharmacol. Exp. Ther.* **168**, 199.

Saphir, J. R., and Ney, R. G. (1966). *J. Amer. Med. Ass.* **195**, 782.

Sasane, A., Matno, T., Nakamura, D., and Kubo, M. (1971). *J. Magn. Resonance* **4**, 257.

Scheiffarth, F., Baenkler, H. W., and Islinger, M. (1970). *Z. Gesamte Exp. Med. Binschl. Exp. Chir.* **152**, 125.

Schindler, W. J., and Liebelt, R. A. (1967). *Endocrinology* **80**, 387.

Secher, K. (1938). *Lancet* **1**, 996.

Sheppard, C. W., Wells, E. B., Hahn, P. F., and Goodell, J. P. B. (1947). *J. Lab. Clin. Med.* **32**, 274.

Sievers, K., Hurri, L., and Sievers, U. M. (1963). *Acta Rheumatol. Scand.* **9**, 56.

Sigler, J. W., Bluhm, G. B., Duncan, H., Sharp, J. T., Ensign, D. C., and McCrum, W. R. (1972). *Arthritis Rheum.* **15**, 125.

Silvestrini, B. (1968). *Inflammation, Proc. Int. Symp., 1967*. pp. 26–36.

Sliwinski, A. J. (1968). *Arthritis Rheum.* **11**, 842.

Smit, P. (1968). *Proc. Mine Officers Ass.* **47**, 90.

Smith, R. T. (1963). *Arch. Interamer. Rheumatol.* **6**, 60.

Smith, R. T., Peak, W. P., Kron, K. M., Hermann, I. F., and Deltoro, R. A. (1958). *J. Amer. Med. Ass.* **167**, 1197.

Snyder, R. G. (1939). *Ann. Intern. Med.* **12**, 1672.

Sorensen, A. W. (1963). *Acta Rheumatol. Scand.* **9**, 122.

Stavem, P., Stromme, J., and Bull, O. (1968). *Scand. J. Haematol.* **5**, 271.

Stewart, S. M., Burnet, M. E., and Young, J. E. (1969). *J. Med. Microbiol.* **2**, 287.

Sutton, B. M., McGusty, E., Walz, D. T., and DiMartino, M. J. (1972). *J. Med. Chem.* **15**, 1095 (1972).

Svanberg, T. (1952). *Ann. Rheum. Dis.* **11**, 209.

Szilágyi, T., Tóth, S., Muszbek, L. Lévai, G., and Laczkó, J. (1968). *Acta Microbiol.* **15**, 331.

Szporny, L., and Ezer, E. (1962). *Arch. Int. Pharmacodyn. Ther.* **136**, 153.

Thomas, L. (1970). *Annu. Rev. Med.* **21**, 179.

Thomas, P. (1967). *Rheumatology* **1**, 29.

Tripi, H. B., and Kuzell, W. C. (1947). *Stanford Med. Bull.* **5**, 98.

Umber, F. (1929). *Med. Welt* **3**, 593.

vanden Broek, H., and Han, M. G. (1966). *N. Engl. J. Med.* **274**, 210.

Vykydal, M., Klabusay, L., and Trnavsky, K. (1956). *Arzneim. Forsch.* **6**, 568.

Wagner, J. W., and DeGroot, J. (1963). *Proc. Soc. Exp. Biol. Med.* **112**, 33.

Walz, D. T., and DiMartino, M. J. (1972). *Proc. Soc. Exp. Biol. Med.* **140**, 263.

Walz, D. T., DiMartino, M. J., Kuch, J. A., and Zuccarello, W. (1971a). *Proc. Soc. Exp. Biol. Med.* **136**, 907.

Walz, D. T., DiMartino, M. J., and Misher, A. (1971b). *J. Pharmacol. Exp. Ther.* **178**, 223.

Walz, D. T., DiMartino, M. J., and Misher, A. (1971c). *Ann. Rheum. Dis.* **30**, 303.

Walz, D. T., DiMartino, M. J., Sutton, B., and Misher, A. (1972). *J. Pharmacol. Exp. Ther.* **181**, 292.

Ward, J. R., and Cloud, R. S. (1966). *J. Pharmacol. Exp. Ther.* **152**, 116.

Weissmann, G. (1966). *Arthritis Rheum.* **9**, 834.

Weissmann, G. (1967). *Annu. Rev. Med.* **18**, 97.

244   DONALD T. WALZ *et al.*

Weissmann, G. (1972). *N. Engl. J. Med.* **286**, 141.
Whitehouse, M. W. (1965). *Prog. Drug Res.* **8**, 321–429.
Wiesinger, D. (1965). *Int. Symp. Non-Steroidal Anti-Inflammatory Drugs. Proc., 1964* pp. 221–226.
Wilkinson, R., and Eccleston, D. W. (1970). *Brit. Med. J.* **2**, 772.
Winter, C. A., and Nuss, G. W. (1966). *Arthritis Rheum.* **9**, 394.

Chapter 9

Antiinflammatory Steroids

THOMAS L. POPPER AND ARTHUR S. WATNICK

Schering Corporation
Bloomfield, New Jersey

I. INTRODUCTION

This chapter includes a survey of the evolution of corticosteroid therapy from 1962 to early 1972. The most important advance during this period was the development of a rational approach to local corticosteroid therapy. The full impact of local therapy has not been completely realized because research in drug delivery systems to local sites has lagged behind research in chemistry and biology. As research in this field is progressing more rapidly, application of local therapy to diseases responsive to corticosteroids should be forthcoming during the next decade.

More precise clinical assays are required to evaluate both the efficacy and side effects, e.g., osteopenia, for the new corticosteroids. If local application can decrease the liabilities of corticosteroid therapy, then wider use in different diseases can be envisioned for this important class of drugs.

Chemical names of corticoids referred to most frequently in the text are listed below.

Cortisone 17α, 21-Dihydroxy-4-pregnene-3,11,20-trione

Hydrocortisone   Cortisol; $11\beta,17\alpha,21$-Trihydroxy-4-pregnene-3,20-dione

Corticosterone $11\beta,21$-Dihydroxy-4-pregnene-3,20-dione

Prednisone $17\alpha,21$-Dihydroxy-1,4-pregnadiene-3,11,20-trione

Prednisolone $11\beta,17\alpha,21$-Trihydroxy-1,4-pregnadiene-3,20-dione

6α-Methylprednisolone 6α-Methyl-$11\beta,17\alpha,21$-trihydroxy-1,4-pregnadiene-3,20-dione

Triamcinolone 9α-Fluoro-$11\beta,16\alpha,17\alpha,21$-tetrahydroxy-1,4-pregnadiene-3,20-dione

Dexamethasone 9α-Fluoro-16α-methyl-$11\beta,17\alpha,21$-trihydroxy-1,4-pregnadiene-3,20-dione

Betamethasone 9α-Fluoro-16β-methyl-$11\beta,17\alpha,21$-trihydroxy-1,4-pregnadiene-3,20-dione

Paramethasone 6α-Fluoro-16α-methyl-$11\beta,17\alpha,21$-trihydroxy-1,4-pregnadiene-3,20-dione

Flumethasone $6\alpha,9\alpha$-Difluoro-16α-methyl-$11\beta,17\alpha,21$-trihydroxy-1,4-pregnadiene-3,20-dione

Dichlorisone $9\alpha,11\beta$-Dichloro-$17\alpha,21$-dihydroxy-1,4-pregnadiene-3,20-dione

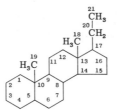

Pregnane

II. EVOLUTION OF THERAPEUTIC AGENTS

The effectiveness of corticosteroids as therapeutic agents for inflammatory diseases is well known. Their usefulness in the treatment of chronic inflammatory conditions is questioned by many clinicians because of the medical complications arising from their long-term use. Some untoward reactions seen with corticosteroids are interference with the pituitary–adrenal relationship, leading to adrenal insufficiency, and effects on electrolyte balance and glucose metabolism; the latter could exacerbate a (pre-existing) diabetic condition. Other serious side effects attributed to corticosteroids are osteoporosis as well as decreased ability to resist bacterial or viral infections.

Early work in corticosteroid research was geared toward the selection of compounds that were more potent antiinflammatory agents but that had a reduced incidence of side effects. As a result of this research effort a number of drugs were found, e.g. prednisolone, with increased antiinflammatory potency (3-5 times cortisol) and less adverse effect on electrolyte balance. The relative ease of separating the electrolyte effects from the antiinflammatory effects should have been predicted because these two activities are not necessarily demonstrable in the same naturally occurring adrenal steroids. For example deoxycorticosterone effects the electrolyte balance but has no antiinflammatory activity.

Very little success has been attained in synthesizing corticosteroids with a better separation of antiinflammatory activity from the other major side effects, e.g., osteoporosis and decreased resistance to infections. Lack of success in this area may be due to (1) the direct relationship between antiinflammatory activity and the side effect or (2) the animal models being used, select only those compounds with the aforementioned side effects.

Most scientists in the major pharmaceutical companies in the United States selected the former reasoning and had begun to look for other types of compounds with the expectation of finding potent antiinflammatory agents without the liabilities of corticosteroids. In their quest for new classes of antiinflammatory drugs, they required new animal models, e.g., carrageenan-induced inflammation. A number of nonsteroidal antiinflammatory agents have been introduced in the last 10–12 years, with indomethacin being the most potent. Although indomethacin has high potency in the animal model(s), its clinical efficacy in patients with rheumatic arthritis has been questioned in a trial comparing indomethacin and aspirin with placebo (Cooperating Clinics Committee of the American Rheumatism Association, 1967).*

The object of this chapter is not to compare the merits of nonsteroidal and steroidal antiinflammatory drugs, but to stress that new approaches to corticosteroid research, both in the clinic and in animal studies, are required to attain the full benefit of this very powerful class of antiinflammatory agents.

Attempts to reduce side effects have led (1) to the successful utilization of corticosteroids that are locally active with little or no systemic activity and (2) to the use of systemically active agents on a less frequent basis, e.g., administered only once a day or on alternate days.

---

*Editors' Note: The clinical evaluation of antiinflammatory agents is very complex. The above-cited study is well worth reading to gain an appreciation of this.

III. METHODS FOR EVALUATING CORTICOSTEROIDS

A. Laboratory

There are extensive reviews of standard laboratory assays used to identify the profile of corticosteroids (Sarett et al., 1963; Ringler, 1964); therefore, they are not described in detail here. However, we describe briefly those assays used to determine the structure–activity relationships reviewed in the following section of this chapter and some of the newer assays that may identify novel antiinflammatory steroids.

In the early days of corticosteroid development the emphasis of research was on high potency in the hope that decreasing the milligram quantity administered would lead to a decrease in side effects. The usefulness of any assay is related to how well the derived drug potencies correlated to clinical efficacy of the drug. Many correlation studies were carried out to provide a historical framework for the synthesizing and selection of new drugs for clinical trial. There are sufficiently large gaps in our knowledge, creating exceptions to any known generalizations, that it is difficult to rely on a single assay on which to base these correlations. In addition to the obvious species difference, the lack of a good animal model for rheumatoid arthritis increases the difficulty of developing qualitatively different corticosteroids. Another complicating factor is that human potencies used in the correlation studies are in fact based on the milligram quantity of drug in the dosage form and not on a potency derived from a true dose-response curve.

Models of inflammation used to determine potencies of corticosteroids were based on placing an irritant, e.g., croton oil or cotton, in contact with the animal. Other corticosteroid assays were empirically derived, e.g., thymolysis or eosinopenia, in which the correlation with inflammation is unknown but which happen to be produced by standard antiinflammatory steroids.

The croton oil-induced granuloma pouch assay (Tolksdorf, 1959) in rats is one of the most widely used screens for corticosteroids. A pneumoderma is formed by injecting air into the subcutaneous space, along with croton oil. The croton oil induces both granuloma tissue and an exudate within the air bleb. Drug is administered systemically (orally or subcutaneously) or locally (intradermally above the pouch or directly into the pouch). The degree of inflammation is measured by the volume of exudate collected and the weight of the granuloma formed.

A modification of the pouch assay is the croton oil ear test (Tonelli et al., 1965). In this test croton oil applied topically to the rat's ear elicits an acute inflammatory response that is quantitated by removing and then weighing the ear. The corticosteroid can be assayed for topical acitivity by applying the drug directly to the ear or for systemic activity by administering the drug orally or parenterally.

Inflammation is also produced by implanting a cotton pellet of known weight into a subcutaneous pocket in rats (Meier *et al.*, 1955). The accumulation of granuloma tissue around the pellet is a measure of the degree of inflammation. Drugs can be absorbed directly on to the pellet to determine local antiinflammatory activity or, as in the previous tests, drugs can be administered systemically. The cotton pellet offers some advantage in that the types and numbers of inflammatory cells can be determined by examining a histological section of the pellet.

Corticosteroids cause thymolysis, and the decrease in the weight of this tissue is used as a measure of a drug's potency. This assay is primarily used for the determination of systemic potency but can be used in conjunction with the assay described above as an end point for systemic effects after local administration of drug.

Corticosteroids also have an effect on glucose metabolism that has led to the development of the liver glycogen deposition assay (Stafford *et al.*, 1956). This assay is carried out either in intact or in adrenalectomized rats and can only be a measure of the systemic activity of a drug. In addition to aiding in the construction of a pharmacological profile for an antiinflammatory corticosteroid, this test is used to evaluate possible effects on glucose metabolism.

Another extensively used assay for antiinflammatory activity of systemically administered corticosteroids is the eosinophil depression test. The pioneering work of Tolksdorf *et al.* (1957) developed this assay in adrenalectomized mice to a point where it could be used to predict the clinical potency of a drug. This end point is used in intact as well as adrenalectomized dogs (Tolksdorf, 1959).

The use of these assays led to a series of corticosteroids with increased antiinflammatory potency but the side effects were not diminished. As investigators began to look for new chemical entities as a means of decreasing side effects, it became apparent that the available assays were not suitable. Thymolysis, eosinopenia, and glycogen deposition appears to be unique to steroidal antiinflammatory drugs and many of the nonsteroids were not very effective in these steroid-sensitive inflammation assays, e.g., croton oil pouch. This necessitated a search for tests in which the activity of such nonsteroid antiinflammatory drugs as aspirin and phenylbutazone could be demonstrated.

Rheumatoid arthritis is now thought to be an immunologically mediated chronic inflammatory disease precipitated by an unknown antigen. The mechanism by which the inflammatory process becomes self-perpetuating is also unknown, but antibodies to γ-globulin (rheumatoid factor) are formed and then complex with its antigen in the synovial space. The immunocomplexes can fix complement, which leads to a series of enzymatic reactions the products of which could sustain the inflammatory process.

Adjuvant-induced polyarthritic rats, antigen-induced arthritis in rabbits, and allergic encephalomyelitis in rats are examples of immunologically mediated inflammatory diseases. The inflammation produced in the rat models is a cell-mediated immunological response, whereas that in the rabbit is produced by immune complexes (Cooke et al., 1972). Corticosteroids are active in these models (Rosenthale and Nagra, 1967; Davis, 1971) but a broad range of corticosteroids have not yet been tested in them. These models will not be described here because they are covered in Chapter 3, Volume II. In these models, however, there is an induction phase in which the immunological mechanisms are primed and then a phase where the immune response elicits an inflammation that causes tissue destruction. A study of the potency of known corticosteroids during each phase is needed to determine whether relative potencies change with phase and whether differences in potency are related to structural types. This kind of information may lead to the synthesis of structural analogs that are more selective in their action and thereby have fewer side effects.

Another reason for using these newer assays is to select one as a primary screen. The major drawback in the prolonged clinical use of corticosteroids has been their side effects. Such effects as suppression of adrenal function, osteoporosis, and thinning of the skin have not been diminished by increasing the antiinflammatory potency of the corticosteroid. Perhaps the old primary screens only selected a particular class of corticosteroids with these inherent drawbacks. A new primary screen based on a new set of presumptions may increase the probability of identifying new steroidal structures with high antiinflammatory activity and fewer side effects.

B. Clinical

The whole spectrum of clinical tests is not reviewed here (see Chapter 1 by Paulus). However, because the topical or locally acting corticosteriods are the subject of much clinical interest at the present time, only those assays which give some idea of topical potency in man are discussed here.

The McKenzie-Stoughton test (1962) is the most popular way of assaying the topical activity of a corticosteroid. The assay is based on the vasoconstriction caused by the corticoid after it is applied to an area of skin, that is then covered by occlusive dressing. The degree and duration of vasoconstriction of the medicated area is used as the measure of topical antiinflammatory activity. This assay has been modified to allow more reliable quantitative data to be obtained. Place *et al.* (1970) outlined a more uniform method for the vasoconstriction assay. The type of glassware, the formulation of drug, the area of skin used, and the duration of drug application are all controlled. All corticosteroids are made up as alcoholic solutions and applied to an area of skin that is outlined by a thin film of silicone grease. After the vehicle evaporates, the area is occluded for 1–2 hours before the skin is evaluated for vasoconstriction. The response is sufficiently variable for the authors to stress the need to use large numbers of subjects.

In the clinical area there is a great need to devise short-term assays for the more important side effects. There are adequate and sensitive measures for determining the effects on adrenal function but, unfortunately, no assays for early recognition of such side effects as osteoporosis are yet available. Only long-term corticosteroid treatment will uncover this untoward reaction. Inability to obtain rapid clinical validation of laboratory findings has undoubtedly been one of the reasons for the slow development of agents exhibiting a separation of therapeutic and untoward activities.

IV. STRUCTURE–ACTIVITY RELATIONSHIPS

As it is beyond the scope of this chapter to present a complete survey of all the developments on new corticoids in the last decade, only the most significant advances in this area are described here.

In the decade since the most comprehensive reviews on structure–activity relationships of corticoids were written (Bush, 1962; Sarett *et al.*, 1963; Ringler, 1964), the principal purpose in synthesizing new corticoids served three purposes: (1) to find antiinflammatory agents with decreased side effects without concomitant significant loss of the antiinflammatory potency; (2) to find agents with local activity without significant systemic effects; (3) to find agents with either increased duration of a activity (so-called "depot-corticoids") or with rapid onset of activity.

A. Search for Corticosteriods with Better Separation of Antiinflammatory Activities from Side Effects

It is the opinion of the authors that the considerable research effort expended in this area during the last decade has not realized the returns or met with the success hoped for. Although novel corticosteroids with extremely high antiinflammatory potencies (often over 10^3 times that of cortisol) were synthesized—a remarkable chemical achievement on any score—the incidences of side effects, unfortunately, at least as indicated by the results of laboratory testing in animals, were also rather high. Therefore, only a few of these new compounds could be successfully introduced into clinical use.

Introduction of new substituents into the cortisol molecule, addition of double bonds, and other relatively simple chemical modifications led to the introduction of many highly potent antiinflammatory agents in the 1952–1962 period. Elimination of at least one of the most significant side effects, electrolyte retention, was effected first by Δ^1 insertion and then by combination of 9α fluorination and 16α hydroxylation or later by 16 methylation. The principal corticoids of the early 1960's, prednisone, prednisolone, triamcinolone, 6α-methylprednisolone, dexamethasone, betamethasone, paramethasone, flumethasone, etc., are still among the most widely used steroidal antiinflammatory agents. Relatively few new structures have appeared since that did not incorporate at least some of the basic structural features of these compounds, i.e., $\Delta^{1,4}$-diene, 6α-, and/or 9α-halogen substitution, or 16-methyl or 16α-hydroxy substitution, the latter often in the form of a cyclic ketal joined with the 17α-hydroxyl group.

Among the more recent developments, attachment of a heterocyclic ring to positions C-2 and C-3, or C-16 and C-17, in the modified cortisol molecule has led to interesting compounds. In 1963 Hirschmann, Fried, and co-workers reported the synthesis of 2'-aryl-4-pregneno [3,2-c] pyrazoles with extremely high antiinflammatory potencies in the rat. In addition, sodium retention appeared to be absent in this series of compounds (Fried et al., 1963). The structure-activity relationship data for the most interesting compounds in this series are listed in Table I. Surprisingly, maximum antiinflammatory activity is reached in the $\Delta^{4,6}$ series, especially in the presence of a 6-methyl group and although the 9α-fluoro substituent increases the antiinflammatory potency, its potentiating effect is much less dramatic than in the absence of the [3,2-c] pyrazole ring. Among the compounds listed on Table I cortivazol (4) is of the greatest interest and was recently introduced as an oral corticoid in Argentina. Table I also lists the activities of a number of 6,7-difluoro-methylene-4-pregneno-[3,2-c] pyrazoles prepared by Harrison, Fried, and co-workers (Harrison et al., 1968). It is noteworthy that the 6,7β-difluoro-methylene compound (13) has extremely high thymolytic activity, even higher than the corresponding 6,7α-difluoromethylene analog (12). Hitherto, no 6β- or 7β-substituted corticoid has shown any activity enhancement as compared to the corresponding unsubstituted compounds.

Another interesting group of heterocyclic steroids with high antiinflammatory activity is the [17α,16α-d]oxazolino corticoids reported by Nathansohn et al. (1969). The presence of [17α,16α-d] oxazolino ring

TABLE I Pregn-4-eno[3,2-c]pyrazoles and Related Compounds

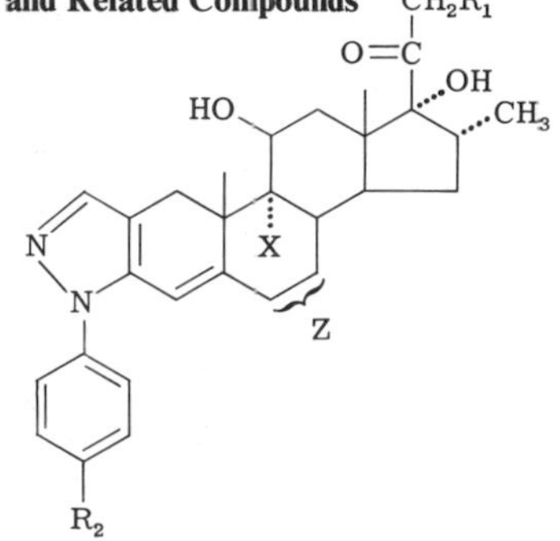

Compound number	R_1	R_2	X	Z	Systemic[a] granuloma	Adrenal[a] atrophy	Thymolysis	Topical anti-inflammatory	Reference
1	OAc	H	H	—	60				Hirschmann et al. (1964a)
2	OAc	F	H	—	100				Hirschmann et al. (1964a)
3	OAc	F	F	—	500	500			Hirschmann et al. (1964b)
4[b]	OAc	H	H	Δ^6-6-Methyl	600	740	400[a]	500–700[a]	Steelman et al. (1971)
5	H	H	H	Δ^6-6-Methyl	350	400	215[a]		Steelman et al. (1971)
6	OH	F	H	Δ^6-6-Methyl	600				Fried et al. (1963)
7	OH	H	F	Δ^6-6-Methyl	2000				Fried et al. (1963)
8	H	H	H	Δ^6-6-Methyl	348				Fried et al. (1963)
9	H	F	H	Δ^6-6-Methyl	464				Fried et al. (1963)
10	OH	H	H	$6\alpha,7\alpha$-CF_2			860[c]	90	Harrison et al. (1968)
11	OH	F	H	$6\alpha,7\alpha$-CF_2			750[c]	153[d,e]	Harrison et al. (1968)
12	OH	F	F	$6\alpha,7\alpha$-CF_2			1400[c]	70[d]	Harrison et al. (1968)
13	OH	F	F	$6\beta,7\beta$-CF_2			1920[c]	110[d]	Harrison et al. (1968)

Biological potency (cortisol = 1)

[a] In normal male rats, according to Steelman et al. (1963). [b] Antirheumatic activity in man is 75 times cortisol (Steelman et al., 1971). [c] Modification of the method of Dorfman et al. (1961). [d] Suppression of ear edema. Modification of the method of Tonelli et al. (1965). [e] One-to-two times as potent as fluocinolone acetonide in the vasoconstrictor assay of McKenzie and Stoughton (1962).

253

affords products with ether-water partition coefficients resembling those of the corresponding $16\alpha,17\alpha$-acetonides. This particular physical constant has been related to topical antiinflammatory activity, as will be seen in Section IV,B,1. The structure–activity data of the more interesting compounds in this series are listed in Table II. Among the $[17\alpha,16\alpha\text{-}d]$ oxazolino steriods, (19), L-6400, was studied in the greatest detail. In rats, the antiinflammatory potency of L-6400 is approximately that of dexamethasone. Like dexamethasone, L-6400 is catabolic and has no effect on electrolyte excretion. L-6400 appears to have a shorter duration of action than dexamethasone, as indicated by its less intense and shorter lasting effect on the pituitary–adrenal axis (as measured by blood corticosterone levels) and on glycemia in response to a glucose load (Restelli and Arrigoni-Martelli, 1971). A compound with this profile can be used in alternate day therapy.

TABLE II

$[17\alpha,16\alpha\text{-}d]$ Oxazolino Steroids

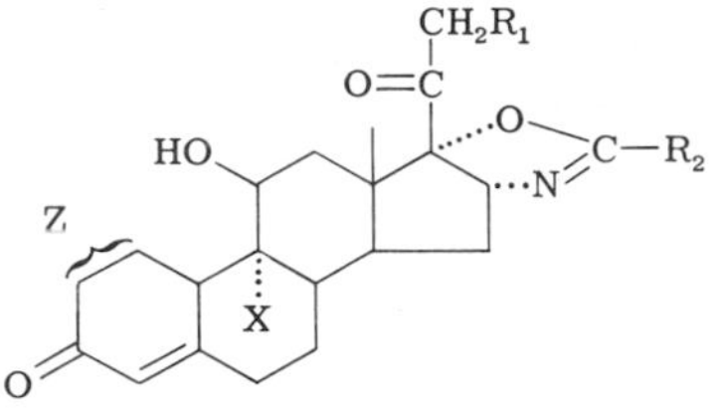

Compound number	R_1	R_2	X	Z	Biological potency (cortisol = 1)		Partition coefficient $(Et_2O\text{–}H_2O)$
					Liver glycogen[a]	Cotton pellet granuloma[b]	
14	OAc	CH_3	H	Δ^1	10	35	9.2
15	OH	CH_3	H	Δ^1	19	35	0.61
16	H	CH_3	H	Δ^1	23	24	6.1
17	OH	CH_3	H	—	2.5	2.4	—
18	OH	CH_3	F	Δ^1	180	250	0.88
19	OAc	CH_3	F	Δ^1	180	250	10.0
20	H	CH_3	F	Δ^1	88	135	7.5
21	OH	H	F	Δ^1	13	14	0.23
22	OH	nC_4H_9	F	Δ^1	15	11	—
23	OH	C_6H_5	F	Δ^1	10	270	38
Dexamethasone	—	—		—	180	270	6.6

[a]Determined on adrenalectomized male rats by the method of Olson *et al.* (1944).
[b]Determined on adrenalectomized male rats by the method of Meier *et al.* (1950).

The advantages of this type of therapy will be discussed in Section V,A. The topical activity of L-6400, measured by vasoconstrictor activity in man, indicates that a 0.1% cream of this compound will have a therapeutic activity at least equal to that of a 0.1% triamcinolone acetonide cream or a 0.025% fluocinolone acetonide cream, and these expectations were verified in using a 0.025% and 0.1% cream of L-6400 in the treatment of psoriasis and eczema (Arrigoni-Martelli et al., 1971; F. B. Nicolis, private communication).

Although corticosterone itself shows no antiinflammatory activity in man and has much lower antiinflammatory potency in animals than cortisol (Sarett et al., 1963, p. 131), 6α-fluoro-Δ^1-16α-methylcorticosterone is a potent antiinflammatory agent in experimental animals and man. Other derivatives of corticosterone have also shown high antiinflammatory activities in animals, and the data are summarized in Table III. Fluocortolone (27) has found therapeutic use in humans as a systemic corticosteroid, whereas fluocortolone caproate (28) is used as a topical antiinflammatory agent. Desoximethasone (26) has been recently introduced into clinical practice as a topical antiinflammatory agent in France.

In view of the high antiinflammatory activities of the 9α-fluoro-16-methylcorticoids, it is not at all surprising that 9α-fluoro-16-methyleneprednisolone is an effective antiinflammatory agent (Kraft and Harting, 1968). Some of the biological activities of 16-methylenecorticoids are listed in Table IV. Fluprednylene acetate (30) is being used as an antiinflammatory agent in man and also as a topical antiinflammatory agent (Schwind, 1968).

Among the $9\alpha,11\beta$-dichlorosteroids (dichlorisone derivatives), a number of new compounds are reported, and although most of these compounds are more interesting for topical application and are discussed in Section IV,B,1,d, their systemic antiinflammatory activities are listed in Table V.

The marked increase of antiinflammatory potency of the water-soluble disodium phosphate (33) over the parent alcohol (32) was demonstrated in the rat, in the dog, and in man. Oral administration of (33) caused eosinopenia in the dog to a much greater extent than equivalent doses of the parent (32). In man, the enhancement caused by 21 phosphorylation of (32) against arthritis and alopecia totalis, was about twofold. This increase in potency is attributed to better absorption of the phosphate (33) (Herzog et al., 1967).

Another interesting group of corticoids synthesized during the last decade was the derivatives of 3-(2'-chloroethoxy)-$\Delta^{3,5}$-6-formylpregnanes (Suchowsky and Baldratti, 1967). A number of these compounds, listed in Table VI, possessed high antiinflammatory potencies. Fluorformylon (44) was the most potent locally acting antiinflammatory agent in this class and was put into clinical use as a topical agent. It is noteworthy that (44), even at low

TABLE III

Corticosterone Derivatives

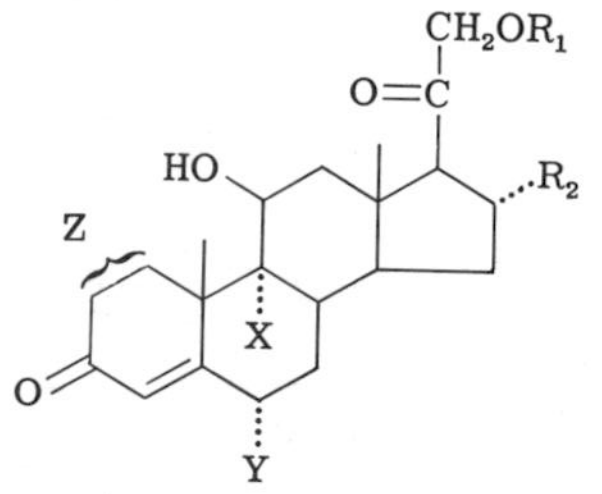

Compound number	R$_1$	R$_2$	X	Y	Z	Biological potency (cortisol = 1)					Reference
						Granuloma pellet[a]	Granuloma pouch local[b]	Eosinopenia[c]	Liver glycogen[d]	Thymolysis	
24	H	H	H	H	—	0.5				0.3	Branceni et al. (1965)
25	H	CH$_3$	H	H	Δ^1	3[e]				3[e]	Branceni et al. (1965)
26	H	CH$_3$	F	H	Δ^1	15[f] (p.o.) 37 (s.c.)				50[f] (p.o.) 37 (s.c.)	Branceni et al. (1965)
27	H	CH$_3$	H	F	Δ^1	50[g] (s.c.) 350 (p.o.)	4	63 (s.c.) 100 (p.o.)	3–10	17 (s.c.)	Domenico et al. (1965)
28	COC$_5$H$_{11}$	CH$_3$	H	F	Δ^1	10 (s.c.) 23 (p.o.)	2				Domenico et al. (1965)

[a] Jequier et al. (1965).
[b] Selye (1953a).
[c] Speirs and Meyer (1951).
[d] Vennig et al. (1946).
[e] Compared to prednisolone = 3 times cortisol in the same test.
[f] Compared to dexamethasone = 150 times cortisol in the same test.
[g] Granuloma pouch test; see footnote b.

TABLE IV

16-Methyleneprednisolone Derivatives

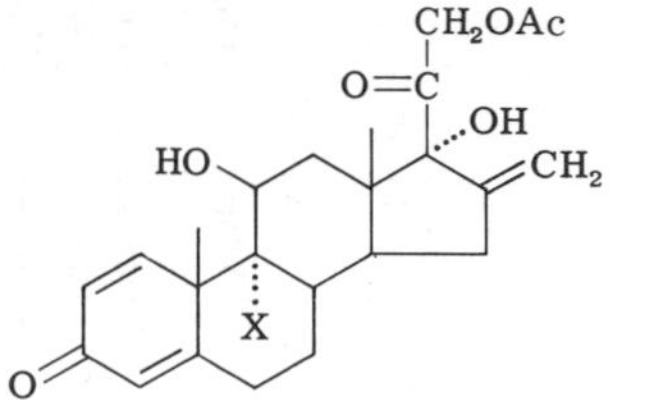

		Biological potency (cortisol $= 1$)		
Compound number	X	Granuloma pouch (s.c.)	Thymolysis	Liver glycogen
29	H	58.7	2.0	38.2
30	F	97.2	17.6	187.0

doses (> 1 mg/kg), protected mice and rats but not guinea pigs from fatal anaphylactic shock. The water-soluble hemisuccinate derivative (**48**) gave an immediate but shorter lasting action in protecting mice or rats (Fregnan and Suchowsky, 1968).

The preparation of 16α-halogenated corticoids was reported for the first time in the early 1960's. The 16α-fluoro group increased the antiinflammatory potency of prednisolone and 6α-substituted prednisolone derivatives to a greater degree than the 16α-chloro group. In the 9α-fluoroprednisolone series, however, the 16α-chloro group enhanced potency to a greater degree than the 16α-fluoro group, regardless of whether there was any 6 substituent present. A comparison of the antiinflammatory potencies of the 16α-chloro and 16α-fluorocorticoids is shown in Table VII.

The introduction of prednisolone and prednisone into medical practice dramatically demonstrated the importance of the Δ^1 double bond for increasing antiinflammatory potency. However, the effect that introducing other double bonds into the corticoid molecule would have on the antiinflammatory potency was not predictable. For example, the introduction of the Δ^6 double bond can either enhance, decrease, or leave unaffected the antiinflammatory activity. A number of 8(9)-dehydroprednisolone derivatives have shown marked thymolytic potency in experimental animals as can be seen in Table VIII (Heller *et al.*, 1966). In general, the $\Delta^{8(9)}$ compounds are of somewhat lower potency than the corresponding 8,9-dihydro compounds (prednisolone derivatives). The large decrease in activity of the

TABLE V

Dichlorisone Derivatives

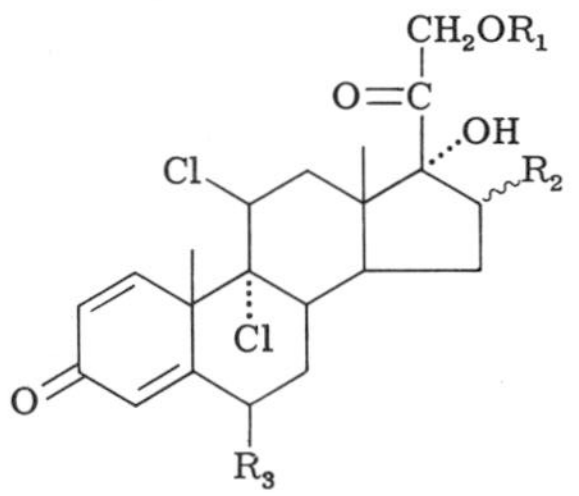

Compound number	R$_1$	R$_2$	R$_3$	Biological potency (prednisolone acetate = 1)			Human potency (prednisolone = 1)			Reference
				Granuloma pouch	Thymolysis	Adrenal atrophy	Dermatitis (topical)	Arthritis (p.o.)	Colitis (p.o.)	
31	COCH$_3$	H	H	—	—	—	0.25[a]	0.01	0.05	Herzog et al. (1967)
32	H	α-CH$_3$	H	1.1	0.9	1.5	—	0.16	0.25	Herzog et al. (1967)
33	PO$_3$Na$_2$	α-CH$_3$	H	8.2	4.1	7.5	—	0.33	—	Herzog et al. (1967)
34	PO$_3$H$_2$	α-CH$_3$	H	7.3	3.9	6.8	—	—	—	Herzog et al. (1967)
35	H	H	H	0.1	0.08	—	—	—	—	Collins et al. (1967)
36	H	H	CH$_3$	0.7	0.8	1.5	—	—	—	Collins et al. (1967)
37	H	H	F	1.7	3.3	1.7	—	—	—	Collins et al. (1967)
38	H	β-CH$_3$	H	0.09	0.07	—	—	—	—	Collins et al. (1967)
39	H	α-CH$_3$	F	7.0	7.7	9.1	—	—	—	Collins et al. (1967)

[a] Compared to cortisol.

TABLE VI

Derivatives of 3-(2′-Chloroethoxy)-$\Delta^{3,5}$-6-formylpregnanes

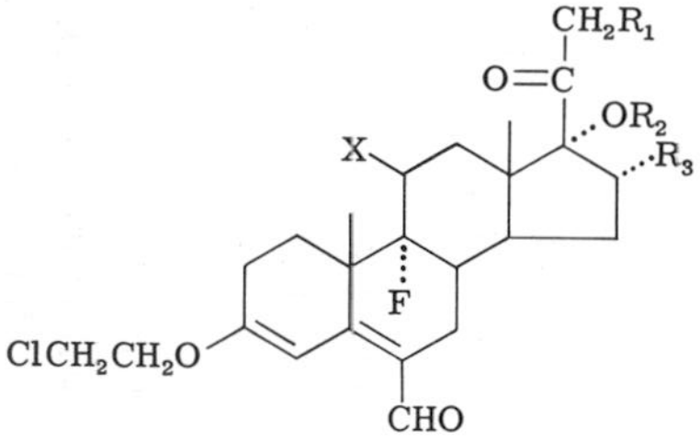

Compound number	R_1	R_2	R_3	X	Biological potency (cortisol acetate = 1): Granuloma pouch[a] Local[d]	Granuloma pouch[a] Oral	Granuloma pouch[a] s.c.	Cotton pellet (local)[b]	Liver glycogen[c]
40	H	16α,17α-Acetonide		β—OH	61.4	<37.5	<16.5	0.8	1
41	OH	H	H	β—OH	3.4	—	—	—	<0.5
42	OAc	H	H	=C	113.3	57.7	78.6	7.7	4.0
43	OAc	H	H	β—OH	10.3	46.9	—	0.5	—
44	OAc	16α,17α-Acetonide		β—OH	680.0	35.7	22.9	6.5	20.0
45	OAc	16α,17α-Acetonide		=C	13.3	23.4	—	2.4	—
46	$OCOC_4H_9$	16α,17α-Acetonide		β—OH	130.0	12.5	<16.5	24.0	4.0
47	OAc	H	CH_3	β—OH	130.0	70.8	—	<0.8	—
48	$OCO(CH_2)_2COONa$	16α,17α-Acetonide		β—OH		—	—	—	—

[a] Robert and Nezamis (1957).
[b] Hershberger and Calhoun (1957).
[c] Stafford *et al*. (1955).
[d] Fregnan and Suchowsky (1968).

TABLE VII

16α-Halogenated Prednisolone Derivatives

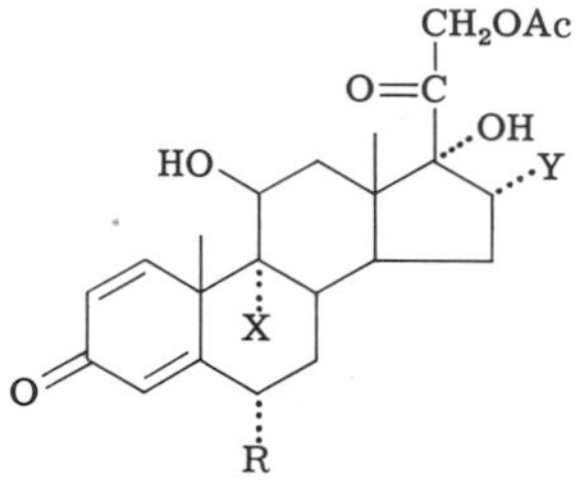

| Compound number | Y | R | X | Biological potency (cortisol = 1) | | Reference |
				Granuloma pouch[a]	Liver glycogen[b]	
49	H	H	H	3	4	Kagan et al. (1964)
50	F	H	H	16	—	Magerlein et al. (1960)
51	Cl	H	H	8	9	Kagan et al. (1964)
52	F	H	F	75	—	Magerlein et al. (1960)
53	Cl	H	F	313	360	Kagan et al. (1964)
54	H	CH₃	H	10	15	Kagan et al. (1964)
55	F	CH₃	H	20	25	Magerlein et al. (1961)
56	Cl	CH₃	H	19	15	Kagan et al. (1964)
57	F	CH₃	F	190	250	Magerlein et al. (1960)
58	H	F	H	25	100	Kagan et al. (1964)
59	F	F	H	100	116	Magerlein et al. (1961)
60	Cl	F	H	58	100	Kagan et al. (1964)
61	F	F	F	480	425	Magerlein et al. (1961)
62	Cl	F	F	1100	1030	Kagan et al. (1964)

[a] Robert and Nezamis (1957).
[b] Stafford et al. (1955).

16α-methyl compound (**64**) compared to that of 16α-methylprednisolone clearly shows the fallacy of projecting biological relationships of one series into another series.

Another corticoid with additional double bonds is the $\Delta^{1,4,6,15}$-tetraene, EMD 8995 (**67**) (Harting and Kraft, 1971), which is listed in Table IX together with other miscellaneous corticoids with significant antiinflammatory potencies.

Finally, during the last decade synthetic ACTH (corticotrophin) analogs have been introduced into therapy. Although the corticosteroids have the advantage of being orally active, whereas corticotrophin must be given by intramuscular injection and because of its antigenecity may produce hyper-

TABLE VIII

8(9)-Dehydroprednisolone Derivatives

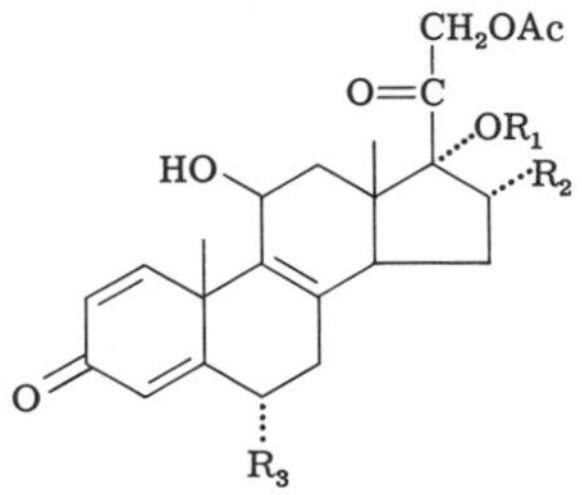

Compound number	R_1	R_2	R_3	Thymolysis (cortisol = 1)[a]
63	H	H	F	2.34
64	H	CH_3	H	0.36
65	16α,17α-Acetonide		H	2.8
66	16α,17α-Acetonide		F	11.4

[a] Mauer et al. (1962).

sensitivity reactions, in certain cases there are definite advantages to the use of ACTH analogs. There is no growth-restricting effect with the use of ACTH analogs (Friedman and Strang, 1966) and withdrawal from ACTH treatment is claimed to be easier (Savage et al., 1971). Several ACTH analogs are currently available for human use (and reviewed in more detail in Chapter 11 by Fisher). Tetracosactrin, a synthetic polypeptide containing the first 24 amino acids of the peptide chain, is reported to maintain its biological activity with a reduced incidence of allergic reactions relative to natural porcine ACTH. A depot form of this hormone (0.5 mg twice a week) does not cause significant suppression of the pituitary–adrenal axis (Geyer and Reimer, 1970; Irvine et al., 1971). Combination of synthetic corticotrophins with a corticoid has been sometimes used in an attempt to preserve adrenal function but without much evident success (Carter and James, 1970b).

B. Search for Agents with High Local Antiinflammatory Activity without Significant Systemic Effects

Ever since discovery of antiinflammatory effects of cortisone and cortisol, investigators have sought for more potent analogs that are active only at the site(s) of inflammation, to avoid the undesirable side effects observed with systemic administration. We shall rather arbitrarily consider "local" administration under the following headings: (1) topical administration,

TABLE IX

Miscellaneous Novel Corticoids

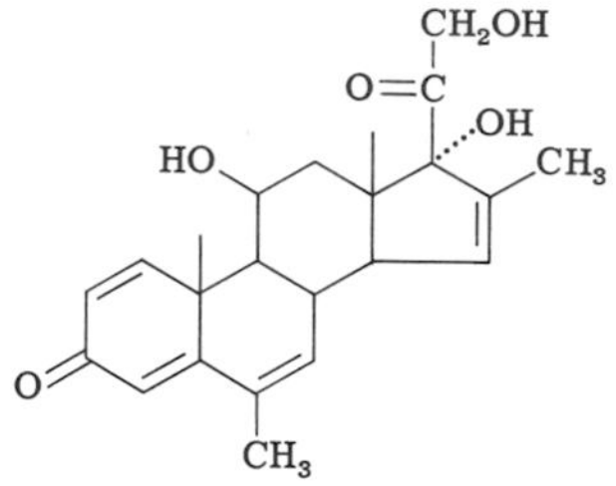

6 7

	Biological potency (cortisol = 1)			
Compound	Granuloma Pouch	Thymolysis	Adrenal suppression	Liver glycogen
Prednisolone	2	3.3	1.8	3.9
Dexamethasone	480	238	391	333
67	337	128	138	172

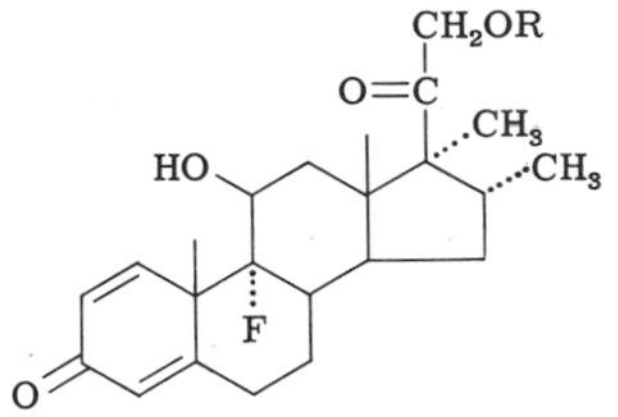

67a (R = COCH$_3$) (Schaub and Weiss, 1967).
     Thymolysis, 14.5 times cortisol. Increased Na$^+$ excretion.

67b (R = H) (Woods *et al.*, 1971)
     Thymolysis, 0.6 times betamethasone.
     Granuloma pouch, 0.75 times betamethasone.

(2) intraarticular administration, (3) intraocular administration, and (4) locally acting corticoids in allergy and asthma.

1. TOPICAL CORTICOSTEROIDS

Although cortisone and cortisone 21-acetate were devoid of topical activity, cortisol and cortisol 21-acetate were reported to be effective in various inflammatory dermatological disorders (Goldman *et al.*, 1952; Sulzberger and Witten, 1952). The more potent analogs of cortisol, i.e., prednisolone,

6α-methylprednisolone, triamcinolone, dexamethasone, or betamethasone, were synthesized principally for treating such systemic diseases as rheumatoid arthritis and asthma but were useful topically when formulated in appropriate vehicles. It should be stressed that these compounds were chosen for their high systemic potency, and their topical application was considered as only of secondary importance. These corticoids were relatively safe when administered by the topical route, with little, if any, irritating or sensitizing properties. In addition they were free or odor or staining and when applied in suitable vehicles were successful in the treatment of various dermatological inflammations.

Nevertheless, even in the late 1950's there was no deliberate effort made by scientists working in the steroid field to develop corticosteroids principally for topical use. During the 1960's the enormous advancement in the development of highly effective topical corticoids with little or no systemic effects could be traced to three principal factors.

The first was the early observation that triamcinolone acetonide was ten times as active topically as triamcinolone but only equiactive systemically (Sarett et al., 1963, p. 137). The related 6α-fluoro derivative, fluocinolone acetonide, possessed even higher topical activity although it was ineffective systemically.

Second, the development of relatively simple biological assays, both in experimental animals and man, afforded a greater ability to predict topical activity of steroids. Particular attention has to be given to the development of the Stoughton-McKenzie test.

The third factor was a better understanding of the relationship between certain physicochemical parameters of the steroid and its efficacy when administered topically.

Before the structure–activity relationships among topical corticosteroids are discussed, a few basic concepts concerning their mode of action in human skin must be mentioned.

A steroid, to be topically effective, must penetrate through the fully formed keratin (horny) layer of the stratum corneum (Fig. 1). The lower boundary of the stratum corneum offers a barrier to penetration. Once a compound penetrates through the stratum eorneum, it will readily reach the squamus cell layer of the epidermis. An additional barrier exists between the epidermis and the dermis. Those compounds which penetrate through this second barrier will reach the systemic circulation, giving rise to undesirable side effects. For a topical agent to be useful, it is desirable that the drug remain in the epidermis and migrate only slowly into the dermis.

If the keratin layer of the stratum corneum is properly hydrated (i.e., with an occlusive dressing), the penetration of some antiinflammatory steroids is greatly increased, sometimes by a factor of 100. Under ordinary

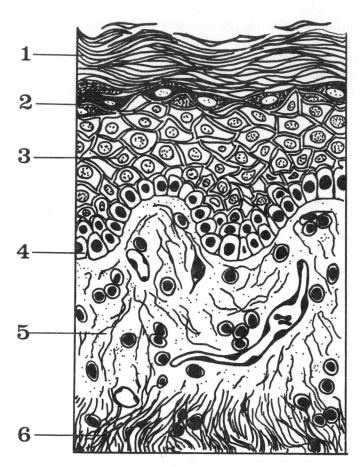

Fig. 1 Section of human skin. (1) Stratum corneum. The outer layers of these keratinized epithelia are loosely arranged and relatively easy to penetrate with steroids. Cells at the lower boundary of this layer are compressed and are difficult to penetrate. (2) Stratum granulosum. (3) Stratum spinosum. (4) Stratum germinativum. (5) Dermis, papillary layer. (6) Dermis, reticular layer.

conditions (i.e., without prior hydration or occlusive dressing), the factors determining absorption through the skin are (1) the nature of the steroid and (2) the vehicle in which the steroid is dissolved. A relatively high lipid solubility that can be correlated with a high ether (lipid)–water partition coefficient (see discussion of L-6400 in Section IV,A), certainly enhances absorption of the steroid. It is essential for effective absorption through the horny layer, and thus for good topical activity, that the steroid be soluble in the vehicle. Therefore under idealized conditions, the steroid will pass from the vehicle into the skin because of favorable partitioning of the steroid between its vehicle and the skin lipids. Even very fine particles in a suspension will not partition efficiently into skin lipids, making the preparation ineffective. The solvent of choice varies to a great extent; it can be lipophilic, e.g., various waxes, Vaseline, or mineral oil, or hydrophilic, e.g., propylene glycol, polyethylene glycol, dimethyl sulfoxide (DMSO), and glyceryl monostearate.

The formulation of the steroid can be in ointment form (Vaseline based), cream (aqueous emulsion), or solution (propylene glycol, etc.). The form used depends largely on the nature and stability of the compound. It is beyond the scope of this chapter to discuss in any detail the very important pharmaceutical factors governing the formulation of topical corticosteroids. The influence of formulation on topical corticosteroid activity has been repeatedly emphasized by a number of investigators (Sarkany et al., 1965; Sarkany and Hadgraft, 1969; Stoughton and Fritsch, 1964; Burdick et al., 1970).

It was pointed out above that triamcinolone acetonide is a much more effective topical agent than the parent $16\alpha,17\alpha$-diol, triamcinolone. The 16,17-acetonide group renders the steroid more lipophilic then the parent 16,17-diol, and therefore its penetration into the skin is greatly enhanced. In general, many of the significant systemically effective corticosteroids have been converted to highly active topical antiinflammatory agents by relatively simple structural changes. Usually conversion of one or two of the hydroxyl groups to less polar, more lipophilic derivatives, such as esters, diesters, or ketals, is sufficient to transform an effective systemic corticoid to a more active topical antiinflammatory agent.

For comparative purposes the topical corticosteroids are considered here under the following chemical classes:

    a. Acetonides, ketals, and related compounds
    b. 17-Monoesters
    c. 21-Monoesters
    d. 17,21-Diesters and orthoesters
    e. Miscellaneous compounds

Before these individual classes of topical corticosteroids are discussed a few general comments must be made concerning clinical data.

A comparative analysis of the large number of publications dealing with the therapeutic efficacy of topical corticosteroids is very difficult. Many of these reports deal with studies that are designed simply to demonstrate the clinical efficacy of particular topical agents in various dermatoses. Most of the studies carried out before 1964 involve the comparison of the compounds with cortisol or cortisol 21-acetate as a reference standard, whereas more recent studies use fluocinolone acetonide, triamcinolone acetonide, or betamethasone valerate as standards. In trying to rank the relative potencies of various topical corticosteroids, one must not overlook the different circumstances under which the various compounds have been evaluated, e.g., the absence of controlled quantitation of drug, and the area on which it was applied to the patient. In many instances, particularly in the early tests the minimal effective concentration has not been ascertained or reported. Furthermore, there are difficulties in comparing the relative topical potencies of steroids in animals because of the differences between the various assay methods used in different laboratories. Schlagel (1965) has written an excellent review on the comparative efficacy of some topical antiinflammatory steroids.

a. ACETONIDES, KETALS, AND RELATED COMPOUNDS. *i. 16α,17α-Acetonides.* Triamcinolone acetonide (**68**) is the first corticoid in which dissociation between topical and systemic activity has been observed (Sarett *et al.*, 1963, p. 137) and is one of the most frequently used topical antiinflammatory agents. The animal pharmacology (Ringler, 1964, p. 270) of (**68**) and its topical activity in man has been reviewed by Schlagel (1965). The preparation of a number of 21-esters of triamcinolone acetonide has recently been reported and among them the β-benzoylaminoisobutyrate (**69**) was found to be the most active. This compound, when administered topically or subcutaneously, is approximately 3-4 times more potent than (**68**), but when given orally it is about equal in potency to (**68**) (Ordonez, 1971). The increased topical activity may be again explained by decreased polarity and increased lipid solubility.

Fluocinolone acetonide (**71**) is another widely used topical corticosteroid. Fluocinolone acetonide is frequently used as the standard for determining the potency of new corticosteroids in man. In over 400 cases of dermatoses, a 0.025% fluocinolone acetonide cream has been about as effective as a 0.1% triamcinolone acetonide cream (Fishman, 1965). Recently, fluocinonide (**72**), the 21-acetate of (**71**), has been introduced into clinical practice. In a modification of the Stoughton-McKenzie assay, (**72**) had about 5 times the potency of (**71**), whereas the latter compound was about equipotent with triamcinolone acetonide and betamethasone 17-valerate (Place *et al.*, 1970). Limited clinical evaluation of fluocinonide cream (0.05%) has shown this compound to be better than betamethasone valerate cream (0.1%) in a number of cases (Rosenberg, 1971; Binder and McCleary, 1972).

Fluclorolone acetonide (73) is an effective topical corticosteroid in the vasoconstrictor assay (Garnier, 1971) and has recently been introduced into clinical use in South Africa. In rabbits treated systemically with this compound negligible bone effects were observed (Berliner *et al.*, 1970). Tralonide (74), the 21-deoxy-21-fluoro derivative of (73) (0.005% ointment) has been compared in a limited trial with flurandrenolone acetonide (75) in psoriasis and atopic dermatitis. Although there is no significant difference between the two drugs in psoriasis, tralonide is more effective than (75) in atopic dermatitis (Cullen, 1971).

Fluorformylon (44), described in Section IV,A, has high topical antiinflammatory activity, and has recently been introduced into clinical practice in Europe. 16α-Hydroxyprednisolone 16,17-acetonide (desonide, 76), recently introduced into clinical practice, is equipotent to triamcinolone acetonide when administered into the granuloma pouch of rats (Mascietti-Coriandoli and Fraia, 1970). Recently, a 0.05% cream of (76) has produced comparable results to a 0.025% cream of fluocinolone acetonide in a variety of dermatological conditions (Donsky, 1972).

A number of 16,17-acetonides related to 3β,11β-dihydroxy-4-pregnen-20-one are reported to possess significant topical antiinflammatory activity in experimental animals. The most active compounds and some of their biological activities are summarized in Table X (Deghenghi *et al.*, 1966). Although some of the allylic esters are quite potent in the rat, (81), the 21-deoxy derivative of flurandrenolone acetonide, and (77), its 9α-fluoro derivative, have shown the highest topical antiinflammatory activities.

ii. 17α,21-Acetonides. Although only the 16α,17α-acetonides of corticosteroids have found clinical application in man, acetonides of other steroidal vicinal diols have also been prepared and tested for their antiinflammatory activities. For example, 6α,7α-dihydroxyprednisolone 21-acetate 6,7-acetonide (Zderic *et al.*, 1959) and 12β-hydroxyprednisolone 21-acetate 11,12-acetonide (Zderic *et al.*, 1960) have been prepared and found to be essentially devoid of antiinflammatory activity. More interesting are the 17,21-acetonides derived from 1,3-diols. The structures and topical antiinflammatory activities of some 9α-chloro-17α,21-acetonides, and those of the corresponding 17α,21-diols, are listed in Table XI (Robinson *et al.*, 1961). The 17,21-acetonide moiety enhances the topical potency especially with the 9α-chloro-11β-formates.

iii. Miscellaneous derivatives. The topical antiinflammatory activity of L-6400 (19), structurally similar to a 16,17-acetonide, was discussed in Section IV,A.

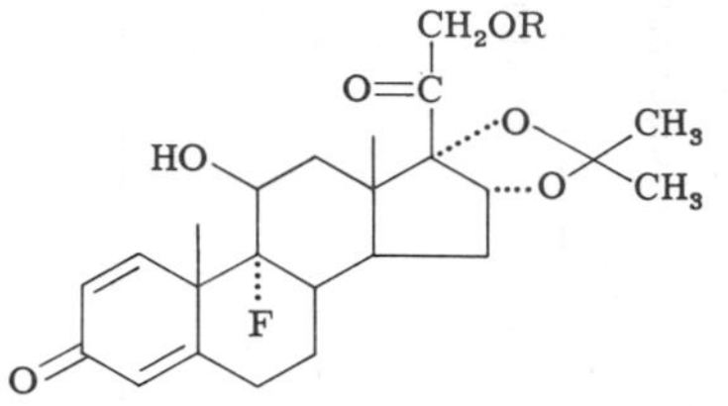

68 R = H

69 R = COCH—CH₂NHCOC₆H₅
        |
        CH₃
70 R = COCH₂C(CH₃)₃

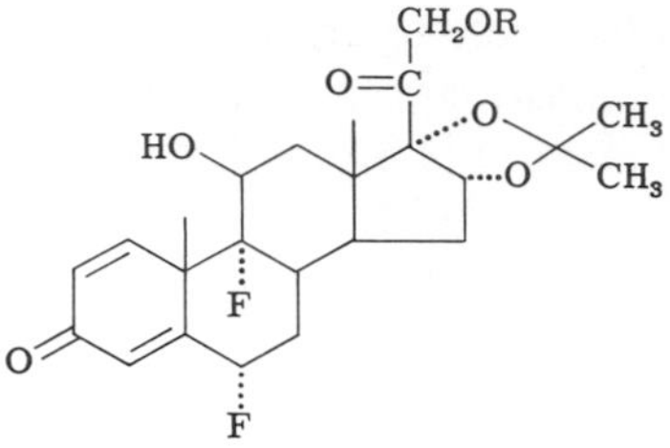

71 R = H
72 R = COCH₃

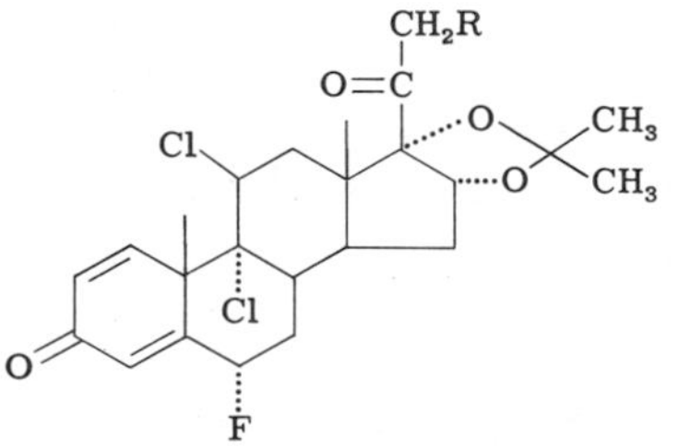

73 R = OH
74 R = F

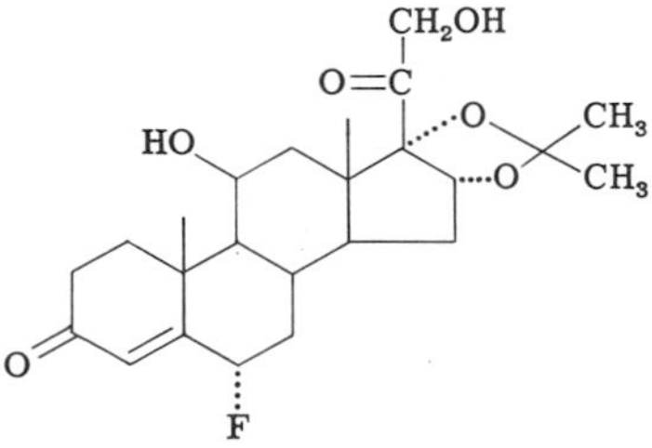

75

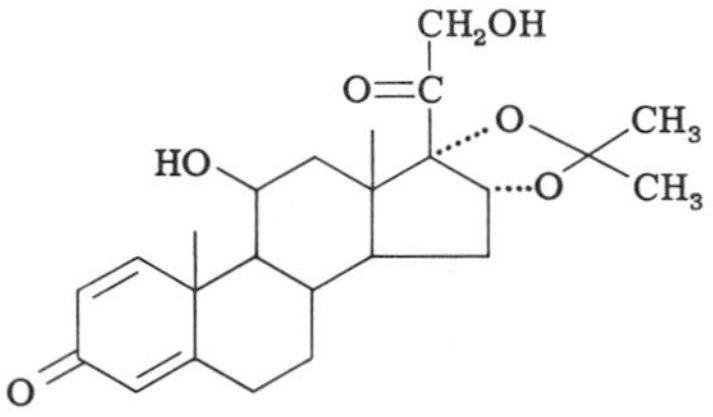

76

$16\alpha, 17\alpha$-Acetonides

b. 17-MONOESTERS. The use of the vasoconstriction assay in humans made it possible to screen a large variety of steroids for topical anti-inflammatory activity (McKenzie and Stoughton, 1962). The earliest comparative study was carried out by McKenzie and Atkinson (1964) on a variety of esters and orthoesters of betamethasone. Some of their findings are presented in Table XII.

Although betamethasone alcohol has only 1% of the activity of the standard, fluocinolone acetonide, the straight chain esters at C-21 have high activity, with the hexanoate being the most potent. Some of the 17,21-

TABLE X

Δ^4-Pregnenolone Derivatives

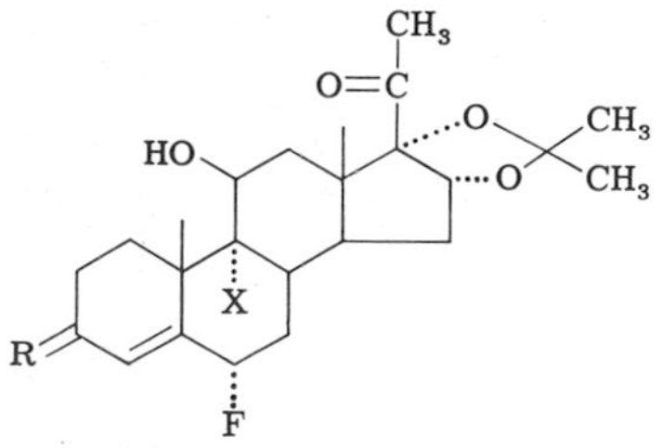

Compound number	R	X	Antiinflammatory potency (cortisol = 1): Granuloma pouch[a] Local	Granuloma pouch[a] Systemic	Adjuvant arthritis[b] Topical	Adjuvant arthritis[b] Systemic	Thymolysis	Liver glycogen	Ether–water partition coefficient
68	Triamcinolone acetonide		200	60	200	200	30	18	11.4
77	O	F	200	40	30	50	30	15	—
78	β-CH_3COO—	F	50	15	12	—	2	2	—
79	β-CH_3COO—	H	40	<1	3	20	<1	<1	3.1
80	β-C_6H_5COO—	H	8	—	—	10	<1	<1	7.8
81	O	H	200	15	20	50	9	5	—

[a] Robert and Nezamis (1957).
[b] Newbould (1963).

TABLE XI

17,21-Acetonides of 9α-Chlorocorticosteroids

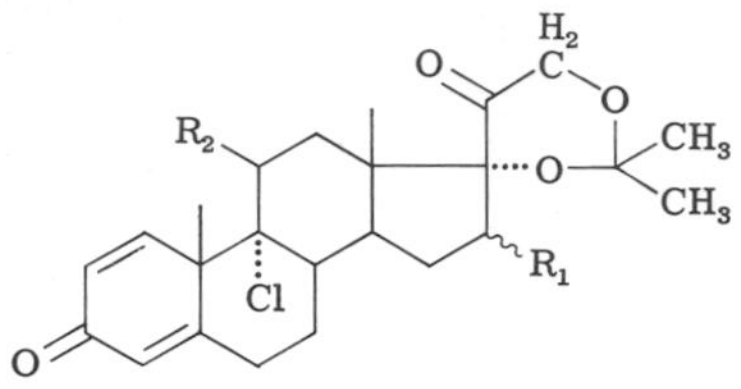

Compound number	R_1	R_2	Antiinflammatory potency (prednisolone acetate = 1)[a]	
			Of acetonide	Of 17α,21-diol
82	H	Cl	11.1	8.5
83	$\alpha-CH_3$	Cl	13.8	5
84	$\beta-CH_3$	Cl	14	13
85	$\alpha-CH_3$	OCHO	11.6	1.3
86	$\beta-CH_3$	OCHO	7	0.5

[a] Local granuloma pouch.

TABLE XII

Relative Potencies of Betamethasone and Some of Its Esters in Vasoconstriction Assays against Fluocinolone Acetonide

Compound number	Compound	Relative potency[a]
87	Betamethasone alcohol	0.8
88	Betamethasone 21-acetate	18
89	Betamethasone 21-butyrate	85
90	Betamethasone 21-valerate	26
91	Betamethasone 21-hexanoate	123
92	Betamethasone 21-palmitate	0.1
93	Betamethasone 21-disodium phosphate	0.9
94	Betamethasone 17,21-ethylorthoformate	1
95	Betamethasone 17,21-ethylorthopropionate	402
96	Betamethasone 17,21-ethylorthovalerate	150
97	Betamethasone 17,21-diethylorthocarbonate	166
98	Betamethasone 17-acetate	114
99	Betamethasone 17-butyrate	168
100	Betamethasone 17-valerate	360

[a] Fluocinolone acetonide = 100.

orthoesters have high vasoconstrictor potency, and this class of compounds is discussed in Section IV,B,1,d. The 17-esters are very potent, with maximum activity reached with the valerate. Betamethasone valerate (100) ointment (0.1%) was compared to a number of topical corticosteroid ointments, notably fluocinolone acetonide (0.025%) and triamcinolone acetonide (0.1%). Compound (100) had comparable or better results in a large number of patients with psoriasis, eczema, and other dermatoses (Williams et al., 1964; Mitchell et al., 1964; Björnberg and Hellgren, 1964). Since its introduction into clinical practice, (100) has become one of the most widely used topical antiinflammatory agents.

Recently, betamethasone 17-benzoate (101) has been reported as a very potent topical corticosteroid in the rat (DiPasquale et al., 1970b), but some systemic effects were observed with this compound both in rats (DiPasquale et al., 1970a) and in man (Mikhail, 1972). The vasoconstrictor effect of (101), using a white, soft paraffin–propylene glycol base, was comparable to that of a betamethasone 17-valerate ointment (Pepler et al., 1971).

Dexamethasone 17-valerate (102) was recently reported to possess high topical antiinflammatory activity in various dermatoses. The steroid alone, or in combination with antibacterial agents (e.g., neomycin or iodochlorhydroxyquin), was clinically effective (Rasponi, 1971; Cozzi, 1971) and was introduced into clinical practice in Italy.

Using the same vehicle, hydrocortisone 17-butyrate (103) (0.1%) was as effective as triamcinolone acetonide (0.1%), and significantly superior to hydrocortisone acetate (1%), in treatment of psoriasis under plastic occlusion (Polano et al., 1970). This observation indicates again that esterification at C-17 enhances the topical activity of most corticoids, even those of relatively low potency.

21-Deoxybetamethasone 17-propionate (104) was found to be more active than betamethasone 17-valerate (100) (3.31 and 13.1 times, depending on the formulation) in a variation of the McKenzie test (Busse et al., 1969). Another 21-deoxycorticoid, 21-deoxyprednisolone-17-propionate (105) in an aqueous gel vehicle (0.1%) was found to be less effective in the treatment of eczema and psoriasis than betamethasone valerate cream (0.1%) (Stahle, 1969). It is remarkable that 17-esterification changes an otherwise essentially inactive corticosteroid (21-deoxyprednisolone has 25% of the systemic activity of cortisol; Ringler, 1964, p. 261) to a clinically useful agent. Compound (105), although a somewhat weaker topical corticosteroid than other 17-esters, is under extensive clinical study under the name desolone propionate. It is apparent that in less severe dermatological conditions it is useful to employ topical corticosteroids of lower potency, such as (105), or more dilute preparations of those with higher potency.

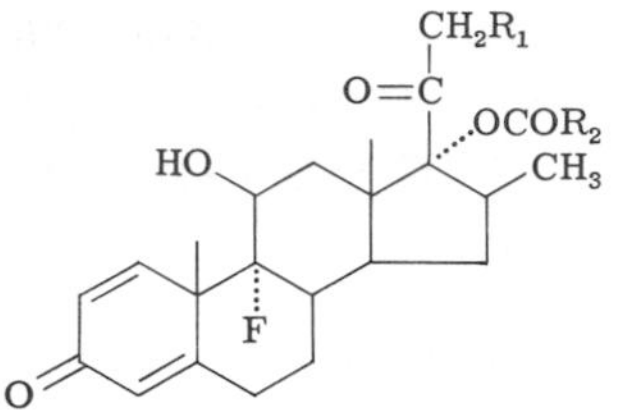

100 R_1 = OH; R_2 = n-C_4H_9
101 R_1 = OH; R_2 = C_6H_5
104 R_1 = H; R_2 = C_2H_5
110 R_1 = $OCOC_2H_5$; R_2 = C_2H_5

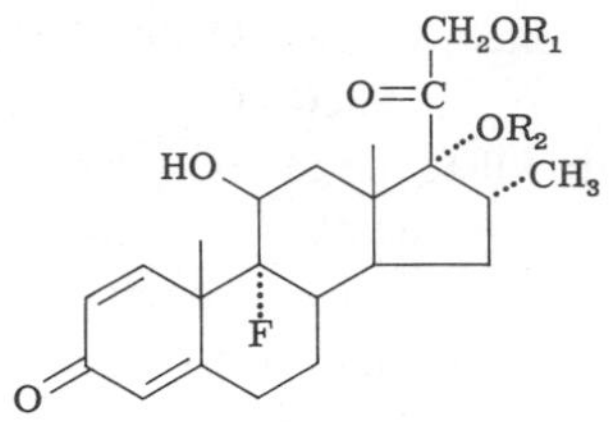

102 R_1 = H; R_2 = COC_4H_9-n
138 R_1 = $COC(CH_3)_3$; R_2 = H
139 R_1 = $\overset{\text{C}}{\underset{\text{O}}{\parallel}}$—⟨pyridyl⟩N; R_2 = H

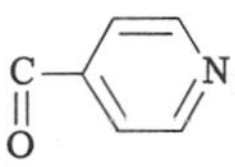

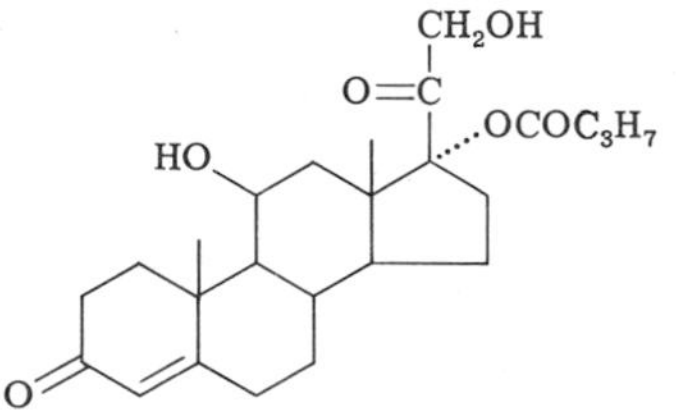

103

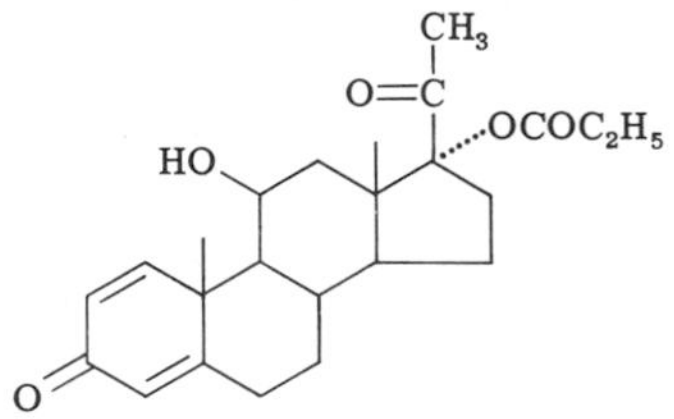

105

Miscellaneous esters

C. 21-MONOESTERS. Monoesters of corticoids at C-21 were the first derivatives to be introduced into topical therapy. Most corticoids, beginning with cortisol, were converted to a variety of C-21 esters, and some were tested clinically as topical (or local) agents. Although the earliest compounds were usually 21-acetates and are not reviewed here, since 1962 a considerable number of other esters has been made, usually with larger, more lipophilic acid residues. Quite often α or β branching has been introduced into the acyl portion to prevent rapid hydrolysis of the ester bond. Some of these latter esters are discussed in more detail in connection with steroids used for intra-articular or depot administration in Section IV,B,2.

Some 21-esters have been discussed in Sections IV,A and IV,B, among them fluocortolone caproate (28), fluprednylene acetate (30), and the various esters of 16,17-acetonides, such as (19), (44), (69), and (72). Most of these compounds have been introduced into clinical practice or are under intensive investigation.

In this section only those 21-esters are reviewed that are related to corticoids which have significant systemic activities.

A literature search has failed to disclose any reports of 21-esters

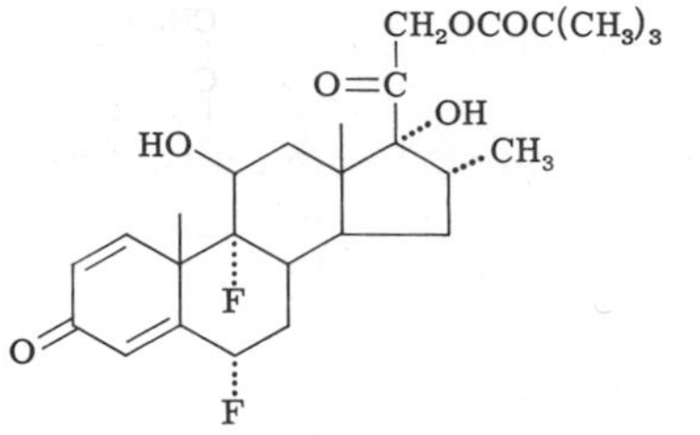

106

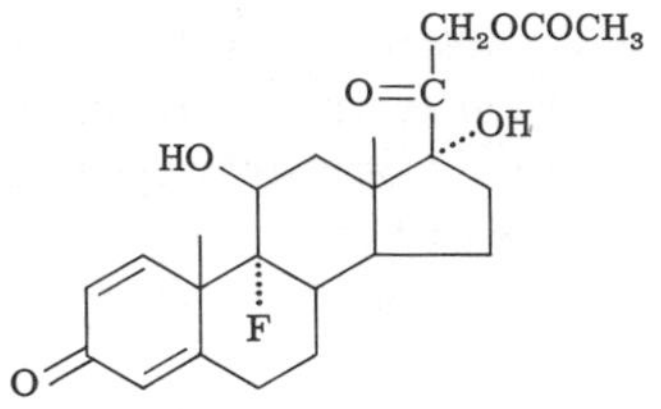

107

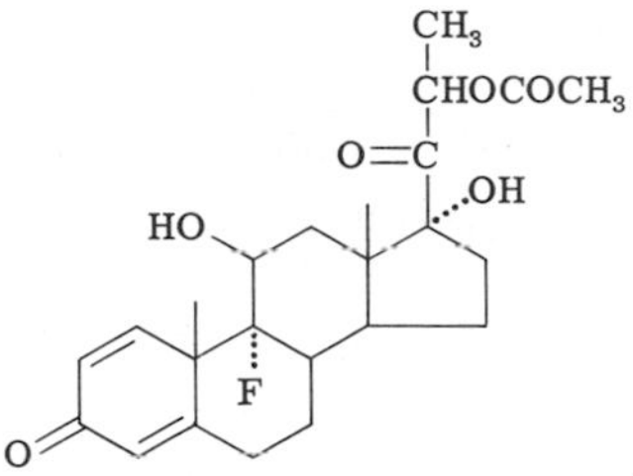

108

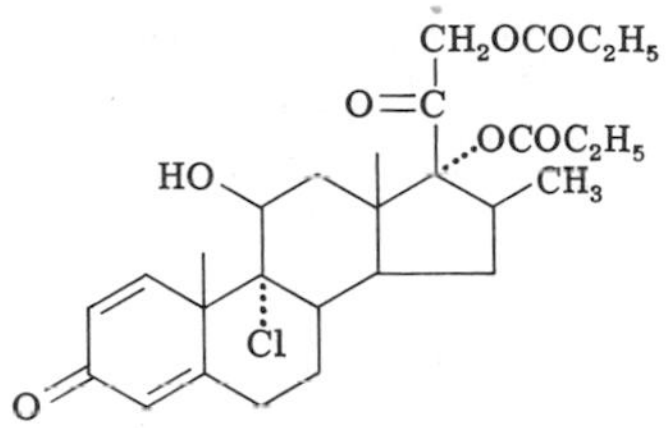

109

Miscellaneous esters

of dexamethasone being used topically, although a number of 21-esters of dexamethasone have found application in intraarticular preparations and in other local applications.

Flumethasone 21-trimethylacetate (106) as a 0.02% ointment was effective in treating several types of dermatoses (van der Meersch and Simons, 1966). This preparation, combined with coal tar and salicylic acid, was reported to be effective in psoriasis (Krebs *et al.*, 1967).

Other 21-esters of corticoids found to be clinically active as topical antiinflammatory agents include 9α-fluoroprednisolone 21-acetate (107) (Andreassi and Valentino, 1971; Piovano and Mazzocchi, 1970) and fluperolone acetate (108) (Campanella, 1964; Teik *et al.*, 1964). Fluperolone acetate, 0.1%, is used as a topical corticoid in a number of countries. An interesting structural feature of the two latter compounds is that they are 16-unsubstituted 9α-fluorocorticoids and thus "unacceptable" for systemic use because of their effect on electrolyte retention. Apparently on topical application this side effect is not particularly significant, although most topical corticoids, when used in usually large quantities, will provoke systemic effects (Scholtz and Nelson, 1965).

d. 17,21-DIESTERS AND ORTHOESTERS. A number of 17,21-diesters with either two different or two same acyl residues attached to both the 17- and the 21-hydroxy group are reported to be potent topical corticoids. Although only a few of these compounds are used clinically, animal experiments indicate that this class of corticoids may well find excellent use in clinical practice.

Beclomethasone 17,21-dipropionate (109) ointment at a concentration of 0.025% in a propylene glycol–paraffin base was found clinically equivalent to fluocinolone acetonide ointment. In the McKenzie vasoconstrictor assay, using fluocinolone acetonide as standard, (109) was five times as potent as standard, whereas betamethasone 17-valerate was 3.6 times standard (Caldwell et al., 1968). Compound (109) has been introduced into clinical practice in England. Another interesting application of (109) will be discussed in section IV,B,4. In the clinic, betamethasone 17,21-dipropionate (110) is a very effective topical corticosteroid and it is currently undergoing extensive testing in several countries (Frederiksson and Gip, 1972; Viglioglia, 1972).

A number of 17,21-diesters and 17-monoesters of 16α-methyldichlorisone have been tested for their topical potencies in rats, and the results are summarized in Table XIII (Shapiro et al., 1967). The most potent agents among the 17,21-diesters are the dipropionate (116), the dibutyrate (117), and the 17-butyrate-21-acetate (119). However, the dipropionate has significant systemic activity, of interest because it is greater than that of the parent (111), whereas the dibutyrate is essentially devoid of systemic activity. Among the 17-monoesters the 17-butyrate (113) and the 17-valerate (114) were the most potent. Compound (113), in addition to its high topical activity in the rat, shows ten times more potency than (111), its parent alcohol, in preventing exudate formation in the rat systemic pouch. In the dog eosinophil assay (113) is about three times as active as (111) by either oral or intravenous administration. Furthermore, after the compounds are administered orally or intravenously only (113) depresses the eosinophils over 24 hours, indicating a prolonged duration of activity (Collins et al., 1973).

A number of 17,21-diesters and orthoesters related to $6\alpha,9\alpha$-difluoroprednisolone have been reported to have high topical antiinflammatory potencies, and the results are summarized in Table XIV (Gardi et al., 1972). $6\alpha,9\alpha$-Difluoroprednisolone 17-butyrate-21-acetate (131) is a very potent topical agent in the local cotton pellet and the local granuloma pouch assay (DiPasquale et al., 1970b). In systemic granuloma pouch (131) is about twice as potent as betamethasone 17-benzoate on subcutaneous administration (DiPasquale et al., 1970a).

The high vasoconstrictor potency of a number of 17,21-orthoesters related to betamethasone was demonstrated (Table XII). The 17,21-methyl-

TABLE XIII

16α-Methyldichlorisone Esters

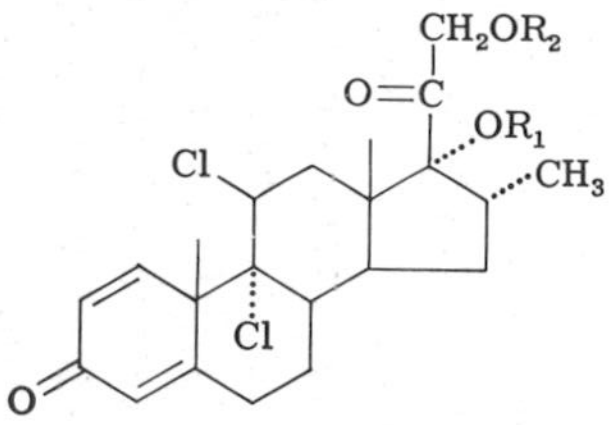

| Compound number | R_1 | R_2 | Biological potency (prednisolone acetate = 1) | | | | | | |
| | | | Topical pouch rat[a] | | Systemic pouch rat (Collins et al., 1967) | | | Mean survival time[b], (days) (Collins et al., 1967) |
			Exudate suppression	Thymolysis (Collins et al., 1967)	Exudate suppression	Thymolysis	Adrenal atrophy	
111	H	H	0.7	0.3	1.4	1.0	1.5	14.0
112	CH_3CO	H	1.2	—	—	—	—	—
113	$n\text{-}C_3H_7CO$	H	27.0	—	—	—	—	—
114	$n\text{-}C_4H_9CO$	H	20.9	—	—	—	—	—
115	CH_3CO	CH_3CO	0.8	0.4	0.4	0.4	1.1	9.0
116	C_2H_5CO	C_2H_5CO	22.6	Inactive	4.2	5.3	8.6	22.3
117	$n\text{-}C_3H_7CO$	$n\text{-}C_3H_7CO$	19.4	Inactive	0.3	0.6	0.5	34.9
118	$n\text{-}C_4H_9CO$	$n\text{-}C_4H_9CO$	0.9	—	—	—	—	—
119	$n\text{-}C_3H_7CO$	CH_3CO	24.7	—	—	—	—	—
120	$n\text{-}C_4H_9CO$	CH_3CO	5.4	—	—	—	—	—
121	CH_3CO	$(CH_3)_3CCO$	0.4	—	—	—	—	—
122	H	C_2H_5CO	1.9	—	—	—	—	—

[a] Intracutaneous injection, modification of the method of Robert and Nezamis (1957).
[b] Mean survival time of adrenalectomized rats following single subcutaneous administration of 0.25 mg of the compound.

orthovalerates of cortisol and prednisolone have high local activity in the granulome pouch with essentially no thymolytic activity. This dramatic dissociation of local and systemic activities was not observed with the corresponding 11-keto compounds, i.e., with the 17,21-methylorthovalerates of cortisone and prednisone (Ercoli *et al.*, 1971).

Conversion of a number of potent corticosteroids to the 17,21-dialkylorthocarbonates decreased systemic effects while it increased local potency in the rat granuloma pouch on intracutaneous administration (Stache *et al.*, 1971).

e. MISCELLANEOUS COMPOUNDS. Fluorometholone (**137**), a 21-deoxy-9α-fluoroprednisolone derivative, although devoid of a lipophilic ester or ketal group, was found to be an efficacious topical agent when applied in 0.025% formulation to a variety of dermatoses (Schlagel, 1965). Desoximethasone (**26**) described in Section IV,A, was recently introduced into clinical practice as a topical corticosteroid.

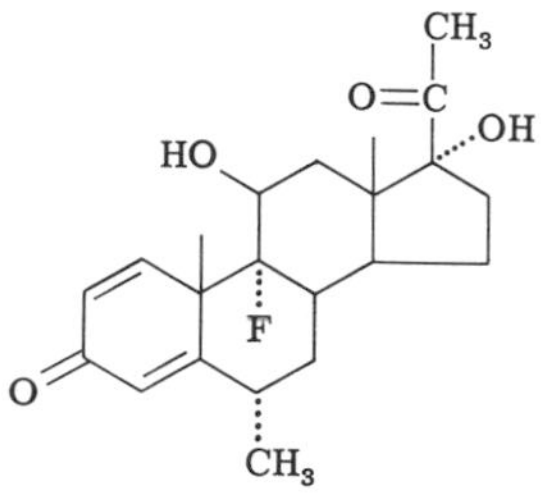

137

2. CORTICOSTEROIDS FOR INTRAARTICULAR ADMINISTRATION

Since 1964 intraarticular injection of corticosteroids into inflamed joints has become the second most frequent use of locally acting corticosteroids after topical application. This type of therapy requires the development of suitable formulations for corticosteroids with high local activity. For such formulations (usually microcrystalline suspensions in water) to be effective, the drug must be released in sufficient quantities to permit local action in the joint but to prevent systemic action by leakage of large quantities. This method of administration is now considered the choice for treatment of inflamed joints, bursae, and tendons and is widely accepted in the overall management of selected patients with rheumatoid arthritis or osteoarthritis. For practical usefulness in intraarticular corticosteroid therapy the duration of antiinflammatory action of the agent(s) administered in this manner is of prime importance. It is not surprising that several of the agents

TABLE XIV

$6\alpha,9\alpha$-Difluoroprednisolone Esters

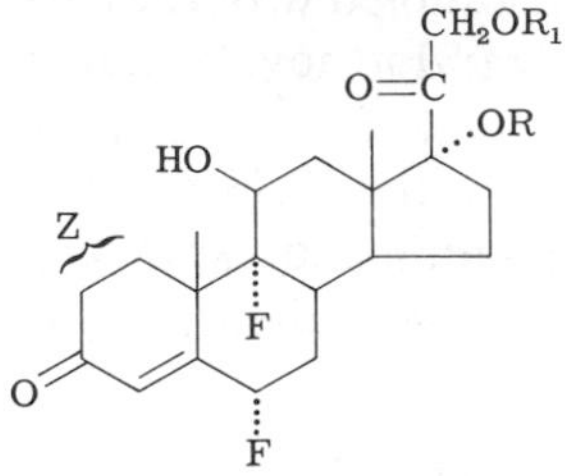

Compound number	R	R_1	Z	Biological potency Granuloma pouch rat[a] (cortisol = 1)	Vasoconstrictor assay man[b] (betamethasone 17-valerate = 1)
123	H	H	Δ^1	—	< 0.1
124	n-C$_4$H$_9$CO	H	—	> 1000	1
125	n-C$_4$H$_9$CO	H	Δ^1	> 1000	1
126	CH$_3$CO	(CH$_3$)$_2$CHCO	Δ^1	—	2
127	C$_2$H$_5$CO	CH$_3$CO	Δ^1	—	3
128	C$_2$H$_5$CO	C$_2$H$_5$CO	Δ^1	—	3
129	C$_2$H$_5$CO	n-C$_3$H$_7$CO	Δ^1	—	3.5
130	C$_2$H$_5$CO	(CH$_3$)$_2$CHCO	Δ^1	—	3
131	n-C$_3$H$_7$CO	CH$_3$CO	Δ^1	—	3.5
132	n-C$_3$H$_7$CO	C$_2$H$_5$CO	Δ^1	—	3
133	n-C$_3$H$_7$CO	(CH$_3$)$_2$CHCO	Δ^1	—	3
134	(CH$_3$)$_2$CHCO	CH$_3$CO	Δ^1	> 1000	2
135	Methylorthobutyrate		Δ^1	> 1000	1
136	Methylorthovalerate		—	> 1000	1

[a] Intrapouch administration, method of Selye (1953b).
[b] Modification of the method of McKenzie and Stoughton (1962).

used in intraarticular therapy are those corticoids or closely related derivatives which have found widespread use as topical antiinflammatory agents. This is so because both therapies require drugs with the same characteristics, i.e., local antiinflammatory activity with relatively little systemic activity.

Triamcinolone acetonide (68) in aqueous suspension (6 to 20-mg dose, depending on the joint size), when administered at 1 to 3 month intervals intraarticularly to patients with arthritic joints or with bursitis, gave excellent relief of pain, swelling, and stiffness in over 60% of the cases (Keagy and Klein, 1967). Triamcinolone hexacetonide (70), a branched chain ester of triamcinolone acetonide, was recently introduced into clinical practice in the United States. This compound, when administered in an aqueous suspension (20 mg) into the inflamed joint, showed a duration of action of about 3 weeks (Kendall, 1967). Other investigators also made similar observations on the intraarticular administration of this compound but they found a marked, temporary, systemic effect 2–4 days after administration (Astorga et al., 1970).

6α-Methylprednisolone acetate, in a depot preparation (40 mg), was found to be effective for 4 weeks when administered intraarticularly (Pearlgood, 1971). Paramethasone acetate (20 mg) in microcrystalline suspension was also effective on intraarticular administration (Valdiserri and Gualtieri, 1970).

A number of dexamethasone derivatives are reported to be useful antiinflammatory agents on intraarticular administration. Dexamethasone 21-trimethylacetate (138) has been found more effective intraarticularly in patients with chronic inflammatory diseases than dexamethasone phosphate, 6α-methylprednisolone acetate, or hydrocortisone acetate (Verhaeghe et al., 1965). Further studies have demonstrated that (138), 10 mg, intraarticularly, can give relief from pain for 3–4 weeks (Kalliomäki, 1967). Dexamethasone 21-isonicotinate (139), 2 mg, in microcrystalline suspension, is very effective on intra-articular administration in a variety of chronic arthritic conditions (Nonhoff and Zeth, 1971). Judged by the administered dose, this compound appears to be one of the most potent corticosteroids tested so far for intraarticular use. Recently, (139) has been introduced into clinical practice in Germany, both as an oral and as an injectable corticoid preparation.

Administration of a single dose (2.5, 5, or 10 mg) of betamethasone 17,21-dipropionate (110) intramuscularly resulted in eosinopenia in the dog persisting for 15–40 days (Collins et al., 1972). Administration of a single dose of (110) to man (2.5–10 mg, intramuscularly) resulted in significant eosinopenia for 6–10 days (Smith et al., 1970). The high local antiinflammatory potency of (110) and its prolonged duration of activity suggested that this compound might be useful for intraarticular administration.

3. STEROIDS FOR OPHTHALMIC ADMINISTRATION

Corticosteroids have been used as ophthalmic preparations since 1953. These agents reduce the extent of permanent scarring from some inflammatory conditions and can prevent loss of vision. These drugs are also of value in ocular inflammations induced by allergy and surgery.

The severe reactions associated with systemically administered corticoids do not occur when corticoids are applied topically to the eye, but local complications may be quite serious. Repeated administration of

topical corticoids may raise the intraocular pressure by reducing out-
flow facility. A number of systemically potent corticoids exert a glauco-
matous response (e.g., dexamethasone, betamethasone). Less potent
corticoids, e.g., cortisol, are used in high concentration and are less
likely to cause serious local adverse reactions, particularly glaucoma,
perhaps because the dosage administered can be better controlled.

Medrysone (**140**), an 11β-hydroxylated progesterone derivative, has good
antiinflammatory activities with relatively little effect on intraocular pressure and has been recently introduced into clinical use. A 1% suspension of
this compound is reported not to significantly increase the intraocular
pressure of patients known to respond to other corticoids with a rise of
intraocular pressure (Spaeth, 1966), whereas it was found to be effective in
the treatment of a number of inflammatory conditions affecting the eye
(Anonymous, 1971b). Fluorometholone (**137**) has shown substantially less
tendency to increase intraocular pressure in 0.1% and 0.25% solution, whereas it was effective in mild to severe noninfectious inflammatory ocular
diseases (Fairbarn and Thorson, 1971).

Dexamethasone 21-phosphate, although highly effective for treating
ocular inflammation, is also known to increase intraocular pressure in
rabbits (Lorenzetti, 1970) and in man (Paterson, 1965). This has also been
reported for prednisolone 21-phosphate (0.5%), dexamethasone (0.1%),
and betamethasone (0.1%) (Ramsell *et al.*, 1967). Further work is required to show whether very low concentrations (< 0.05%) of these potent
corticosteroids can inhibit inflammation without significantly increasing
intraocular pressure.

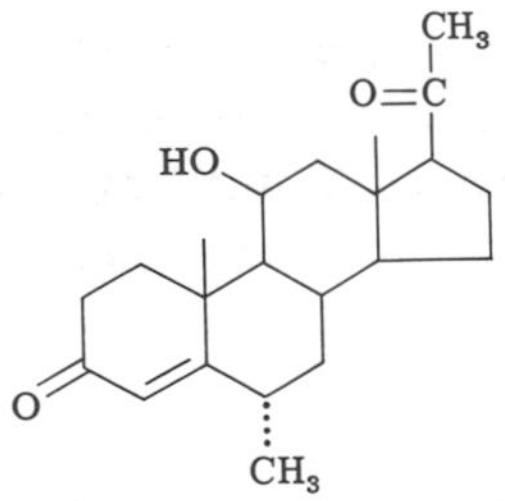

140

4. LOCALLY ACTING CORTICOSTEROIDS FOR ALLERGY AND BRONCHIAL ASTHMA

The use of corticosteroid aerosols for treatment of perennial allergic
rhinitis was reported in 1965. Dexamethasone phosphate aerosol, applied
intranasally, effectively controlled the symptoms of allergic rhinitis on
short-term administration (less than 2 weeks) (Smith, 1965). However, administration of the aerosol for less than a week also exerted a strong systemic

effect, resulting in adrenal suppression, as measured by several biochemical parameters (Aaron and Muttitt, 1965). The same precautions are needed in using corticoids delivered by this method as for other systemic corticoid therapy (Chervinsky, 1966).

In contrast, dexamethasone 21-isonicotinate (**139**) aerosol produced good to excellent effects in bronchial asthma with 89% of the 46 cases studied (Biedermann, 1971). Although systemic administration of corticoids could be partially or fully eliminated during the treatment with (**139**), the authors did not indicate whether any systemic corticoid effect (adrenal suppression) occurred when the drug was administered to the patient in this manner over extended periods of time.

The most encouraging development in the use of aerosolized corticosteroids was that 400 μg/day beclomethasone dipropionate (**109**), described in Section IV,B,1,d, relieved the symptoms of bronchial asthma in five patients. Even after a month of treatment, no adrenal suppression was indicated in any of the patients (Smith *et al.*, 1971). In a more extensive trial in 60 patients this steroid controlled asthmatic symptoms without systemic effects. Before treatment with (**109**) was initiated, 37 of the 60 patients in this study had to be on constant systemic corticoid therapy, with consequent side effects, in order to control their symptoms over the previous 1–16 years. After transfer to beclomethasone dipropionate aerosol treatment, steroid withdrawal symptoms were seen, which provided further evidence that (**109**) was not systemically absorbed (Brown *et al.*, 1972). In 1972 beclomethasone dipropionate aerosol was introduced into clinical practice in England for the treatment of asthma.

We conclude that corticosteroid aerosols can provide a useful alternative therapy to those perennial asthmatics who do require long-term corticosteroid therapy. To be useful in this type of administration the corticoids should have high local potency with little or no oral activity. A further use of aerosolized corticosteroids for the treatment of various asthmatic conditions is described in Section V,B,2.

C. Depot Corticosteroids and Corticosteroids with Rapid Onset of Activity

In this section two types of corticosteroids are discussed.

First are depot corticosteroids that are usually administered intramuscularly and exert a systemic action for a prolonged time. The prolongation of the biological effect may be caused by the characteristics of the drug itself or by the formulation, or as is more likely, by a combination of both of these factors.

Second are corticoids that by virtue of their chemical structure, water solubility, and good absorption characteristics exert their biological (again systemic) action very rapidly.

The importance of the proper formulation in prolonging the local action of a corticosteroid was discussed in detail in the preceding sections. Such formulations were accomplished for intraarticular corticosteroid preparations by using aqueous microcrystalline suspensions. The depot preparations have also been formulated as microcrystalline suspensions in water. In treating rheumatoid arthritis the actual steroid requirement to control symptoms appears to be almost the same whether steroids are administered daily by mouth or by depot injection. The latter method of administration, however, has certain advantages, for example, certainty of administration or decreasing the incidence of ulceration because the gastrointestinal tract is bypassed (Cochrane, 1971).

A widely used depot preparation, 6α-methylprednisolone acetate, gives relief of inflammatory symptoms for about 2–3 weeks after injection. The actual duration of this drug in the tissue may be for a shorter period, however, because after intramuscular administration the plasma cortisol levels were lowered for only 17 days (Bain et al., 1967). The onset of activity with depot preparations varies; in children with allergies or contact sensitivity reactions, it is between 3 and 18 hours (Dugger, 1962).

The depot form of paramethasone acetate has a duration of activity of 2 weeks (20 mg) or 3 weeks (40 mg). Rausch-Strooman and Petry (1969) measured the duration of suppressed cortisol production to determine the onset, intensity, and duration of antiinflammatory effect of this depot corticoid. Dexamethasone 21-isonicotinate (139) is useful as a depot preparation (10 mg), administered weekly (one or two doses), in relieving the symptoms of chronic bronchitis. In the treated patients side effects are insignificant, whereas relief of symptoms is obtained in 75% of the cases (Wieser and Wintenberg, 1970). Triamcinolone acetonide (68) administered intramuscularly as a microcrystalline suspension to rheumatoid arthritics is effective for 2–3 weeks and reduces the oral requirement of triamcinolone by 50% (Katona and Gil, 1964). A similar form of the drug (50, 80, or 100 mg, single intramuscular dose) was effective in providing symptomatic relief in allergic rhinitis for 1–8 months (Siegel, 1965). Injection of (68) into the inflamed acne pustules ameliorated the condition, not only at the injection sites but also in comedones distant from the injection. This suggests a systemic activity, which has been verified by suppressed levels of plasma cortisol (Potter, 1971). The duration of systemic activity was compared after administering a depot preparation of triamcinolone acetonide (40 mg) to healthy subjects either intramuscularly or intraarticularly. Intramuscular administration of the drug suppressed adrenal function for 3 weeks, whereas by the intraarticular route this effect was of short duration and less intense, indicating a predominantly local effect (Rausch-Strooman *et al.*, 1971).

Triamcinolone acetonide as a depot preparation is also used for treating pulmonary emphysema in conjunction with other drugs. In some severe cases of pulmonary emphysema intramuscularly administered triamcinolone acetonide gives symptomatic relief lasting for several weeks, with fewer side effects than obtained from higher doses of oral corticoids (Johnston and Lee, 1966).

The onset of activity with depot preparations varies to a considerable extent, so there has been a growing trend toward adding a "fast-acting" corticosteroid to the intramuscular preparation. Before these combinations are discussed the structures and biological characteristics of the "fast-acting" corticoids should be mentioned. It is known that water-soluble 21-esters of corticosteroids administered intravenously give prompt therapeutic effect, because the drug is immediately available to the tissues. Among the water-soluble esters of corticosteroids the 21-phosphates (disodium salt) are the most important, whereas the 21-hemisuccinates (sodium salt) are of lesser importance. Although corticosteroid 21-phosphates are active on oral administration (Herzog *et al.*, 1967), their principal use is by the parenteral route, either alone (intravenous administration) in cases of acute traumatic shock or in combination with slower acting corticoids (intramuscular or intraarticular administration). There is much evidence that the 21-phosphates rapidly hydrolyze to the active 21-alcohols and the inorganic acid residue attached to C-21 is essential only for quick delivery and good absorption of the compound.

The use of dexamethasone 21-phosphate in ocular inflammations (Lorenzetti, 1970; Paterson, 1965) and in various allergies (Smith, 1965; Aaron and Muttitt, 1965; Chervinsky, 1966) is described in Section IV,B,3. In addition, this compound is also used by intravenous or intramuscular injection in the treatment of acute disorders responsive to corticoid therapy.

A novel application of corticosteroid 21-phosphates (and hemisuccinates) is the combination of a water-soluble (fast-acting) phosphate and insoluble (slow-acting) 21-acetate of the same steroid, in about equimolar concentrations. A combination of betamethasone 21-disodium phosphate and betamethasone 21-acetate administered intramuscularly to patients with acute and long-term allergic disorders gives excellent alleviation of symptoms (Davis, 1966). The therapeutic effect is maintained when the same combination of two corticoids (administered intramuscularly) provides an antiinflammatory action within 2–3 hours after injection, which reached its peak after 4–6 days and then decreased gradually after 8–10 days (Antonescu, 1970; Carpio *et al.*, 1965).

The duration of action, as measured by biochemical parameters, was compared by administering single intramuscular injection of triamcinolone acetonide (40 mg), triamcinolone 16,21-diacetate (50 mg), and betamethasone acetate–betamethasone phosphate combination (9 mg). Triamcinolone acetonide suppressed the adrenals for 4 weeks, whereas the other two preparations affected adrenal function for only 1 week.

These results indicate that in selecting a corticoid for intramuscular administration, one must keep in mind the relatively prolonged adrenal suppression that occurs with triamcinolone acetonide as compared with the other two drugs (Mikhail *et al.*, 1969).

A combination of 6α-methylprednisolone acetate (slow acting) and 6α-methylprednisolone sodium succinate (fast acting) has been compared to the commercially available depot preparation of 6α-methylprednisolone acetate in patients with contact dermatitis and urticaria. The patients on the combination drug, compared with those on the depot preparation, have shown significantly less itching on the day of injection (Wexler, 1972). It appears to us that extending the combination of slow-acting and fast-acting corticoids to other depot preparations and to intraarticular therapy may offer some significant advantages in the future.

V. NEW APPROACHES TO CORTICOSTEROID THERAPY

A. Once-a-Day and Alternate Day Therapy

The failure to discover corticosteroids with a separation of activities has led physicians to alter the therapeutic regimen in order to reduce side effects. Instead of giving low doses of drug several times a day, the corticosteroid is given at a higher dose once a day or on alternate days, the rationale being that the interval between treatments should be sufficient for various physiological processes, e.g., adrenal function, to recover while the symptoms of the disease are still being controlled at a manageable level. For the most part this form of therapy has been successful except in cases of severe arthritis in which the inflammatory symptoms may return before the next treatment is due.

Diminished adrenal responsiveness to ACTH in patients receiving corticosteroids can be dangerous in stressful situations (Carter and James, 1970a). This danger may exist long after discontinuing treatment because the adrenals may be suppressed for as long as 6–9 months thereafter (Adams *et al.*, 1966).

Fluctuations in adrenal function occur normally in man over a 24-hour period with the highest plasma cortisol levels occurring between 8 am and 10 am and the lowest level at about 4 pm (Faiman and Winter, 1971). The high cortisol level will decrease adrenal function by inhibiting the release of ACTH from the pituitary. However, as the circulating cortisol level decreases, there is less blockade of ACTH release resulting in increased adrenal secretion. In the classical therapeutic regimen where the drug is given throughout the day, the normal circadian rhythm is obscured by the continual blockade of pituitary ACTH release with exogenous corticosteroids. Under the new regimen corticosteroid is given between 8 am and 10 am daily or on alternate days to permit the normal afternoon rise in ACTH to stimulate the adrenal.

Myles *et al.* (1971) tested prednisolone in patients with various chronic diseases requiring long-term corticosteroid therapy. The drug (8–20 mg/day) was given as a single dose at 10 am or twice a day at 10 am and 10 pm for 8 weeks. The daily total dose was the same regardless of whether it was given once or twice. Prednisolone was therapeutically effective given in a divided or a single dose, but the latter regimen had less effect on adrenal function. The patients on the single-dose regimen had a blood cortisol level at the lower limits of normal, suggesting some inhibition of adrenal function. All individuals given the divided dose had a plasma cortisol level well below the normal range. Nugent *et al.* (1965) gave a single daily dose of 30 mg prednisolone to patients with rheumatoid arthritis. The single-dose regimen produced less side effects than 50 mg of prednisolone on alternate days or 100 mg of prednisolone for three successive days a week. The single dose regimen was only slightly less effective against rheumatoid arthritis than the other two regimens. Bethge (1970) found that human adrenal function was more sensitive to the action of prednisolone than Nugent did. Prednisolone at up to 3 mg/day caused no suppression of adrenal function, whereas higher doses increased the likelihood of adrenal suppression. Ceresa *et al.* (1969) studied the effect of time of dosing on the adrenal suppression by dexamethasone and 6α-methylprednisolone after intravenous administration. Dexamethasone given at a rate of 10–50 μg/hour from 10 pm to 12 noon partially suppressed plasma cortisol levels, whereas increasing the infusion rate to 100 μg/hour caused complete suppression. Infusion of 6α-methylprednisolone at a constant rate of 660 μg/hour did not affect plasma cortisol level when given from 8 am to 4 pm but suppressed adrenal function at other times, i.e., when started after 4 pm. If dexamethasone was infused from 8 am to 4 pm, it did not affect adrenal function but Bethge (1970) found that this corticosteroid, as well as betamethasone, was not suitable for once-a-day therapy.

Paramethasone acetate had little effect on adrenal function at a 5-mg dose given once a day or every other day (Ortega, 1967). The same total dose, given daily in three equally divided doses, caused a decrease in plasma cortisol levels.

Triamcinolone at 4 mg given once a day had less effect on the adrenal circadian rhythm than did an equipotent antiinflammatory dose of dexamethasone at 0.75 mg (Radvila et al., 1969). Triamcinolone as a single dose of 4–6 mg was effective in patients with either dermatosis or allergies but was ineffective in rheumatoid arthritis with doses up to 16 mg (Demos et al., 1964).

Alternate day therapy is another means of decreasing side effects while maintaining therapeutic efficacy of systemic corticosteroids. Prednisone, given every 48 hours at a dose of 90 mg/m² of body surface gives good clinical results with few side effects in patients with nephrotic syndrome (Saxena et al., 1966). It is important to note that the growth rate of these patients resumes. The hypertension associated with this syndrome ameliorates and the plasma cortisol levels return to normal.

In another study, severely asthmatic children were treated every other day with either 10–30 mg of prednisone or 1.5–4.5 mg dexamethasone (Easton et al., 1971). Prednisone and dexamethasone brought symptomatic relief but the former drug did not affect the adrenal function, whereas the latter did, especially at the higher dose. Children with moderately severe asthma responded well to lower doses of prednisolone or prednisolone 21-stearoylglycolate (Kuzemko and Lines, 1971). All children on 2.5–5 mg prednisolone or 6–7 mg prednisolone 21-stearoylglycolate, given on alternate days, had normal adrenocortical reserves and resumed growing. In patients with idiopathic nephrotic syndrome, prednisone at 75 mg given on alternate days caused a moderate depression of plasma cortisol, but the adrenals were responsive to ACTH and when exposed to stress the plasma cortisol levels rose to the same degree as that of normal subjects (Ackerman and Nolan, 1968). Prednisone and triamcinolone, in cases of pemphigus vulgaris, gave good therapeutic effects with alternate day therapy but only prednisone was shown to have little effect on adrenal function (Rabham and Kopf, 1971). In this study betamethasone and dexamethasone were not effective when given every other day.

The plasma cortisol levels were temporarily lowered in normal patients given 0.5 mg of dexamethasone at 8 am, but these levels were suppressed for 24 hours when the drug was given at 4 pm (Nichols et al., 1965). Dexamethasone was given in other regimens in an attempt to decrease side effects (Adams et al., 1966). Patients with glomerulonephritis or nephrotic syndrome were given dexamethasone (8 mg) for three consecutive days each week.

This regimen produced all the signs of hypercortisonism but during the fourth day after withdrawal the plasma cortisol returned to near normal levels.

Robles-Gil (1967) reported on the duration of suppressed adrenal function after therapy with a number of corticosteroids. Cortisone, cortisol, prednisone, and 6α-methylprednisolone affected adrenal functions for up to 18 hours, whereas triamcinolone and paramethasone suppressed adrenal function for the longest period of time, 54 hours.

These various clinical studies demonstrate that once-a-day and alternate day therapy is helpful in reducing side effects. None of the drugs presently being used in this way has been specifically synthesized for this type of therapy. The important task facing scientists working with corticosteroids is the development of assay systems to characterize and identify agents that do not alter the adrenal circadian rhythm but have the required antiinflammatory potency. Plasma half-life of a corticosteroid is not directly correlated with its usefulness in once-a-day or alternate day therapy. Triamcinolone, with the longest plasma half-life, 300 minutes (Demos et al., 1964), can be used successfully in this type of therapeutic regimen, whereas dexamethasone and betamethasone cannot. 6α-Methylprednisolone also has a relatively long plasma half-life of 221 minutes (Ceresa et al., 1969) and can also be used in this new form of therapy.

How long the corticoid is retained at the cell receptor may be the important factor for therapeutic effects with resulting adrenal suppression. It is apparent from the above discussion that antiinflammatory activity and adrenal suppression can be separated. If the corticosteroid receptors in normal and inflammatory cells are the same, it follows that the former recovers its function more quickly than the latter. Gerlach and McEwen (1972) have demonstrated that corticosterone, the naturally occurring corticosteroid in rats, localizes to the greatest extent in the hippocampus. This may be the area of the brain receptors controlling release of corticotropin releasing factor. Future research should be directed toward synthesizing novel antiinflammatory corticosteroids that are less likely to cross the blood–brain barrier and are therefore less likely to affect adrenal function. Such a novel drug may be used more successfully given once a day or on alternate days, which leads to a decrease in the other side effects associated with the normal use of corticosteroids.

B. The Effect of Steroids on the Immune Response

The so-called "immunosuppressive action" of corticosteroids is used extensively to prevent homograft rejection and to alleviate the symptoms of allergies.

1. ORGAN TRANSPLANTATION

During the past decade, the most widely utilized immunosuppressive therapy for subjects with organ transplants has been corticosteroids and azathioprine (Anonymous, 1971a). The dose of azathioprine is kept at the maximum level that the patient can tolerate, whereas the steroid dosage is initially high and then tapered, i.e., reduced over a period time. The desire to decrease the corticosteroid dose stems from the side effects associated with these drugs, e.g., delayed healing and increased incidence of infection. The inclusion of corticosteroids into the immunosuppressive regimen, however, has helped to keep renal allografts functioning for about 2 years (Friedman, 1970).

Corticosteroid suppression of both humoral and cell-mediated immune responses in such experimental animals as mice, rats, and rabbits is the result, in part, of its lympholytic effects (Friedman, 1970). Thymolysis, in the past, has served as a parameter for assaying antiinflammatory potencies (see Section IIIA) and as a rough guide to possible immunosuppressive activity of corticosteroids. The work of Cohen and Claman (1971) suggests that thymolysis as an indicator of immunosuppression may be misleading, however. These investigators have clearly shown that up to 90% of all thymocytes are cortisol sensitive but these are not the cells primarily involved in inducing an immune response. The thymocytes that are required for an immune response are corticosteroid resistant. Furthermore, Segal et al. (1972) has demonstrated that thymus-derived lymphocytes that have come in contact with antigen are also corticosteroid resistant. In addition, Claman et al. (1971) demonstrated that human thymocytes are more resistant to lysis than those of the rat and mouse.

As described in Section IV,B,1, the steroids that are principally used in the clinic are primarily selected for their antiinflammatory potency. The recent rapid developments in the field of immunology have now begun to provide the necessary techniques to identify corticosteroids that may be more selective in their action and, therefore, perhaps more effective clinically.

2. ALLERGY

It is universally accepted that corticosteroids are efficacious in allergic diseases. The main drawback to their use here, as in other disease states, is the number of side effects encountered after chronic administration. Topically active corticosteroids have been used successfully in allergic eczemas, as indicated in Section IV,B,1. The problems arise when corticosteroids must be given systemically to treat such diseases as allergic asthma.

In children who have not reached puberty such treatment is likely to retard growth.

Aviado and Carrillo (1970) found that corticosteroids affected asthma in a variety of ways. The corticosteroid inhibited the inflammation resulting from an antigen–antibody reaction or inhibited the level of circulating antibody. Cortisone (10 mg/kg) and dexamethasone (4 mg/kg) reduced the formation of histamine by the lung. Cortisone also caused a fall in pulmonary resistance and inhibited agonist activity by blocking acetylcholine-induced bronchial spasms.

Miller (1971) used the long-acting depot preparation, 6α-methylprednisolone, for treating patients with asthma and hay fever. This treatment relieved both the acute episodes of asthma for up to 24 days and the symptoms of hay fever without any untoward reactions. The same results were obtained with oral doses of 6α-methylprednisolone.

Since the early days of steroid therapy for allergic asthma, it was obvious that it would be advantageous to deliver the drug directly to the bronchial mucosa. This could lead to high local concentrations and give symptomatic relief from asthma while preventing the attainment of significant systemic levels that would lead to side effects. The initial studies with cortisol (Gelfand, 1951) were of only limited success. Siegel et al. (1964) tested dexamethasone phosphate but the systemic absorption of dexamethasone led to the typical corticosteroid side effects.

A major advance may be at hand with the use of aerosolized beclomethasone dipropionate (Brown et al., 1972), which is briefly described in Section III,B,4. This preparation effectively controls asthma with no evidence of systemic absorption or corticosteroid side effects. In fact, corticosteroid withdrawal symptoms are apparent using the corticoid aerosol in patients who had previously been using systemic corticosteroids. Aerosol therapy is particularly beneficial to juvenile asthmatics because its presence is limited to the lung and, therefore, does not retard growth.

Aerosolized corticosteroids might also be useful in cases of emphysema. Beerel and Vance (1971) demonstrated that systemic prednisone did have benificial effects on pulmonary gas diffusing capacity but many side effects were observed. Continuous treatment with locally acting aerosolized corticosteroids might arrest or delay the changes seen in the lung of emphysematous patients.

Corticosteroid therapy has also proved useful in allergies of the ear, nose, and throat (Rawlins, 1966). Development of delivery systems that restrict topically effective agents to discrete areas in the ear, nose, and throat is a useful research endeavor. Corticosteroids that are devoid of oral activity may be extremely beneficial in such delivery systems.

VI. CONCLUSIONS

The discovery of the antiinflammatory activity of cortisol, coming hard on the heels of the acclaim given to penicillin, has led many people to place it in a similar category as a "wonder drug." As with the penicillins, however, this description has had to be modified because of the untoward reactions associated with its beneficial effects. Scientists are able to stay ahead in the antibiotics field by isolating or synthesizing new agents that are effective against bacterial strains resistant to penicillin. In the corticosteroid field after one initial success, the separation of antiinflammatory activity from effects on electrolyte balance, no substantial advances have been made toward separating other activities. The general lack of success in attaining this goal, despite very extensive chemical manipulations of the parent oxypregnane structure, may reflect the fact that both the desired and untoward activities are only different biological expressions of a common mechanism of corticosteroid action.

There is some experimental evidence indicating that a single activity may account for the entire spectrum of biological responses. Munck (1971) claims that corticosteroids decrease the utilization of glucose by peripheral tissue by blocking its transport into the cell, possibly by preventing phosphorylation. Rat thymus cells exposed to cortisol ($10^{-6} M$) are less active metabolically, taking up less glucose and producing less lactic acid (Munck, 1968). There is some indication that the corticosteroid effect on glucose uptake may be related to the former's antiinflammatory potency. In this particular *in vitro* system cortisone is inactive, because thymocytes cannot reduce it to cortisol, whereas the 9α-fluoro group enhances the effect on glucose uptake to the same extent as it amplifies the antiinflammatory potency *in vivo* (Kattwinkel and Munck, 1966).

Schayer (1964) suggested that both the physiological and pharmacological action of corticosteroids is caused by the passive attachment of the steroid to the microvascular smooth muscle cells, which interferes with the dilation of small blood vessels. This effect on blood flow to the tissues decreases the available substrate and leads to a catabolic action.

It is clear that if either the Munck or Schayer hypothesis is indeed the basis for the antiinflammatory activity of corticosteroids, then it will be difficult to synthesize a corticosteroid with the long sought for separation of activities. This is because either of these proposed mechanisms causes extensive tissue catabolism and therefore results in such important corticosteroid side effects as osteopenia, thinning of skin, and loss of cartilage.

Because of the low probability of synthesizing a corticosteroid with such a separation of activities, research in the corticosteroid area must have both short-range and long-range goals. The short-range goal of corticosteroid research must be directed to areas where a separation of activity is not an absolute requirement, e.g., better compounds for once-a-day or alternate day therapy. The continued development of compounds and delivery systems (mechanical devices or unique formulations) permitting drugs to localize at a desired site also falls into this category. In order to attain long-range goals, further attempts must be continually made to identify compounds with a separation of activity utilizing new screening procedures, both in laboratory animals and in the clinic. Until these new agents become available, the classical corticosteroids will remain in the clinicians' armamentarium because they promptly suppress many forms of inflammation and are life saving in conditions in which the inflammatory process per se is life threatening, as in lupoid glomerulonephritis.

ACKNOWLEDGMENTS

The authors gratefully acknowledge helpful criticism by Drs. H. L. Herzog, P. L. Perlman, and I. I. A. Tabachnick. We are also indebted to Mrs. Lisette Curry and Mrs. Sarah Haines for their expert preparation of the manuscript, and to Mr. Charles Casmer for his drawing of Fig. 1.

REFERENCES

Aaron, T. H., and Muttitt, E. L. C. (1965). *Ann. Allergy* **23**, 100.
Ackerman, G. L., and Nolan, C. M. (1968). *N. Eng. J. Med.* **278**, 405.
Adams, D. A., Gold, E. M., Gonick, H. C., and Maxwell, M. H. (1966). *Ann. Intern. Med.* **64**, 542.
Andreassi, L., and Valentino, A. (1971). *Minerva Med.* **62**, 42.
Anonymous (1971a). *Lancet* **2**, 901.
Anonymous (1971b). *Drugs* **2**, 5.
Antonescu, S. (1970). *Dermato-Venerologia* **15**, 47.
Arrigoni-Martelli, E., Bonollo, L., Schiatti, P., and Nicolis, F. B. (1971). *Abstr. Int. Congr. Horm. Steroids, 3rd, 1970* Int. Congr. Ser. No. 210, Abstract No. 371.
Astorga, G., Rossi, G., Campodonico, M., and Munoz, A (1970). *Rev. Med. Chile* **98**, 610.
Aviado, D. M., and Carrillo, L. R. (1970). *J. Clin. Pharmacol. J. New Drugs* **10**, 3.
Bain, L. S., Jacomb, R. G., and Wynn, V. (1967). *Ann. Phys. Med.* **9**, 49.
Beerel, F. R., and Vance, J. W. (1971). *Amer. Rev. Resp. Dis.* **104**, 264.
Berliner, D. L., Bartley, M. H., Kenner, G. H., and Jee, W. S. S. (1970). *Brit. J. Dermatol.* **82**, Suppl. 6, 53.
Bethge, H. (1970). *Klin. Wochenschr.* **48**, 317.
Biedermann, A. (1971). *Wien. Med. Wochenschr.* **121**, 331.
Binder, R., and McCleary, J. (1972). *Curr. Ther. Res.* **14**, 35.
Björnberg, A., and Hellgren, L. (1964). *Acta Dermato-Venereol.* **44**, 333.
Branceni, D., Rousseau, G., and Jequier, R. (1965). *Steroids* **6**, 451.

Brown, H. M., Storey, G., and George, W. H. S. (1972). *Brit. Med. J.* **1**, 585.

Burdick, K. H., Poulsen, B., and Place, V. A. (1970). *J. Amer. Med. Ass.* **211**, 462.

Bush, I. E. (1962). *Pharmacol. Rev.* **14**, 317.

Busse, M. J., Hunt, P., Lees, K. A., Maggs, P. N. D., and McCarthy, T. M. (1969). *Brit. J. Dermatol.* **81**, Suppl. 4, 103.

Caldwell, I. W., Hall-Smith, S. P., Main, R. A., Ashurst, P. J., Kirton, V., Simpson, W. T., and Williams, G. W. (1968). *Brit. J. Dermatol.* **80**, 111.

Campanella, P. (1964). *Minerva Dermatol.* **39**, 273.

Carpio, M. G., Kandora, H., and Royas, L. (1965). *Rev. Med. Chile* **93**, 168.

Carter, M. E., and James, V. H. T. (1970a). *Ann. Rheum. Dis.* **29**, 73.

Carter, M. E., and James, V. H. T. (1970b). *Ann. Rheum. Dis.* **29**, 409.

Ceresa, F., Angeli, A., Boccuzzi, G., and Molino, G. (1969). *J. Clin. Endocrinol.* **29**, 1074.

Chervinsky, P. (1966). *Ann. Allergy* **24**, 150.

Claman, H. N., Moorhead, J. W., and Benner, W. H. (1971). *J. Lab. Clin. Med.* **78**, 499.

Cochrane, G. (1971). *Rheum. Phys. Med.* **11**, 89.

Cohen, J. J., and Claman, H. N. (1971). *J. Exp. Med.* **132**, 1026.

Collins, E. J., Aschenbrenner, J., Nakahama, M., and Tabachnick, I. I. A. (1967). *Proc. Int. Congr. Horm. Steroids, 2nd, 1966* p. 530.

Collins, E. J., Aschenbrenner, J., and Nakahama, M. (1972). *Steroids* **20**, 543.

Collins, E. J., Aschenbrenner, J., and Nakahama, M. (1973). *Steroids* **21**, 443.

Cooke, T. D., Hurd, E. R., Ziff, M., and Jasin, H. E. (1972). *J. Exp. Med.* **135**, 323.

Cooperating Clinics Committee of the American Rheumatism Association. (1967). *Clin. Pharmacol. Ther.* **8**, 11.

Cozzi, R. (1971). *Minerva Dermatol.* **46**, 273.

Cullen, S. I. (1971). *Curr. Ther. Res.* **13**, 595.

Davis, B. (1971). *Ann. Rheum. Dis.* **30**, 509.

Davis, W. G. (1966). *Curr. Ther. Res.* **8**, 94.

Deghenghi, R., Boulerice, M., Rochefort, J. G., Sehgal, S. H., and Marshall, D. J. (1966). *J. Med. Chem.* **9**, 513.

Demos, C. H., Krasner, F., and Gorel, J. T. (1964). *Clin. Pharmacol. Ther.* **5**, 721.

DiPasquale, G., Rassaert, C. L., and McDougall, E. (1970a). *Steroids* **16**, 663.

DiPasquale, G., Rassaert, C. L., and McDougall, E. (1970b). *Steroids* **16**, 679.

Domenico, A., Gibian, H., Kerb, U., Kieslich, K., Kramer, M., Neumann, F., and Raspe, G. (1965). *Arzneim.-Forsch.* **15**, 46.

Donsky, H. J. (1972). *Cutis* **9**, 46.

Dorfman, R. I., Kinel, F. A., and Ringold, H. J. (1961). *Endocrinology* **68**, 616.

Dugger, J. A. (1962). *Clin. Med.* **69**, 10.

Easton, J. G., Busser, R. J., and Heimlich, E. M. (1971). *J. Allergy Clin. Immunol.* **48**, 355.

Ercoli, A., Gardi, R., Celasco, C., and Falconi, G. (1971). *Abstr. Int. Congr. Horm. Steroids, 3rd, 1970* Int. Congr. Ser. No. 210, Abstract No. 363.

Faiman, C., and Winter, J. S. D. (1971). *J. Clin. Endocrinol. Metab.* **33**, 186.

Fairbarn, W. D., and Thorson, J. C. (1971). *Arch. Ophthalmol.* **86**, 138.

Fishman, H. C. (1965). *West. Med.* **6**, 270.

Frederiksson, T., and Gip, L. (1972). *Abstr. Int. Congr. Dermatol., 14th, 1972* Int. Congr. Ser. No. 248, Abstract No. 666.

Fregnan, G. B., and Suchowsky, G. K. (1968). *Eur. J. Pharmacol.* **3**, 251.

Fried, J. H., Mrozik, H., Arth, G. E., Bry, T. S., Steinberg, N. G., Tishler, M., and Hirschmann, R. (1963). *J. Amer. Chem. Soc.* **85**, 236.

Friedman, E. A. (1970). *Transplantation* **10**, 552.

Friedman, M., and Strang, L. (1966). *Lancet* **2**, 568.

Gardi, R., Vitali, R., Falconi, G., and Ercoli, A. (1972). *J. Med. Chem.* **15**, 556.

Garnier, J. P. (1971). *Clin. Trials J.* **8**, 55.

Gelfand, M. L. (1951). *N. Engl. J. Med.* **245**, 293.

Gerlach, J. L., and McEwen, B. S. (1972). *Science* **175**, 1133.

Geyer, G., and Reimer, E. E. (1970). *Wien. Klin. Wochenschr.* **82**, 324.

Goldman, L., Preston, R., and Rockwell, L. (1952). *J. Invest. Dermatol.* **18**, 89.

Harrison, I. T., Beard, C., Kirkham, L., Lewis, B., Jamieson, I. M. Rooks, W., and Fried, J. H. (1968). *J. Med. Chem.* **11**, 868.

Harting, J., and Kraft, H. G. (1971). *Abstr. Int. Congr. Horm. Steroids, 3rd, 1970* Int. Congr. Ser. No. 210, Abstract No. 366. We are indebted to Dr. H. G. Kraft for sending us the complete manuscript.

Heller, M., Lenhard, R. H., and Bernstein, S. (1966). *Steroids* **7**, 381.

Hershberger, L. G., and Calhoun, D. W. (1957). *Endocrinology* **60**, 153.

Herzog, H. L., Neri, R., Symchowicz, S., Tabachnick, I. I. A., and Black, J. (1967). *Proc. Int. Congr. Horm. Steroids, 2nd 1966* p. 525.

Hirschmann, R., Buchschacher, P., Steinberg, N. G., Fried, J. H., Ellis, R., Kent, G. J., and Tishler, M. (1964a). *J. Amer. Chem. Soc.* **86**, 1520.

Hirschmann, R., Steinberg, N. G., Schoenewaldt, E., Paleveda, W. J., and Tishler, M. (1964b). *J. Med. Chem.* **7**, 352.

Irvine, W. J., Cullen, D. R., Khan, S. A., and Ratcliffe, J. G. (1971). *Brit. Med. J.* **1**, 630.

Jequier, R., Plongeron, R., Verro-Orloff, A. M., and Branceni, D. N. (1965). *Therapie* **20**, 445.

Johnston, T. G., and Lee, F. (1966). *S. Med. J.* **59**, 241.

Kagan, F., Birkenmeyer, R. D., and Magerlein, B. J. (1964). *J. Med. Chem.* **7**, 751.

Kalliomäki, J. L. (1967). *Curr. Ther. Res.* **9**, 327.

Katona, G., and Gil, R. J. (1964). *Arch. Interamer. Rheumatol.* **7**, 93.

Kattwinkel, J., and Munck, A. (1966). *Endocrinology* **79**, 387.

Keagy, R. D., and Klein, H. A. (1967). *Amer. J. Med. Sci.* **253**, 45.

Kendall, P. H. (1967). *Ann. Phys. Med.* **9**, 55.

Kraft, H. G., and Harting, J. (1968). *Arzneim.-Forsch.* **18**, 15.

Krebs, A., Mischler, M., and Kuske, H. (1967). *Schweiz. Med. Wochenschr.* **97**, 151.

Kuzemko, J. A., and Lines, J. G. (1971). *Arch. Dis. Childhood* **46**, 366.

Lorenzetti, O. J. (1970). *J. Pharmacol. Exp. Ther.* **175**, 763.

McKenzie, A. W., and Atkinson, R. M. (1964). *Arch. Dermatol.* **89**, 741.

McKenzie, A. W., and Stoughton, R. B. (1962). *Arch. Dermatol.* **86**, 608.

Magerlein, B. J., Birkenmeyer, R. D., and Kagan, F. (1960). *J. Amer. Chem. Soc.* **82**, 1252.

Margerlein, B. J., Birkenmeyer, R. D., Lincoln, F. H., and Kagan, F. (1961). *Chem. Ind. (London)* p. 2050.

Mascietti-Coriandoli, E., and Fraia, A. (1970). *Arzneim.-Forsch.* **20**, 111.

Mauer, S., Heyder, E., and Ringler, I. (1962). *Proc. Soc. Exp. Biol. Med.* **111**, 345.

Meier, R., Schuler, W., and Desaulles, P. (1950). *Experientia* **6**, 469.

Meier, R., Desaulles, P., and Schar, B. (1955). *Naunyn-Schmiedeberg's Arch. Exp. Pathol. Pharmakol.* **224**, 104.

Mikhail, G. R. (1972). *Excerpta Med.* **26**, 111. (Abstr. No. 583).

Mikhail, G. R., Livingood, C. S., Mellinger, R. C., Paige, T. N., and Salyer, H. L. (1969). *Arch. Dermatol.* **100**, 263.

Miller, J. (1971). *Curr. Ther. Res.* **13**, 188.

Mitchell, D. M., Heany, S. H., and Eakins, T. S. J. (1964). *J. Ir. Med. Assoc.* **55**, 45.

Munck, A. (1968). *J. Biol. Chem.* **243**, 1039.

Munck, A. (1971). *Perspect. Biol. Med.* **14**, 265.

Myles, A. B., Bacon, P. A., and Daly, J. R. (1971). *Ann. Rheum. Dis.* **30**, 149.

Nathansohn, G., Pasqualucci, C. R., Radaelli, P., Schiatti, P., Selva, D., and Winters, G. (1969). *Steroids* **13**, 365.

Newbould, B. B. (1963). *Brit. J. Pharmacol. Chemother.* **21**, 127.

Nichols, T., Nugent, C. A., and Tyler, F. H. (1965). *J. Clin. Endocrinol.* **25**, 343.

Nonhoff, R., and Zeth, K. F. (1971). *Arzneim.-Forsch.* **21**, 382.

Nugent, C. A., Ward, J., MacDiarmid, W. D., McCall, J. C., Baukel, J., and Tyler, F. H. (1965). *J. Chronic Dis.* **18**, 323.

Olson, R. E., Jacobs, F. A., Richert, D., Thayer, S. A., Kopp, L. J., and Wade, N. J. (1944). *Endocrinology* **35**, 430.

Ordonez, E. T. (1971). *Anzneim.-Forsch.* **21**, 248.

Ortega, E. (1967). *Proc. Panamerican Congr. Rheumatol., 4th, 1969* Int. Congr. Ser. No. 165, pp. 146–156.

Paterson, G. (1965). *Trans. Ophthalmol. Soc. U.K.* **85**, 295.

Pearlgood, M. (1971). *J. Roy. Coll. Gen. Practit.* **21**, 410, and references therein.

Pepler, A. F., Woodford, R., and Morrison, J. C. (1971). *Brit. J. Dermatol.* **85**, 171.

Piovano, P. B., and Mazzocchi, S. (1970). *Minerva Dermatol.* **45**, 279.

Place, V. A., Giner-Velazquez, J., and Burdick, K. H. (1970). *Arch. Dermatol.* **101**, 531.

Polano, M. K., Duurmond, D., van der Lely, M. A., and Warnaar, P. (1970). *Brit. J. Dermatol.* **83**, Jubilee Issue, 93.

Potter, R. A. (1971). *J. Invest. Dermatol.* **57**, 364.

Rabham, N. B., and Kopf, A. W. (1971). *Arch. Dermatol.* **103**, 615.

Radvila, A., Dettwiler, W., Rohner, R., and Studer, H. (1969). *Schweiz. Med. Wochenschr.* **99**, 709.

Ramsell, T. G., Trillwood, W., and Draper, G. (1967). *Brit. J. Ophthalmol.* **51**, 398.

Rasponi, L. (1971). *G. Ital. Dermatol.* **46**, 36.

Rausch-Strooman, J. G., and Petry, R. (1969). *Arzneim.-Forsch.* **19**, 767.

Rausch-Strooman, J. G., Petry, R., Brandt, T., and Thomas, E. (1971). *Arzneim.-Forsch.* **21**, 836.

Rawlins, A. G. (1966). *Ann. Allergy* **24**, 560.

Restelli, A., and Arrigoni-Martelli, E. (1971). *Abstr. Int. Congr. Horm. Steroids, 3rd, 1970* Int. Congr. Ser. No. 210, Abstract No. 364. We are indebted to the authors for sending us their complete manuscript.

Ringler, I. (1964). *Methods Horm. Res.* **3**, 227–349.

Robinson, C. H., Finckenor, L. E., Tiberi, R., and Oliveto, E. P. (1961). *J. Org. Chem.* **26**, 2863.

Robert, A., and Nezamis, J. E. (1957). *Acta Endocrinol. (Copenhagen)* **25**, 105.

Robles-Gil, J. (1967). *Proc. Panamerican Congr. Rheumatol. 4th, 1969* Int. Congr. Ser. No. 165, pp. 157–163.

Rosenberg, E. W. (1971). *Arch. Dermatol.* **104**, 632.

Rosenthale, M. E., and Nagra, C. L. (1967). *Proc. Soc. Exp. Biol. Med.* **125**, 149.

Sarett, L. H., Patchett, A. A., and Steelman, S. L. (1963). *Progr. Drug. Res.* **5**, 13–153.

Sarkany, I., and Hadgraft, J. W. (1969). *Brit. J. Dermatol.* **81**, Suppl. 4, 98.

Sarkany, I., Hadgraft, J. W., Caron, G. A., and Barrett, C. W. (1965). *Brit. J. Dermatol.* **77**, 569.

Savage, O., Chapman, L., Robertson, J. D., Davis, P., Popert, A. J. and Copeland, W. S. C. (1971). *Brit. Med. J.* **1**, 172.

Saxena, K. M., Crawford, J. D., and Shannon, D. C. (1966). *Clin. Pediat.* **5**, 366.

Schaub, R., and Weiss, M. J. (1967). *J. Med. Chem.* **10**, 789.

Schayer, R. W. (1964). *Perspect. Biol. Med.* **8**, 71.

Schlagel, C. A. (1965). *J. Pharm. Sci.* **54**, 335.

Scholtz, J. R., and Nelson, D. H. (1965). *Clin. Pharmacol. Ther.* **6**, 498.

Schwind, K. (1968). *Arzneim.-Forsch.* **18**, 31.

Segal, S., Cohen, I. R., and Feldman, M. (1972). *Science* **175**, 1126.

Selye, H. (1953a). *Recent Progr. Horm. Res.* **8**, 117.

Selye, H. (1953b). *Proc. Soc. Exp. Biol. Med.* **82**, 328.

Shapiro, E. L., Finckenor, L. E., Pluchet, H., Weber, L., Robinson, C. H., Oliveto, E. P., Herzog, H. L., Tabachnick, I. I. A., and Collins, E. J. (1967). *Steroids* **9**, 143.

Siegel, C. (1965). *Curr. Ther. Res.* **7**, 625.

Siegel, S. C., Heimlich, E. M., Richards, W., and Kelley, V. C. (1964). *Pediatrics* **33**, 245.

Smith, A. P., Booth, M., and Davey, A. J. (1971). *Brit. Med. J.* **3**, 705.

Smith, H. M., Collins, E. J., Aschenbrenner, J., and Wood, M. (1970). *Abstr., Int. Congr. Pharmacol., 4th, 1969* p. 452.

Smith, R. E. (1965). *Ann. Allergy* **23**, 273.

Spaeth, G. L. (1966). *Arch. Ophthalmol.* **75**, 784.

Speirs, R. S., and Meyer, R. K. (1951). *Endocrinology* **48**, 316.

Stache, U., Haede, W., Fritsch, W., Radscheit, K., and Schroder, H. G. (1971). U.S. Patent 3,621,014.

Stafford, R. O., Barnes, L. E., Bowman, B. J., and Meinzinger, M. M. (1955). *Proc. Soc. Exp. Biol. Med.* **89**, 371.

Stafford, R. O., Barnes, L. E., Bowman, B. J., and Meinzinger, M. M. (1956). *Proc. Soc. Exp. Biol. Med.* **91**, 67.

Stahle, I. O. (1969). *Australas. J. Dermatol.* **10**, 148.

Steelman, S. L., Morgan, E. R., and Silber, R. H. (1963). *Steroids* **1**, 163.

Steelman, S. L., Morgan, E. R., and Glitzer, M. S. (1971). *Steroids* **18**, 129.

Stoughton, R. B., and Fritsch, W. (1964). *Arch. Dermatol.* **90**, 512.

Suchowsky, G. K., and Baldratti, G. (1967). *Proc. Int. Congr. Horm. Steroids, 2nd, 1966* p. 536.

Sulzberger, M. B., and Witten, V. H. (1952). *J. Invest. Dermatol.* **19**, 101.

Teik, K. O., Poh, F. W., and Yam, K. K. (1964). *Singapore Med. J.* **5**, 69.

Tolksdorf, S. (1959). *Ann. N. Y. Acad. Sci.* **82**, 829.

Tolksdorf, S., Battin, M. L., Cassidy, J. W., MacLeod, R. M., Warren, F. H., and Perlman, P. L. (1957). *Proc. Soc. Exp. Biol. Med.* **92**, 207.

Tonelli, G., Thibault, L., and Ringler, I. (1965). *Endocrinology* **77**, 625.

Valdiserri, L., and Gualtieri, G. (1970). *Minerva Ortop.* **21**, 550.

van der Meersch, J. J., and Simons, R.D.G.P. (1966). *Dermatologica* **132**, 460.

Vennig, E. J., Kazmin, V. E., and Bell, J. C. (1946). *Endocrinology* **38**, 79.

Verhaeghe, A., Lebeurre, R., Hennion, M., and Cheval, P. (1965). *Lille Med.* **10**, 211.

Viglioglia, P. A. (1972). *Semana Med* (*B. Aires*) **140**, 325.

Wexler, L. (1972). *Clin. Med.* **79**, 30.

Wieser, O., and Wintenberg, H. (1970). *Med. Welt* **39**, 1707.

Williams, D. I., Wilkinson, D. S., Overton, J., Milne, J. A., McKenna, W. B., Lyell, A., and Church, R. (1964). *Lancet* **1**, 1177.

Woods, G. F., Hewett, C. L., and Buckett, W. R. (1971). *Abstr. Int. Congr. Horm. Steroids, 3rd, 1970* Int. Congr. Ser., No. 210, Abstract No. 152.

Zderic, J. A., Carpio, H., and Djerassi, C. (1959). *J. Org. Chem.* **24**, 909.

Zderic, J. A., Carpio, H., and Djerassi, C. (1960). *J. Amer. Chem. Soc.* **82**, 446.

Chapter 10

Colchicine and Allopurinol

THOMAS J. FITZGERALD*

Department of Pharmacology
University of Kansas Medical Center
Kansas City, Kansas

I. INTRODUCTION

Gout, the "forgotten disease" in 1946 (McKracken *et al.*, 1946), has received a considerable amount of attention since then, especially in the last decade, and the effort expended has been quite fruitful. In fact, this

---

*Present address: School of Pharmacy, Florida Agricultural and Mechanical University, Tallahassee, Florida.

extensive research on gout has made it the most thoroughly understood of the inflammatory diseases. The etiologic role of sodium urate has been elucidated, a spinoff of which has been the development of animal models of gout. Although the steps preceeding and following deposition of monosodium urate crystals have not been clarified, a foothold has been established and a better understanding of not only gout but of other types of inflammation as well must result.

Not surprisingly, the pharmacology of antigout agents has witnessed a parallel development. The ancient and empirically used but highly effective agent colchicine has been the subject of much research, and its mechanism in gout seems well on the way to being clarified. Recent years have also seen the introduction and acceptance of allopurinol in gout therapy. This agent was specifically designed as an inhibitor of xanthine oxidase and has been used to check the production of urate.

This chapter seeks to collect and correlate the chemical and biological aspects of the antigout agents, colchicine and allopurinol, in light of new information about this very old disease. A number of other agents also used in gout are absent from this chapter. Those which are general antiinflammatory agents, such as indomethacin and phenylbutazone, are treated in other chapters in this book. Such nonsteroidal antiinflammatory drugs are also reviewed elsewhere (Weiner and Piliero, 1970; Coyne, 1970). Still other drugs, such as probenecid and sulfinpyrazone, which are not antiinflammatory agents as such but are used in the treatment of gout for their uricosuric activity, are included in the Appendix at the end of this chapter. For a review of uricosuric agents, see Gutman (1966).

II. GOUT

A. Purine Metabolism

The end product of purine metabolism in man is uric acid, which exists in plasma as the singly ionized urate anion.* Because this substance (as microcrystalline monosodium urate) has been implicated as the etiologic factor in gout its formation and removal from the body are of interest.

---

*In this review the expressions "urate" and "sodium urate" will be used interchangeably with "monosodium urate." In previous monographs these terms have also been used interchangeably with "uric acid." To avoid confusion, the term "uric acid" is used here only to indicate the free, un-ionized acid.

Purines may enter the metabolic scheme through ingested food, by *de novo* synthesis, or by degradation of nucleic acids. The *de novo* synthesis of purines begins with the reaction of glutamine and 5-phosphoribosyl-1-pyrophosphate (**1**) to give 5-phosphoribosylamine (**2**), which is committed to formation of purine molecules and has no other known function. The ring system is then built up in a series of reactions to give inosinic acid (**3**), the first purine formed, which can be converted to other purine ribotides and thence to RNA. Some of the inosinic acid thus produced does not go into synthesis of

nucleic acids but is converted directly to urate (**6**) through the intermediates hypoxanthine (**4**) and xanthine (**5**) by the enzyme xanthine oxidase. This pathway is the only known mechanism for the production of urate. Seegmiller (1967) cites a case that provides strong evidence against the possibility of alternate pathways for the production of urate. A patient congenitally deficient in xanthine oxidase was found to excrete no urate in the urine; instead, xanthine and hypoxanthine were excreted.

Urate may be removed from the body by various pathways but the kidney provides the major route. Glomerular filtration is followed by virtually complete reabsorption of the filtered urate in the proximal convoluted tubule. Tubular secretion of urate therefore accounts for all the uric acid appearing in the urine. It is the acidity of the fluid in the collecting tubule that converts urate to the even less soluble uric acid that appears in the urine.

The uricosuric agents, probenecid and sulfinpyrazone, increase urinary uric acid excretion by inhibiting tubular reabsorption on the filtered urate. In this way the plasma urate concentration is lowered. This appears to be accomplished by competitive inhibition for the common "organic acid system" (Gutman, 1966). The salicylates in large doses also exhibit uricosuric activity, presumably through the same mechanism as probenicid and sulfinpyrazone. This uricosuric action, however, is only seen with high doses (4 gm/day or more); lower doses (1–2 gm/day) tend to suppress uric acid excretion through an inhibitory action on tubular secretion of urate. Large doses of salicylates also inhibit tubular secretion of urate but this is more than compensated for by the inhibition of tubular reabsorption. The net result is the observed uricosuric action.

Although man is deficient in uricase, the enzyme responsible for degrading urate to allantoin in other species, [^{15}N]-labeled urate appears in human urine as urea, ammonia, or allantoin. Some of this destruction of urate is performed by intestinal bacteria on urate secreted in the bile, the products being reabsorbed and excreted in the urine. A less significant site of uricolysis takes place in leukocytes through the action of peroxidase on urate (Seegmiller, 1967).

B. Acute Gout

1. HYPERURICEMIA

The characteristic manifestation of gout is hyperuricemia. This condition may arise from a variety of causes but of greatest significance is overproduction or urate. The nature of urate overproduction, is not clear, however. Kelley et al. (1969) have studied 18 hyperuricemic patients with gout caused by a phosphoribosyltransferase deficiency. Familial studies suggest that the enzyme deficiency in these patients is the result of a mutation involving a structural gene. One possible mechanism leading to the overproduction of urate may be related in part to the increased concentrations of phosphoribosylpyrophosphate (PRPP) or of the free bases hypoxanthine and guanine. It should be noted that all patients with the enzyme defect produced excess quantities of urate but that not all patients with gout or even excess urate production exhibit the enzyme deficiency.

Pagliara and Goodman (1969) reported finding that about 50% of patients with primary gout have significantly elevated plasma levels of glutamate (but not glutamine). Because the rate-limiting step in the biosynthesis of purines is condensation of glutamine and PRPP, intracellular concentration of glutamate may be a factor in determining the rate of this reaction.

The fact that neither of these defects is found in all gouty patients suggests that searching for a single metabolic defect to account for hyperuricemia is unrealistic. More likely the term "gout" collectively represents a group of purine metabolism defects, each resulting in an overproduction of urate. Also included in this term are deficiencies in urate elimination that have the same effect as overproduction of urate, i.e., hyperuricemia.

Those forms of gout arising from hyperuricemia produced by a mechanism other than a metabolic defect or impaired urate elimination are often classified as "secondary gout." A long list of the sources of secondary gout has been compiled (McLaughlin et al., 1970, and references therein). Included in this list are lead poisoning, which causes hyperuricemia as a result of renal damage, and myeloproliferative diseases, which result in hyperuricemia through a high rate of nucleic acid turnover. Any condition that impairs renal handling of urate or that results in an over-production and catabolism of purines may give rise to hyperuricemia. Certain drugs may also increase blood levels of urate. The tuberculostatic drug, pyrazinamide, leads to hyperuricemia by inhibiting tubular secretion of urate. The same mechanism is apparently responsible for the hyperuricemia produced by the widely used diuretic, diazoxide. These few examples serve to illustrate the variety of factors that may influence blood levels of urate and thereby give rise to gout.

2. FACTORS INITIATING AN ACUTE ATTACK

Onset of an acute attack of gout is characterized by a progressively increasing pain in a joint of the extremities, often afflicting the metatarsalphalangeal joint of the big toe. Within a short time the pain becomes excruciating and is accompanied by swelling, warmth, and discoloration of the joint.

Although a number of factors have been indicted as initiating agents in acute gout, such as overindulgence in rich foods, alcohol, and sex, there is no evidence to support these contentions. However, there does appear to be an association between acute attacks of gout and such factors as trauma (surgery is a common precipitating factor), emotional tension, and changes in the weather, among others (Talbott, 1967). The mechanism by which these conditions induce acute attacks of gout is not known.

By whatever mechanism the above-mentioned external factors may precipitate an acute attack of gout, the actual symptomatology is a result of the intrasynovial presence of microcrystalline monosodium urate (McCarty and Hollander, 1961). Examination of gouty joints has consistently revealed the presence of sodium urate in microcrystalline form, and when synthetic crystalline urate is injected into the synovial joints of gouty or normal humans an inflammatory response is produced (Seegmiller *et al.*, 1962; Faires and McCarty, 1962). Amorphous sodium urate produces no inflammatory response; however, injection of microcrystalline sodium orotate or calcium phosphate is accompanied by inflammation, thereby suggesting that although the chemical nature of a material is not the decisive factor in determining its phlogistic properties, its physical state is. That the inflammation is not species specific is illustrated by development in dogs of goutlike inflammation on intrasynovial injection of microcrystalline sodium urate. More recently it has been suggested that classical gout should actually be considered but one member of a family of "crystal deposition diseases" (Phelps and McCarty, 1969). Another crystal deposition disease is pseudo-gout, in which calcium pyrophosphate is the irritating agent.

The discovery of microcrystalline sodium urate as the inflammatory agent in gout was originally disclosed by His (1900) and Freudweiler (1901). However, this concept became sidetracked, and a role for urate in gout was generally denied for 60 years until its rediscovery in 1961.

3. ROLE OF POLYMORPHONUCLEAR LEUKOCYTES

In addition to the presence of sodium urate crystals in gouty synovial fluid, large numbers of polymorphonuclear leukocytes (PMN) are also observed, many of them containing crystals of sodium urate. The presence of these cells is essential to an acute attack of gout. Phelps and McCarty (1966) have shown that if a dog is depleted of its PMN's (which is accomplished by pretreatment of the animals with vinblastine) no response to intrasynovially administered sodium urate crystals can be elicited. In fact, the extent of response appears to be related to the white blood cell population of the joint fluid. It has therefore been suggested (Seegmiller *et al.*, 1962) that gouty inflammation may involve a cyclic process wherein precipitated sodium urate crystals are phagocytized by PMN's and lactic acid produced by the phagocytic process lowers the local pH, resulting in further precipitation of sodium urate. A more detailed scenario of events has since evolved and has been elegantly presented by Weissmann (1971). The vacuole containing the ingested crystal fuses with lysosomes, which release their contents into the vacuole. The lysosomal enzymes strip the crystal of its plasma-protein coating and the crystal then interacts by hydrogen bonding with the phagolysosomal membrane causing it to rupture. The lysosomal enzymes spill into the cell causing its death and dissolution and the release of toxic and inflammation-mediating substances into the joint space. Thus, damage wrought by the hydrolytic lysosomal enzymes appears to be primarily responsible for gouty inflammation.

Significant participation of kinins in gouty arthritis appears unlikely in light of the findings of Phelps *et al.* (1966). These workers have shown that although injections of carboxypeptidase B into canine joints inhibit the response to injected bradykinin, they do not alter the response to urate crystals. Nevertheless, as the authors point out, this may not be the final word with regard to inflammatory mediators in gout because these experiments do not rule out the possibility of a peptide resistant to carboxypeptidase B.

Although it has been generally accepted that urate crystals find their way into PMN's by a phagocytic process, Bluhm *et al.* (1969) have presented an alternative concept. These workers suggest that urate crystals may form within the leukocyte by precipitation from a saturated medium. Therefore, the presence of urate crystals may not be an essential prerequisite for an acute attack of gout and a causative role for noncrystalline urate may be possible. It should be noted that these experiments have been conducted on synovial fluid *in vitro* at 4°C. Whether intracellular crystal formation can take place *in vivo* has not been established.

Factors affecting PMN motility and the mechanism by which these cells are mobilized into the joint have been studied by Phelps and co-workers. It has been found that urate in solution stimulates PMN motility but is not chemotactic (Phelps, 1969a). Later experiments, however, have strongly suggested that following phagocytosis of urate by PMN's a chemotactic substance is released by the cells (Phelps, 1969b). In this manner PMN's may be attracted to a location of urate crystals in the joint fluid after a chance meeting between cells and crystals. Because diamond dust neither produces inflammation upon intrasynovial injection in dogs nor causes release of chemotactic factor after phagocytosis, some property of urate other than its crystallinity is responsible for its inflammatory effects. The process of phagocytosis itself therefore does not seem to be responsible for release of the chemotactic factor (Tse and Phelps, 1970). These same workers have examined a number of purine and pyrimidine analogs on PMN motility (Tse and Phelps, 1971). They conclude that a substituent at the 5 position of the pyrimidine nucleus is important for stimulation of random motility. Thus, whereas uracil (7) has no effect on PMN motility, 5-methyluracil (thymine, 8) is as effective a stimulant as urate. Their results also suggest that motility may be inversely related to intracellular levels of cyclic AMP.

7 R = H
8 R = CH_3

A review of past and present knowledge of gout has appeared (Gutman, 1973).

C. Animal Models of Acute Gout

Once it became apparent that microcrystalline sodium urate was responsible for initiating an attack of gout, the next step was to employ this knowledge in the development of animals models of gout. The obvious benefits deriving from such model systems included the possibility of examining heretofore untried agents for their antigout activity as well as providing a means of evaluating new antigout agents. In addition, the nature of the inflammation could be investigated in a manner not previously possible.

1. THE CANINE MODEL: INTRAARTICULAR INJECTION

Intrasynovial injections of sodium urate in dogs as a potential model of gout were first employed by Faires and McCarty (1962). An inflammatory reaction was obtained and was characterized at its peak by a typical three-legged gait. Somewhat later McCarty *et al.* (1966) were able to quantitate this model by measuring intraarticular pressure, pH, and leukocyte concentration in the knees of anesthesized dogs. Crystals of calcium pyrophosphate were also used to induce inflammation. Subsequently, urate-induced inflammation in dogs was employed to assess the role of the PMN in crystal-induced synovitis (Phelps and McCarty, 1966) and to investigate the mechanism of action of indomethacin (Phelps and McCarty, 1967). This drug was found to be quite effective in suppressing the inflammation and appeared to do so by inhibition of leukocyte motility.

Rosenthale *et al.* (1966) used the canine model of urate-induced inflammation to evaluate the effectiveness of a number of antiinflammatory drugs. Both indomethacin and phenylbutazone completely suppressed the inflammation (as measured by their effect on the three-legged gait), whereas aspirin and soluble hydrocortisone, among other agents, were inactive. Colchicine was not tested.

Although this system appears to mimic the human situation in many respects, it suffers from the disadvantages of employing rather expensive animals and of the relatively large size of the animal, which requires a fair amount of drug.

2. SUBPLANTAR INJECTIONS OF SODIUM URATE CRYSTALS IN RODENTS

Models of inflammation based on irritant-induced paw edema in rodents have been used for many years. The rat paw seems to have found the widest application in inflammation research, employing a large number of diverse irritants. However, the carrageenan-induced paw edema in rats as developed by Winter et al. (1963) has become the system of choice for evaluating anti-inflammatory drugs. Recent evidence suggests that the carrageenan rat paw edema is mediated by the release of kinins (Briseid et al., 1971; Crunkhorn and Meacock, 1971). Willis (1970) has demonstrated that prostaglandins are released into rat paw exudate induced by carrageenan. A mouse model of carrageenan-induced paw edema has also been described (Levy, 1969).

The first attempt to use urate-induced paw swelling in rats as a model of gout was reported by Trnavský and Kopecký (1966). Suspensions of monosodium urate were injected into the subplantar region of the hind paw and the extent of inflammation was evaluated by measuring the swelling of the talocrural joint and paw edema with a contact measuring device. Both the acute phase (first 4 hours after injection of the urate crystals) and the subacute phase (the following 5 days) were evaluated. Paw swelling subsided rather quickly (within 24–48 hours). The authors also employed a subcutaneous injection of urate crystals in the interscapular region to induce formation of a granuloma, which was removed 7 days later and weighed. A number of antiinflammatory agents were evaluated using these inflammatory responses. Histological examination revealed that the inflammation was manifested by leukocytic and histocytic cellular reaction.

Denko and Whitehouse (1970) also used a subplantar injection of urate crystals to induce swelling in the hind paw of rats. The opposite hind paw received either saline or sodium urate solution as a control; the latter had no phlogistic activity. This urate-induced inflammation was used to explore the pharmacological effects of colchicine. The extent of swelling was quantitated between 4 and 6 hours after administering the urate crystals by severing the foot above the ankle and weighing the feet wet and after drying. Inflammation was induced in a similar manner with carrageenan and Freund's adjuvant. Although pretreatment of the animals with colchicine reduced the urate-induced paw swelling, no such action by colchicine was recorded in the carrageenan- or Freund's adjuvant-induced inflammation.

Urate-induced paw swelling has also been used in mice as a model of acute gout (Fitzgerald et al., 1971a). The inflammation, as expressed by paw swelling that is measured by a paw immersion technique (Uyeki et al., 1969), is dose dependent and reached a maximum about 6 hours after administration of the urate. As in the case of the rat model, urate-induced paw swelling in mice is considerably reduced by pretreatment of the animals with colchicine.

The relationship between various models of acute gout and the actual human condition is, of course, questionable, and considerable caution should be exercised in extrapolating results from models to human gout. To illustrate this point, the response of the various model systems to drugs can be considered. For instance, McCarty (1970) points out that the rank order of effectiveness of antiinflammatory drugs in suppressing urate-induced inflammation in humans is different (aspirin > corticosteroid > phenylbutazone > colchicine) than that observed in clinical treatment of gout (phenylbutazone > colchicine > corticosteriod > aspirin). How much different, then, is the response to drugs among different species? It has been found, for instance, that phenylbutazone is an effective antiinflammatory agent against both carrageenan-induced (Winter *et al*., 1963) and urate-induced (Trnavský and Kopecký, 1966) paw swelling in rats at doses of 90 and 125 mg/kg, respectively. Against carrageenan-induced paw swelling in mice, however, phenylbutazone is only weakly effective at a dose of 200 mg/kg (Levy, 1969), and in urate-induced paw swelling in mice phenyl-butazone is completely ineffective, even at doses of 250 mg/kg (Fitzgerald *et al*., 1971b). In contrast, Rosenthale *et al*. (1966) have found phenylbutazone to be a highly effective antiinflammatory agent in the canine model of gout, completely suppressing the inflammation in low doses (6 mg/kg).

Additional examples are provided by deacetylcolchiceine (TMCA) and podophyllotoxin. A colchicine derivative, deacetylcolchiceine is claimed to be as effective against human gout as colchicine (Wallace, 1961) but is far less effective than colchicine in the mouse model (Fitzgerald *et al*., 1971a). Podophyllotoxin, an antimitotic agent similar to colchicine, suppressed urate-induced paw swelling in mice (Fitzgerald *et al*., 1971b) but did not do so in rats (Denko and Whitehouse, 1970).

3. URICASE INHIBITION IN RATS

A novel approach toward developing an animal model of gout has been taken by Johnson *et al*. (1969). Most mammals possess the enzyme uricase, which converts urate to the much more soluble allantoin. Man, however, lost this enzyme during his evolutionary development with the result that humans have a much higher blood level of urate than those species possessing uricase. It is this relative hyperuricemia that predisposes humans to gout.

Johnson and co-workers reasoned that chemical inhibition of uricase in experimental animals might lead to a hyperuricemia that could be used as a model of the human disease. Of a number of *s*-triazines that these workers examined as potential uricase inhibitors, potassium oxonate (**9**) exhibited the highest activity, and at the same time proved to be a poor inhibitor of xanthine oxidase, a favorable attribute in this instance. Because of its rapid

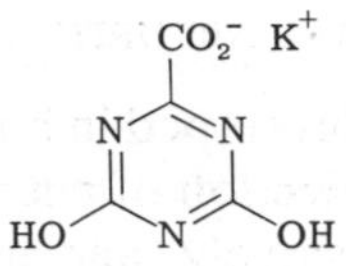

$$CO_2^- \ K^+$$

HO—N=N / N=N—OH structure

9

deactivation, multiple injections of oxonate (250 mg/kg) were necessary at 2.5-hr intervals. After the third injection plasma urate reached a maximum of 2.5 times the control value. The most favorable results, however, were obtained when the diet contained 5% oxonate and 1% uric acid. Serum urate rose to six times the control level after 9 days of this regimen and remained at this value. Urinary output of urate rose to 22 times normal. Microscopic examination of sectioned kidneys at the end of 23 days revealed the presence of crystalline deposits of uric acid in the collecting tubules. From these results it appears that this model effectively simulates hyperuricemia in humans. It will be of interest to observe the effect of oxonate-induced hyperuricemia on urate-induced paw swelling. As the authors point out, an irreversible and noncompetitive inhibitor of uricase will be quite useful.

4. URATE-INDUCED INFLAMMATION IN RABBITS

Spilberg and Osterland (1970) injected monosodium urate crystals into the skin and knee joints of male albino rabbits in order to examine the effect of trypsin–kallikrein (T-K) inhibitor on the resulting inflammation. Cutaneous inflammation was determined by measuring, at 18 hours, the diameters of the erythema, induration, and central necrosis produced by sodium urate crystals alone or mixed with T-K inhibitor. Synovial inflammation was appraised, also at 18 hours, by histologic evaluation of the synovium and by leukocyte counts. These parameters were graded on a 0 to 4+ basis. Sodium urate crystals plus T-K inhibitor mixture was injected into one knee joint and the urate suspension alone was injected into the other knee of the same animal. For controls, other animals were given saline in one knee and T-K inhibitor alone in the opposite knee. T-K inhibitor, a polypeptide that inhibits trypsin, chymotrypsin, several kallikreins, plasmin, leukocyte elastase, and spleen cathepsin D, also considerably diminished both the cutaneous and synovial urate-induced inflammation. The inflammatory response in complement-depleted animals was the same as in control animals, which suggested to these workers that normal blood levels of complement were not required for the urate-induced inflammatory response in this system. No antiinflammatory drugs were examined in this model of gout.

5. AVIAN MODEL OF MICROCRYSTAL ARTHRITIS

Floersheim *et al.* (1973a,b) developed in birds models of gout and pseudo-gout based on intraarticular injection of microcrystalline sodium urate and calcium pyrophosphate, respectively, and used these models to evaluate antiinflammatory activity of several substances. Inflammatory response in these systems was related to a one-legged stance produced when the bird lifted the injected leg to relieve the inflammatory reaction. The length of time during which the bird stood on one leg was taken as a measure of extent of inflammatory reaction. Antiinflammatory activity of drugs was determined by noting either an increase in the time of onset of the one-legged stance or a decrease in the total duration of the stance. Usually the birds were observed for 3 hours; in control animals (no drug treatment) the one-legged stance lasted 110–120 minutes. As the authors pointed out, this model of inflammation offers the advantage of assessing the functional aspects of antiinflammatory activity. The authors evaluated a number of cytotoxic agents (s.c.) in the urate system to determine whether these anti-proliferative drugs would have antiinflammatory effects in nonimmuno-logical (i.e., microcrystal) inflammation. It was found that procarbazine and actinomycin D were effective in suppressing the urate-induced inflam-mation but that cyclophosphamide, methotrexate, cytosine arabinoside, 6-mercaptopurine, and BCNU were not effective. Interestingly, neither vinblastine nor vincristine were effective. However, at similar doses these agents did suppress urate-induced paw swelling in mice (Fitzgerald *et al.*, 1971b), and vinblastine was active in rats (Zweig *et al.*, 1972). Colchicine suppressed the urate-induced inflammation at doses (0.5–1.5 mg/kg) similar to those found effective against urate-induced paw swelling in mice (Fitz-gerald *et al.*, 1971a) and in rats (Denko and Whitehouse, 1970; Zweig *et al.*, 1972). Colchicine was not active in suppressing calcium pyrophosphate-induced inflammation, which paralleled a similar finding in human pseudo-gout (Phelps and McCarty, 1969).

D. Models for Assessing Uricosuric Drugs and Xanthine Oxidase Inhibitors

1. URICOSURIC ACTIVITY

Animal models for examination of potential uricosuric activity of drugs in man have not been particularly successful. (For a more complete discussion of this topic and further references, see Gutman, 1966.) The difficulty arises because there are basic differences in the renal mechanisms for handling urate in various species and also because most species other than man possess the enzyme uricase.

The *Cebus* or organ grinder monkey has been employed in an attempt to analyze renal handling of uric acid and to examine the effects of known uricosuric agents (Fanelli *et al.*, 1970; Skeith and Healey, 1968). It has been found that although probenecid is uricosuric, zoxazolamine, the most potent uricosuric agent in man, is inactive. Blanchard *et al.* (1972) have also used this animal in their evaluation of 2-substituted analogs of probenecid.

Fanelli *et al.* (1971) studied renal handling of urate in chimpanzees and found this animal to be quite similar to man in that respect. Probenecid, sulfinpyrazone, zoxazolamine, and salicylate were uricosuric in this species. The chimpanzee was also used to examine the uricosuric properties of the hypolipodemic drugs halofenate and clofibrate (Fanelli *et al.*, 1972). Halofenate, uricosuric in man, was also uricosuric in the chimpanzee. Clofibrate, not uricosuric in man, likewise showed no effect on uric acid excretion in the chimpanzee.

The ability of uricosuric agents to delay renal clearance of Phenol Red (phenolsulfonphthalein) in rats as well as in man has found application in an assay for uricosuric activity (Kreppel, 1959). This method has obvious advantages over the use of either *Cebus* monkeys or chimpanzees, and results obtained with known uricosuric agents in this system have shown good correlation with uricosuric activities in man. The Phenol Red method of assessing uricosuric activity is also discussed by Swingle (Chapter 2, Volume II).

2. XANTHINE OXIDASE INHIBITION

Evaluation of potential inhibitors of xanthine oxidase can be carried out directly using the pure enzyme, as has been done for most substances (Section IV). It is desirable, if not necessary, however, to examine these substances in an *in vivo* system to determine, in addition to their toxicity, the ability of the compounds to reach their locus of action in an active form. The xanthine oxidase inhibitory activity of allopurinol was investigated in this manner in mice (Elion *et al.*, 1963). The animals were injected with solutions of either nonradioactive 6-mercaptopurine or [6-^{35}S]-mercaptopurine. 6-Mercaptopurine and its oxidation product (via xanthine oxidase), 6-thiouric acid, were determined in the urine by an isotope dilution technique. Similar experiments were also conducted in humans. In both cases, the allopurinol-treated subjects showed a marked increase in urinary 6-mercaptopurine compared to 6-thiouric acid, thereby demonstrating an inhibition of xanthine oxidase.

Because the isotope dilution method for measuring 6-mercaptopurine and 6-thiouric acid is lengthy and requires radioactive compounds, it cannot easily be used for screening purposes. However, it may be possible to adapt the method of Johnson *et al.* (Section II,C,3) wherein liver uricase in rats is blocked by administering a specific inhibitor, resulting in hyperuricemia and the excretion of relatively large quantities of uric acid.

III. COLCHICINE

A. Chemistry of Colchicine

Colchicine was isolated from *Colchicum autumnale* in 1820 in the great rush of phytochemical investigations of that era and was identified as the active antigout agent of the plant. The earliest structural work was initiated by Zeisel in the late Nineteenth Century. It was the efforts of Windaus some 40 years later, however, that led to a partially reduced phenanthrene structure (**10**) for colchicine. Subsequent investigations cast doubt on the validity of the Windaus structure and the presently accepted structure (**11**) was

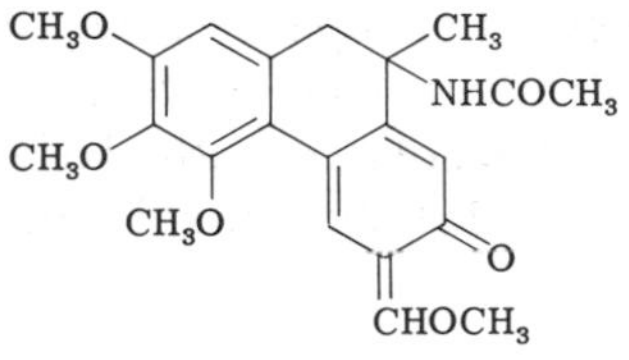

10 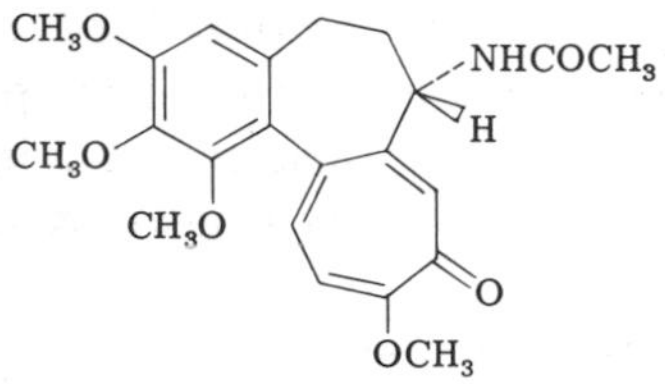　　　　　　　　　　　　　11

formulated by Dewar (1945), who suggested that ring C would be both seven membered and aromatic. This formulation was subsequently substantiated by X-ray diffraction studies (King *et al.*, 1952) on the colchicine–methyl iodide complex and by total synthesis of colchicine achieved through various pathways by a number of workers, as described in Section III,A,4. From a biological point of view, these synthetic schemes were important because a number of interesting analogs and derivatives of colchicine were made available. In addition the way is now open to certain derivatives that cannot be prepared from colchicine itself. An example of this would be the preparation of colchicine analogs, in which the three methoxy groups of the benzene ring would be either absent or replaced with other functional groups, such as methyl or halide.

1. TROPOLONES AND RING C OF COLCHICINE

Many of the biological and chemical properties characteristic of colchicine are associated with the methoxytropone structure comprising ring C. As tropolone chemistry marks its origin in Dewar's imaginative conception of ring C of colchicine, it is not surprising that colchicine chemistry and tropolone chemistry developed concurrently. Therefore, the chemistry of tropolone will be briefly discussed as background for colchicine.

Tropolone (12) is weakly acidic (pK_a = 7), gives a green color with ferric chloride, and on treatment with diazomethane yields the corresponding methyl ether (13, R_1 = R_2 = H) (Nozoe, 1959). Mild hydrolysis of the methyl

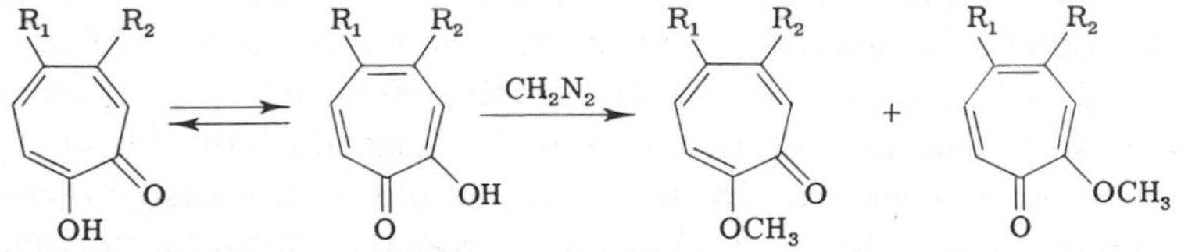

ether with dilute alkali or dilute acid regenerates the parent tropolone in a manner similar to the hydrolysis of esters. If the tropolone is substituted only in the 5 position (R_1) only one methyl ether is obtained. If, however, the molecule is substituted at the 4 position (R_2) treatment with diazomethane yields two methyl ethers as a result of the two tautomeric forms characteristic of tropolones. Methoxytropones, when treated more vigorously with base, undergo rearrangement to give a benzenoid aromatic system (14). Originally, it was supposed that this conversion was mediated through a mechanism strictly analogous to the benzylic acid rearrangement. However, it has been shown that the reaction more likely proceeds through a norcaradiene inter- mediate (15) (Magid et al., 1968). In the presence of amines the methoxyl group of 13 is displaced in a manner similar to amide formation from car- boxylic acid esters.

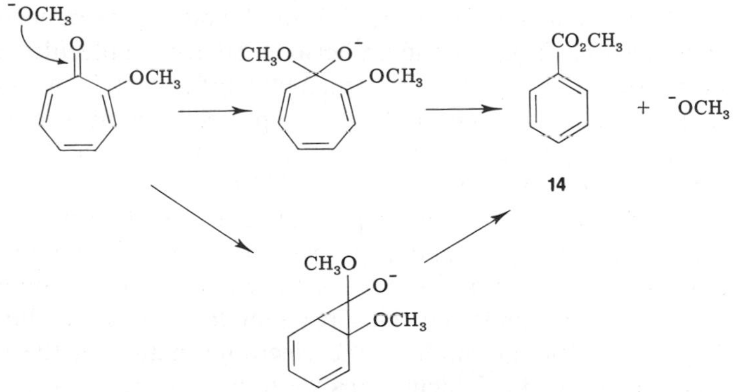

When Dewar introduced the tropolone ring concept as part of colchicine's structure he suggested that this novel system would be aromatic. Subsequent investigations of tropone, tropolone, and their derivatives seemed to confirm

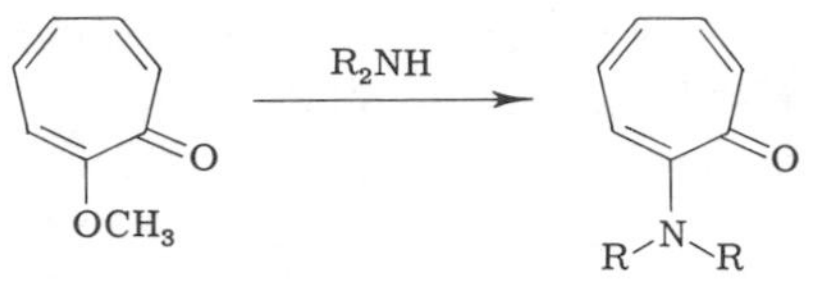

13

the aromatic character, which was attributed to a significant contribution from the dipolar resonance structure (**16**) shown for tropone. Recently, however, Bertelli and Andrews (1969) reevaluated the question of aromatic character in tropone and related compounds using data derived from dipole moment measurements and CNDO/2 calculations. It was their conclusion that tropone and tropolone would be more properly considered polyenones than aromatic systems. This conclusion was supported by analysis of the

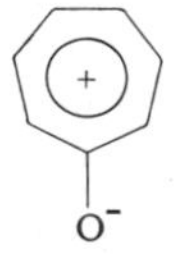

16

NMR spectra of these compounds (Bertelli *et al.*, 1969). The data presented by these authors are consistent, however, with the planarity of tropone as determined by electron diffraction. The π stabilization energy, although only that expected for a polyene system, is apparently sufficient to overcome the strain energy of the planar conformation.

As a result of these studies an X-ray analysis of tropolone was undertaken (Shimanouchi and Sasada, 1970), although similar analysis of various salts and metal complexes had been reported. It was found that the molecule was almost planar, with hydrogen bonding between adjacent molecules to form dimers. Apart from C-1–C-2 bond no apparent bond alternation was seen as would be expected for a polyene and as was reported for some tropone derivatives. The authors pointed out that the average C–C bond length (1.407 Å) agreed with the standard aromatic value (1.392 Å).

Dewar and Trinajstic (1970) have presented results of a semiempirical SCF MO treatment of tropone and tropolone, and derivatives thereof. Their findings again deny aromatic properties to tropone and tropolone and suggest that these compounds more closely resemble polyenones. Therefore, the final answer to the question of the electronic nature of these compounds (and therefore of colchicine) has yet to be settled.

Colchicine itself (**11**) can be considered a substituted 2-methoxytropone, and many of its reactions can be viewed from this standpoint. Thus, mild acid or alkaline hydrolysis yields colchiceine (**17**), which exists as a mixture of tautomers. Treatment of this compound with diazomethane generates a mixture isomeric methyl ethers, colchicine (**11**), and isocolchicine (**18**), as

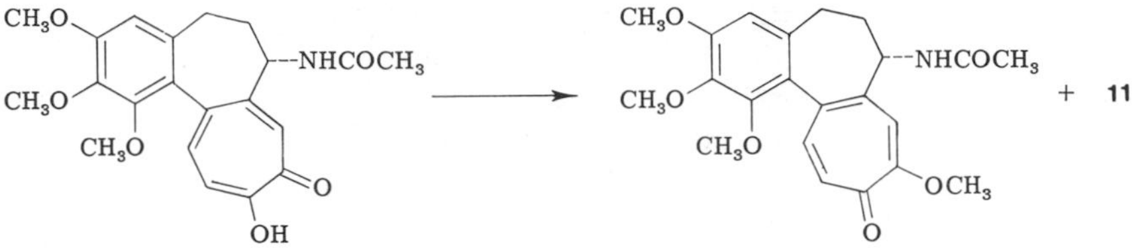

17 → 18 + 11

expected for an unsymmetrically substituted tropolone. Continued hydrolysis of colchiceine produces deacetylcolchiceine (19), often referred to as trimethylcolchicinic acid, or TMCA. As expected, this compound (19) on reaction with diazomethane produces deacetylcolchicine (20) and deacetylisocolchicine (21). Allocolchicine (22) is the benzenoid product obtained from base-catalyzed (⁻OCH₃) rearrangement of either colchicine or isocolchicine and corresponds to methylbenzoate (14) obtained from 2-methoxytropone (13) under similar conditions. Colchicine (and isocolchicine) undergoes displacement reactions with amines to give colchiceinamides (23 , R = (CH₃)₂N, for example). The methoxy group can also be displaced with CH₃SH to give thiocolchicine (23, R = SCH₃). Demethoxycolchicine (also called colchicide; 23, R = H) was obtained by Rapoport and Lavigne (1955) by treatment of thiocolchicine (23, R = SCH₃) with acetone-deactivated Raney nickel. This is, of course, the tropone congener of colchicine.

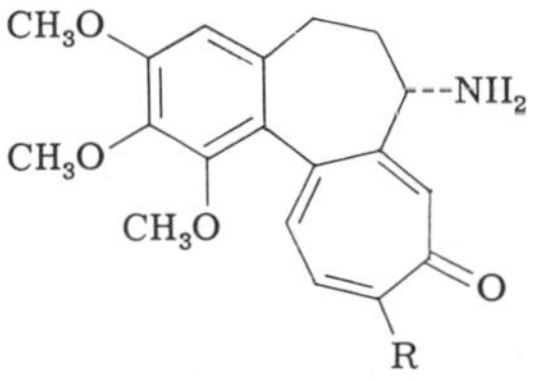

19 R = OH
20 R = OCH₃

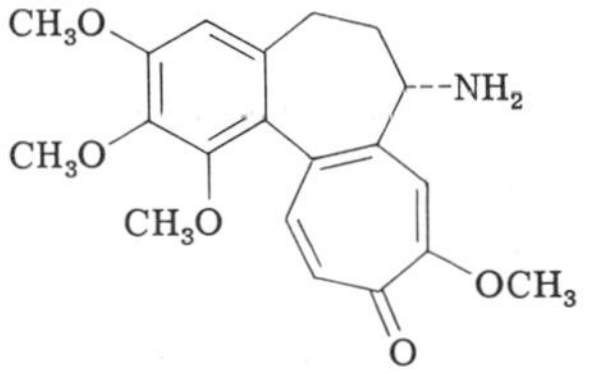

21

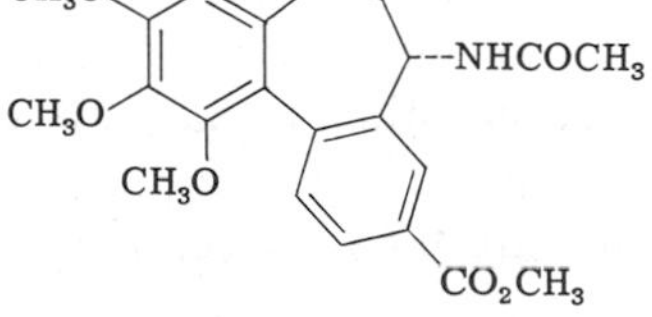

22

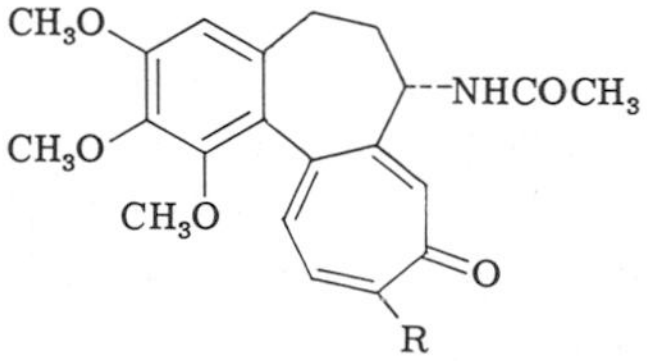

23

Many years ago it was found that chromic acid oxidation of colchicine afforded a substance designated "oxycolchicine." The nature of this compound (24) was elucidated by Buchanan et al. (1964) on the basis of spectral and chemical data. Their formulation clarified the lack of tropone properties and the ketonic behavior of the ring-C carbonyl group observed for this

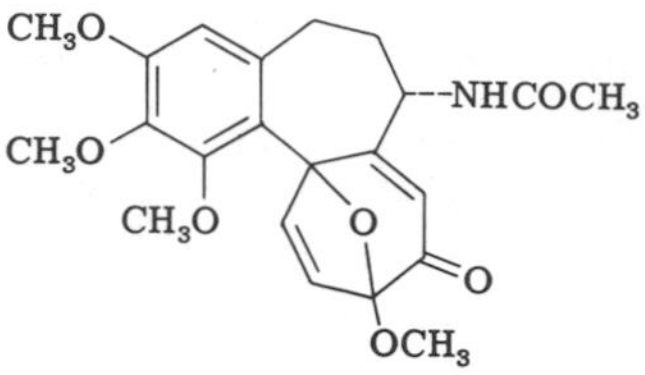

24

compound. That the extra oxygen was located as an ether bridge in ring C was suggested by regeneration of colchiceine (**17**) under the mild reducing conditions of potassium iodide and acetic acid.

An interesting reaction of colchicine with tris(hydroxymethyl) amino-methane (**25**) recently came to light. Margulis *et al.* (1969) observed that tris buffer (of which **25** is a component) solutions of colchicine or demecolcine (Colcemid, **26**) lost their ability to inhibit cilia and flagellar regeneration in *Stentor coeruleus* when allowed to stand for several hours. The products of this reaction were characterized with respect to their melting points and solubility properties. Although no information concerning the structure of these compounds was given, it would seem reasonable to suggest that they might have formed through displacement of the methoxy group on the tropone ring of the colchicine molecule by the amino function of the tris molecule.

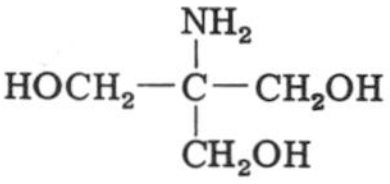

25 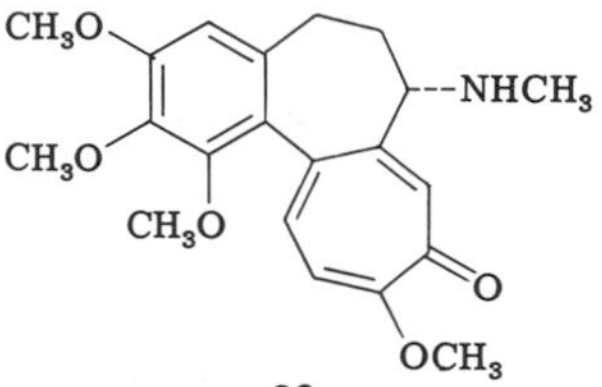   **26**

2. STEREOCHEMISTRY OF COLCHICINE

In contrast to the stereochemical situation encountered in most naturally occurring products, colchicine, with its single asymmetric atom, presents a comparatively simple picture (**11**). The S configuration at this carbon has been defined by ozonolysis of colchicine to yield N-acetyl-L-glutamic acid (**27**) (Corrodi and Hardegger, 1955). The unnatural $(+)$-R-colchicine has

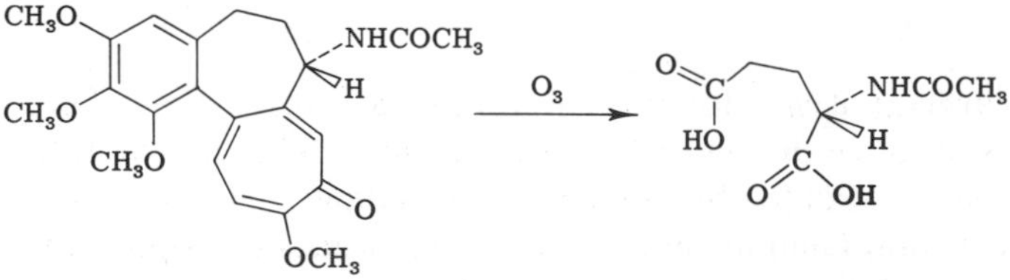

11   **27**

been prepared by these same authors (1957). After racemization of *N*-benzyl-idene-(−)-deacetylcolchiceine in refluxing alkali the Schiff base is hydro-lyzed and the racemic deacetylcolchiceine is resolved. Acetylation of the (+)-deacetylcolchiceine followed by methylation and separation of the isomers gives the unnatural (+)-colchicine.

Hrbek *et al.* (1964) have studied the optical rotatory dispersion of col-chicine and several related compounds. The dispersion curves of a series of colchicine and isocolchicine derivatives all show double negative Cotton effects, the first at about 330 nm and the second at about 280 nm. It has been suggested that the first of these is related to the methoxytropone system because this Cotton effect is not observed in a series of colchinol derivatives. Colchinol (**28**) is a benzenoid rearrangement product of colchicine and may be considered a skewed biphenyl system.

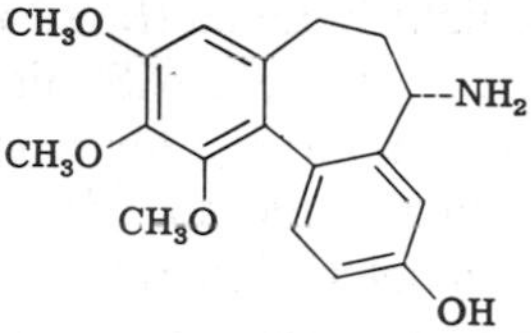

28

The Cotton effect of colchicine and isocolchicine curves at 280 nm was assigned to the K band of the biaryl system and is comparable to the single Cotton effect of the colchinol series. The greater amplitude in the first Cotton effect (330 nm) in the iso series as compared to the colchicine deri-vatives may be caused by different alignment of the tropone system with respect to the phenyl ring. Hbrek *et al.* also point out that differences in the degree of interaction between the lone pair of electrons on the nitrogen and the tropone system may be involved in producing the differences in the dispersion curves. The *S* configuration is assigned to the skewed phenyl-tropone system.

Rapoport and Lavigne (1956) observed that the optical rotation of chloro-form solutions of isocolchicine changed with time, whereas alcohol solutions of this compound as well as alcohol or chloroform solutions of colchicine did not change. After ruling out a number of possible explanations, they suggested that the mutarotation reflected a hindered rotation between rings A and C of isocolchicine. Lack of mutarotation in colchicine solutions was ascribed to a greater rigidity in the colchicine molecule.

3. RADIATION-INDUCED CHANGES IN COLCHICINE

Structural alterations brought about through interaction of the colchicine molecule with light or radiation from radioactive atoms are of importance for at least two reasons. First, the products resulting from exposure of colchicine to light (and probably from exposure to radioactivity also, but these products have not yet been completely identified) have unusual structures not easily obtained by other means. The biological activity of these compounds has not been thoroughly investigated (Section II,B,3). Second, it behooves investigators working with radioactive colchicine (and presumably derivatives thereof also containing the tropone ring system) to be aware of its facile conversion to radioactive breakdown products in order to avoid misinterpreting experimental results. In addition, recent work by Mizel and Wilson (1972) suggests that lumicolchicine may have interesting biological activity of its own. For these reasons a discussion of the chemistry of the effects of radiation on colchicine is presented.

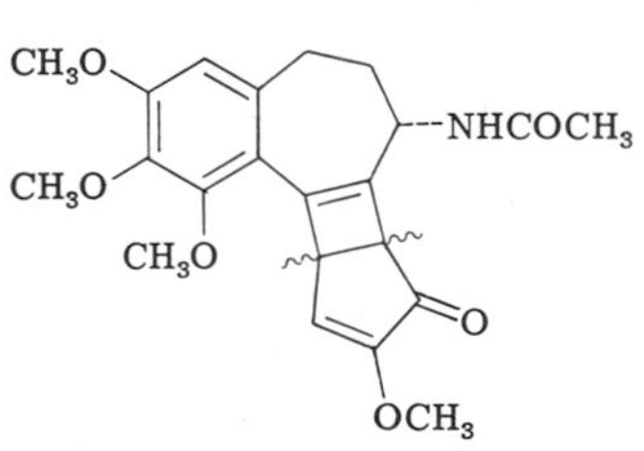

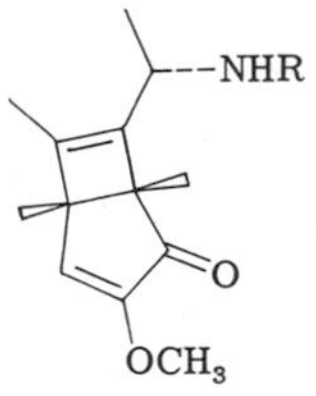

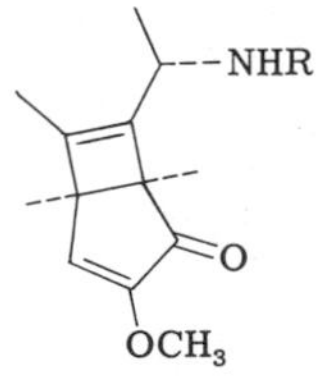

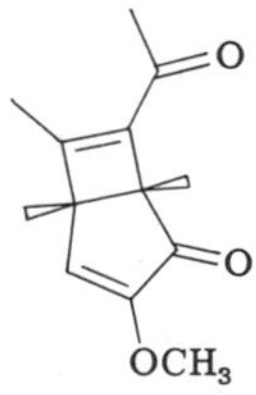

a. PHOTOCHEMISTRY.   Although the sensitivity of colchicine solutions to light had been known for many years it was the work of Grewe and Wulf (1951) that established the light-induced transformations of colchicine. An aqueous solution of colchicine, purged with nitrogen and sealed *in vacuo*, was exposed to sunlight for 2 months, after which time the precipitate was collected and examined. On the basis of fractional crystallization three compounds, all isomeric with colchicine, were isolated and were designated α-, β-, and γ-lumicolchicines, in order of increasing alcohol solubility. On the basis of chemical evidence Forbes (1955) suggested that β- and γ-lumicolchicines had tetracyclic structures (**29**) resulting from rearrangement of the tropone ring and that they were stereoisomers. Nuclear magnetic reasonance studies of β- and γ-lumicolchicines and the alcohols obtained by sodium borohydride reduction of these substances rigorously established (30), R = Ac, as β-lumicolchicine (Chapman *et al.*, 1963a). The structure of γ-lumicolchicine had not been established but evidence favored (31), R = Ac. Direct evidence for the stereoisomeric relationship between β- and γ- lumicolchicines was furnished by Canonica *et al.* (1969a). These authors isolated from *Gloriosa superba* (Liliaceae) a nitrogen-free product, lumicolchicone (32), the structure of which was established by ninhydrin oxidation of *N*-deacetyl-β-lumicolchicine (30, R = H). Through a similar oxidation of *N*-deacetyl-γ-lumicolchicine (31, R = H), γ-lumicolchicone was obtained; it gave identical spectral data and melting point as β-lumicolchicone but showed an equal and opposite optical rotation.

A relationship between α- and β-lumicolchicines had been clear for some time. Irradiation of β-lumicolchine gave the α isomer, whereas heating α-lumicolchicine above 100°C afforded the β compound in nearly quantitative yield. NMR analysis of α-lumicolchicine and its various reduction products established this compound as a dimer of β-lumicolchicine as represented by structure (33) (Chapman *et al.*, 1963b). Although one might have expected that molecular weight determinations would have uncovered the dimeric structure, the usual methods of measurement were difficult or misleading. The tendency of α-lumicolchicine to precipitate at low temperatures precluded the use of cryoscopic methods and the quantitative dissociation of this compound to β-lumicolchicine at temperatures above 100°C led to spurious results with the Rast method.

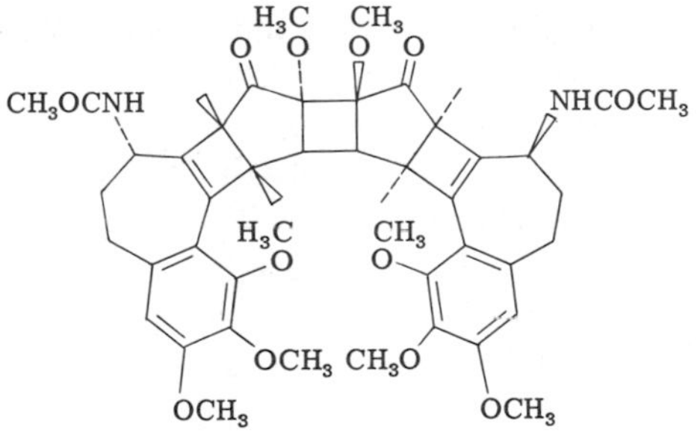

33

The photochemical behavior of isocolchicine (18) was also investigated (Chapman *et al.*, 1963c; Dauben and Cox, 1963). Both groups deduced the structure of the photoisomerization product, lumiisocolchicine, to be (34). This was the sole product isolated from the aqueous reaction medium employed by Chapman's group. However, Dauben and Cox carried out the reaction in methanol and found, in addition to (34), the methanol adduct (35). It was suggested that steric considerations would prefer the stereochemistry of γ-lumicolchicine for structure (**34**). The formation of lumi-isocolchicine as well as the formation of the lumicolchicines appears to be electronically controlled with retention of the styrene chromophore playing a dominant role.

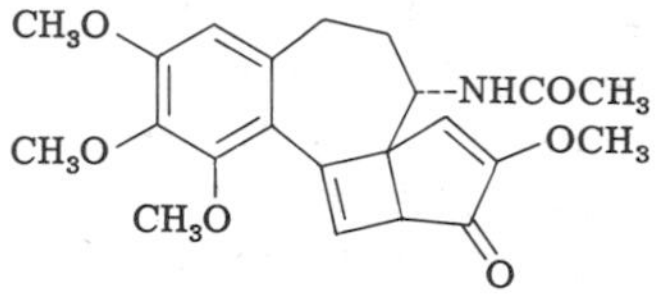

34 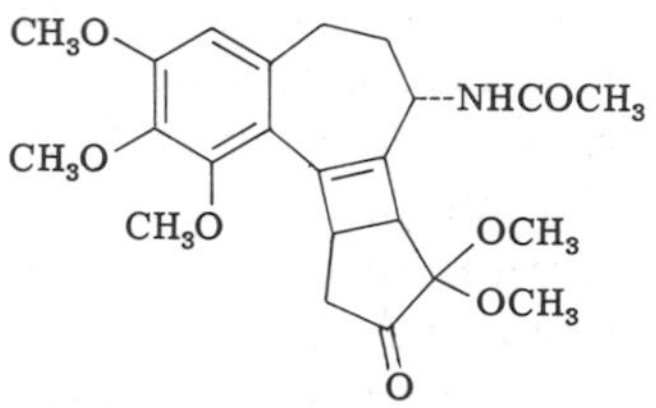   35

Many lumi derivatives have been isolated from natural sources (Potěšilová *et al.*, 1969; Canonica *et al.*, 1967) and their physical, chemical, and spectral properties have been reported.

b. EFFECT OF RADIOACTIVE LABELING. Radioactive colchicine was first prepared by Walaszek *et al.* (1952) by growing *Colchicum autumnalae* in an atmosphere of $^{14}CO_2$ and isolating the labeled compound. This procedure gave randomly labeled [^{14}C] colchicine. Shortly, thereafter, Raffauf *et al.* (1953) prepared colchicine labeled in various positions using [^{14}C] diazomethane and [^{14}C] acetylchloride. A number of labeled colchicine derivatives was also prepared. In neither these nor related reports (Back and Walaszek, 1953; Walaszek *et al.*, 1960) was there any mention of radioactive breakdown products of colchicine. In more recent work, however, there seems to be a special problem involving radiation-induced changes. Taylor (1965) reported preparation of [^3H] colchicine, with the label on the tropone methoxy group, by treatment of colchiceine (**17**) with tritiated diazomethane. Subsequent thin-layer chromatographic analysis of solutions of this material indicated the presence of a second radioactive spot moving faster than the spot corresponding to colchicine (Borisy and Taylor, 1967a). Wilson and Friedkin (1967) prepared [^{14}C] colchicine labeled in the carbonyl carbon of the acetyl group, but although they carried out extensive chromatographic purification no radioactive breakdown products were reported. Ertel and Wallace (1970) used several thin-layer systems for the analysis of solutions of radioactive colchicine. Their results suggested that radioactive colchicine (labeled with ^3H or ^{14}C in the tropone methoxy group) underwent radiation-induced conversion to lumicolchicine(s).

The actual nature of the radiation-induced product has not yet been established. It has been noted that tritiated colchicine degrades at a more rapid rate than colchicine containing ^{14}C (both labels in the tropone methoxy group) (Ertel *et al.*, 1967). No report of the stability of the ^{14}C (carbonyl) label in the acetyl group has appeared. Studies with radioactive colchicine should, therefore, be conducted with these facts in mind, and precautions should be taken to insure that radioactive breakdown products of colchicine do not lead to spurious results.

4. SYNTHETIC APPROACHES TO COLCHICINE AND DERIVATIVES

Although molecules of greater complexity than colchicine had been synthesized, attempts at total synthesis of colchicine during the late 1940's and the 1950's were unsuccessful. Consequently the construction of this molecule posed a serious challenge to organic chemists. Even after the first successful efforts, however, the novelty of the colchicine molecule continued to interest chemists. Furthermore, the discovery that deacetamidocolchicine (37, R = CH_3), the methyl ether of an important relay compound in several of the synthetic schemes, was a more potent antimitotic agent than colchicine itself (Schindler, 1962) maintained interest in the search for improved synthetic methods for the preparation of this compound.

A synopsis of the various successful synthetic pathways to colchicine is presented in Table I.

a. COLCHICINE. Once the relationship between colchicine and tropolone was pointed out (Dewar, 1945) the synthesis of tropone and tropolone followed in short order (Cook *et al.*, 1950; von E. Doering and Detert, 1951). Efforts toward synthesis of colchicine also began and by 1960 had achieved their goal. The first syntheses of colchicine were announced simultaneously (van Tamelen *et al.*, 1959; Schreiber *et al.*, 1959) with details following somewhat later (van Tamelen *et al.*, 1961; Schreiber *et al.*, 1961).

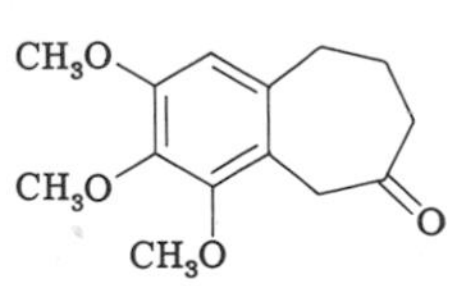

36 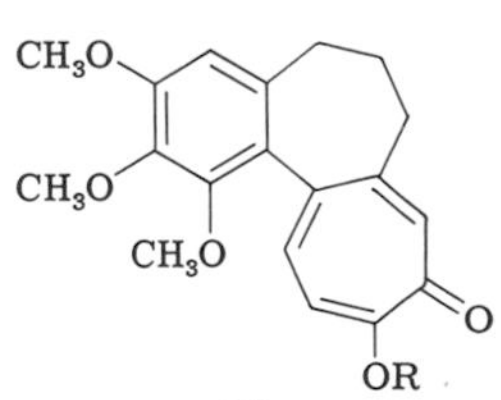   37

Van Tamelen's group initiated their scheme with the trimethoxysuberone (36) and after a sequence of several reactions obtained the key intermediate, deacetamidocolchiceine (37, R = H), which was also prepared by the degradation of colchicine. A short sequence of reactions converted (37, R = H), to racemic deacetylcolchiceine (19). The group led by Eschenmosher

TABLE I

Synopsis of Synthetic Schemes for Colchicine

Starting materials	Eventual product	Reference
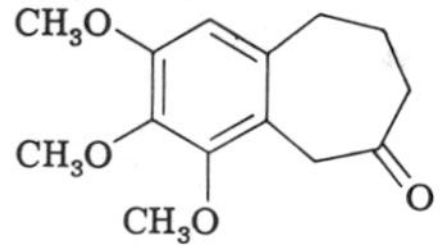	(±)-Deacetylcolchiceine (**19**)	van Tamelen *et al.* (1961).
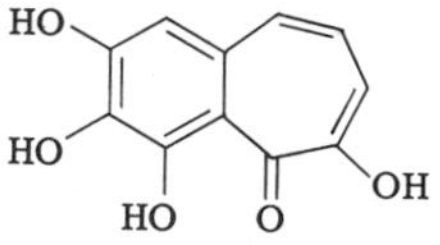	(±)-Deacetylcolchiceine (**19**)	Schreiber *et al.* (1961).
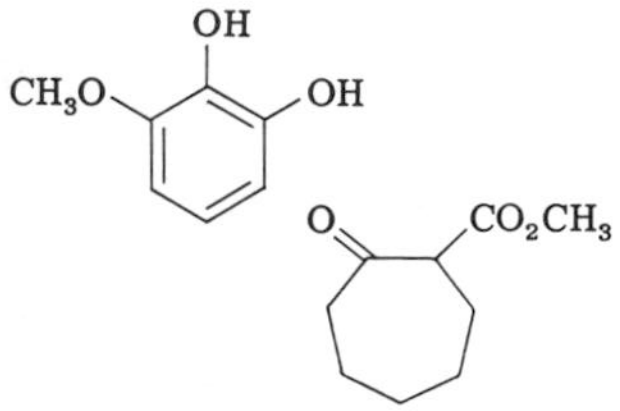	(±)-Deacetylcolchiceine (**19**)	Sunagawa *et al.* (1962).
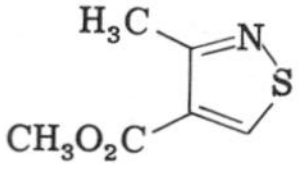	(±)-Colchiceine (**17**)	Woodward (1965).
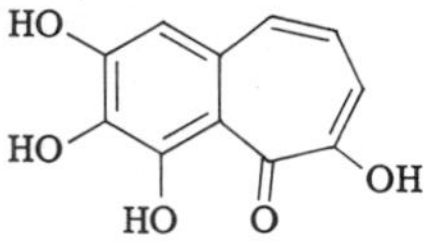	Deacetamidocolchiceine (**37**, R = OH)	Scott *et al.* (1965).

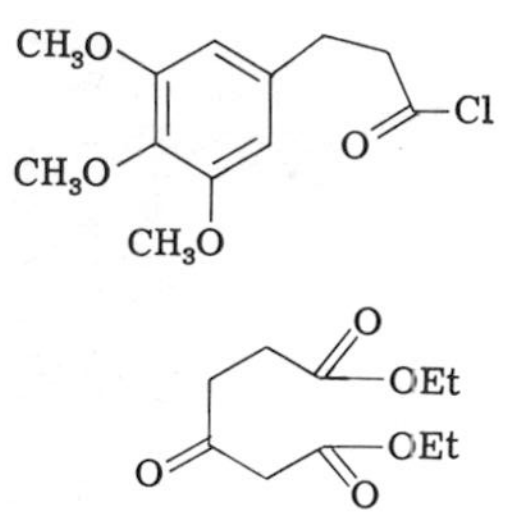

Martel *et al.* (1965).

Kaneko and Matsui (1968).

Hahn (1971).

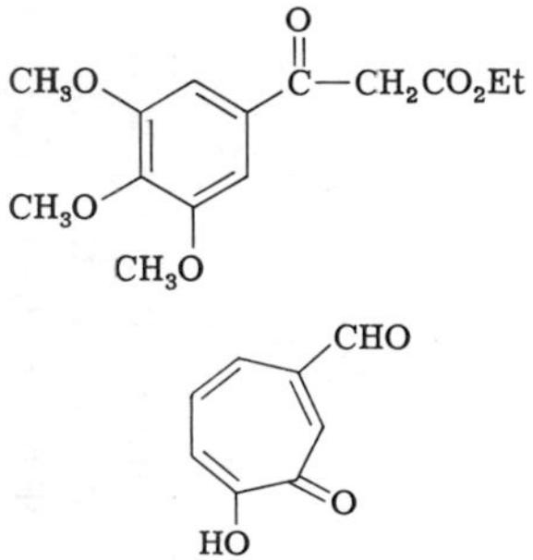

Deacetamidocolchiceine
(**37**, R = OH)

Deacetamidocolchiceine
(**37**, R = OH)

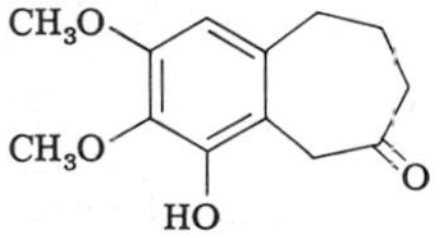

Deacetamidocolchiceine
(**37**, R = OH)

began their synthesis with purpurogallin, and reached relay compound (37, R = H), by a somewhat different series of reactions. Conversion of (37, R = H), to racemic (19) was carried out in a manner similar to that of van Tamelen's group. Because racemic (19) had previously been converted to (−)-colchicine (Corrodi and Hardegger, 1957), the total synthesis of colchicine was thus accomplished.

Since 1961 a number of synthetic approaches to colchicine have been reported. Nakamura's group, instead of constructing a tropolone ring into an already forged A–B ring structure, sought to join rings A and C possessing the proper functional groups for building ring B (Nakamura, 1962; Nakamura et al., 1962; Sunagawa et al., 1962). To accomplish this, the monomethylpyrogallol (38) and the cycloheptanone carboxylate (39) were joined to eventually afford (40). Ring closure in (40) to generate a ketone at the eventual 7 position of colchicine allowed introduction of the nitrogen function through the oxime. After a number of reactions amounting to oxidation of ring C, racemic deacetylcolchiceine (19) was obtained, constituting total synthesis of colchicine.

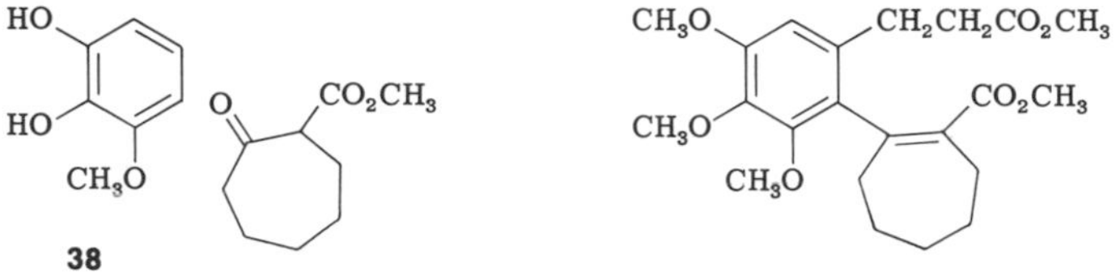

A novel synthesis of colchicine was presented by Woodward (1965). In this scheme racemic colchiceine (17) was obtained after Raney nickel desulfurization and acetylation of (41), which was the eventual product of a synthetic pathway beginning with the substituted isothiazole (42). In contrast to other approaches to the colchicine molecule, the nitrogen atom was carried through the entire synthesis, being inactivated by its participation in the isothiazole ring.

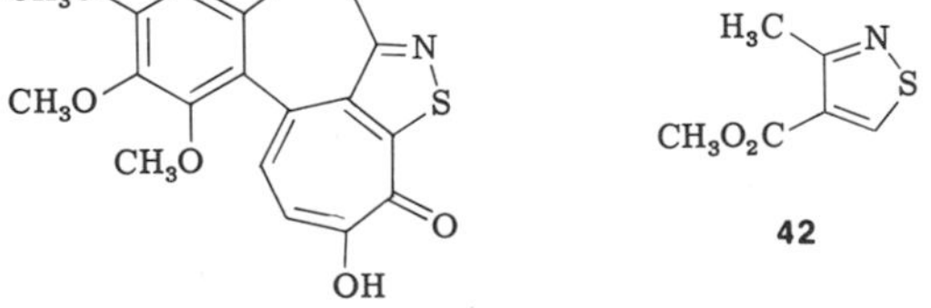

The synthetic route chosen by Scott et al. (1965) was based on a likely biogenetic mode of formation of the alkaloid. The essence of the problem was constructing the polyhydric bicyclic compound (43) and converting this to **44**. Selection of proper reagents to induce this conversion was beset with frustration, and several oxidizing agents led only to unidentifiable products or unchanged starting material. The final choice was one of a delicately balanced mixture of reagents, time, and order of mixing. The reaction, mediated by ferric chloride, most likely proceeded through a radical coupling between the phenyl and tropolone rings. Treatment of **(44)** with CH_3I/K_2CO_3 gave deacetamidocolchiceine (**37**, R = H).

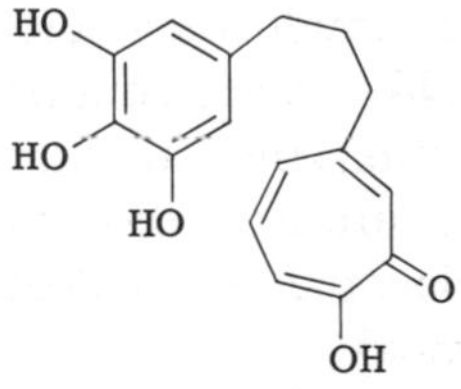

43 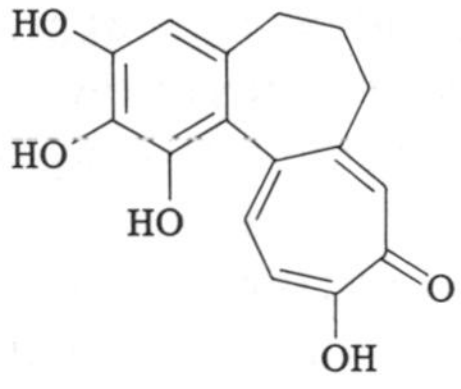   44

Despite the synthesis of colchicine by the five different groups so far described, interest in new synthetic approaches to this substance continues. Primarily, these efforts have been and continue to be aimed at construction of deacetamidocolchiceine (**37**, R = H) both because of its role as a synthetic relay to colchicine itself and because of the interesting biological activity of its methyl ether, deacetamidocolchicine.

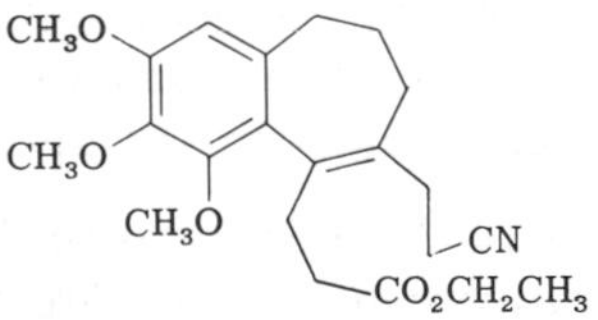

45

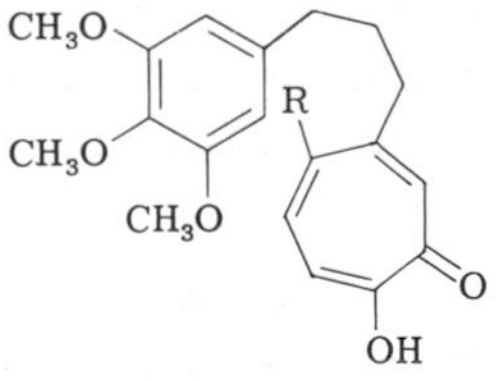

46 R = H
47 R − NH$_2$

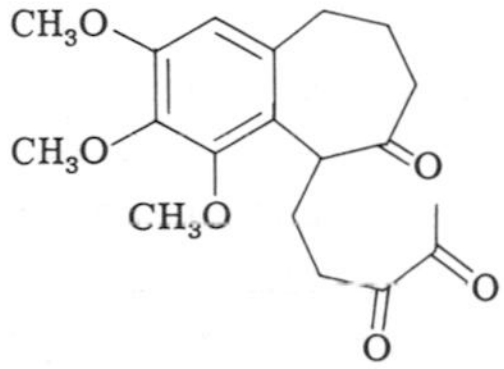

48

Martel *et al.* (1965) developed a synthesis of deacetamidocolchiceine (**37**, R = H) through a cyano ester intermediate (**45**), itself achieved in seven steps from a base-catalyzed condensation of ethyl-β-oxoadipate with 3-(3,4,5-trimethoxyphenyl)propyl chloride. The desired product (**37**, R = H) was obtained after another seven reaction steps. The overall reported yield of (**45**) based on the starting materials was low (about 9% for the seven-step sequence) as was the yield of product (**37**, R = H, 2.8%) from (**45**), as might be expected for a lengthy synthetic pathway. Nevertheless, the authors felt that all the steps up to intermediate (**45**) could be adjusted to proceed quantitatively.

Kaneko and Matsui (1968) prepared deacetamidocolchiceine (**37**, R = H) starting from the phenylpropyltropolone (**46**), which coupled with the *p*-toluidine diazonium salt and gave on reduction, the aminotropolone (**47**). On treatment of (**47**) with isoamylnitrite in sulfuric acid–dioxane and decomposition of the diazonium solution with copper the desired deacetamidocolchiceine (**37**, R = H) was obtained in 5% yield.

The most recent synthetic procedure (Hahn, 1971) involved cyclization of the triketone (**48**) with magnesium methoxide followed by reaction with triethylammonium *N*-carbomethoxysulfamate to give deacetamidocolchiceine (**37**, R = H). Triketone (**48**) was generated by a series of reactions commencing with 1'-hydroxy-2',3'-dimethoxy-2-benzosuberone.

With continuing efforts, such as those described here, toward a practical synthesis of deacetamidocolchiceine (**37**, R = H) it may not be overly adventurous to expect that deacetamidocolchicine (**37**, R – CH$_3$) may eventually become commercially available and at a cost less than that incurred were it prepared from colchicine. The interesting biological properties of this compound can then be studied without the frustration most biologists now experience in attempting to secure even small amounts of this substance.

b. COLCHICINE DERIVATIVES.   Numerous colchicine derivatives have been prepared by various workers either to study structure–activity relationships or in an effort to develop potential antitumor agents. Some of these preparations are mentioned here because either their chemical or their biological properties are of interest.

A group of workers in France developed a number of modifications of the colchicine molecule. Muller *et al.* (1963) observed that the open position on the benzene ring of colchicine would be well suited for electrophilic substitution because of the effect of the methoxy groups. Reasoning that the tropone ring would be deactivated toward electrophilic substitution by complexation with the Lewis acid catalyst and that because of lack of complanarity between the phenyl and tropone rings the effect of the deactivation would not be transmitted to the phenyl ring, these workers carried out selective substitutions at the C-4 position of colchicine by application of a Friedel-Crafts reaction. Treatment of colchicine (**11**, or **49** R = H) with α,α-dichloromethyl ether in the presence of $SnCl_4$ gave the 4-dichloromethyl derivative (**49**, R = $CHCl_2$), which upon hydrolysis afforded 4-formylcolchicine (**49**, R = CHO). Through the versatility of the formyl group various functions were introduced into this position. For example, BF_3/HOAc-catalyzed Beckmann rearrangement of the 4-formyloxime (**49**, R = CH=NOH) generated the 4-formamido derivative (**49**, R = NHCHO) making the amine function available in this position. Acetic anhydride-mediated dehydration of the oxime led to the 4-cyano compound (**49**, R = CN). Other groups introduced at the 4 position of colchicine included CH_2OH, CO_2H, CH_2OCH_3, OH, OCH_3, CH_2Cl, and $CH_2CH=CH_2$ (Blade and Muller, 1964, 1968; Muller, 1963). Derivatives in which the tropone methoxy was replaced by SCH_3 or an alkylamino group were included in the reports by these workers.

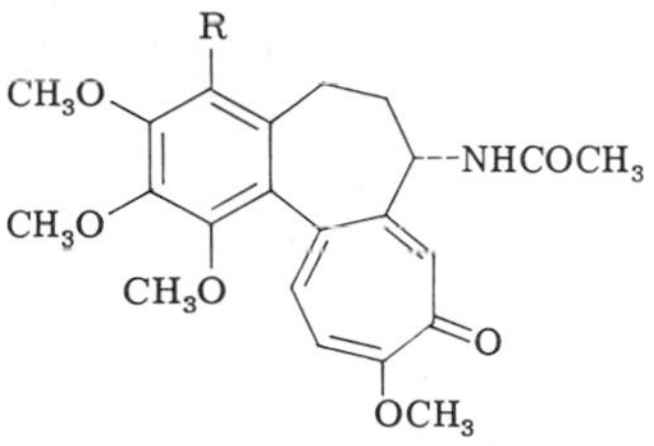

49

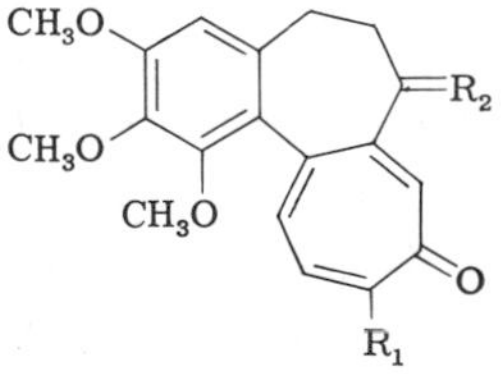

50a

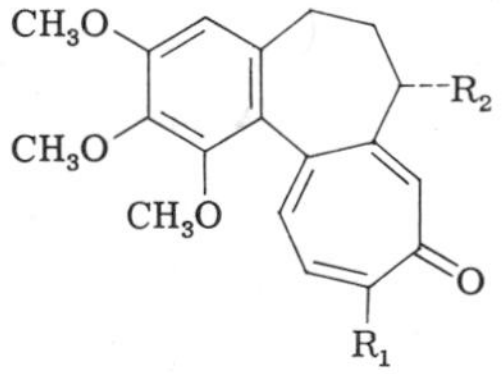

50b

Preparation of a colchicine derivative bearing a keto function in the 7 position (**50a**, R_1 = OCH_3, R_2 = O) in place of the acetamido group was described by Muller and Poittevin (1964). Conversion of deacetylcolchiceine (**19** or **50b**, R_1 = OH, R_2 = NH_2) to the chloramine (**50b**, R_1 = OH, R_2 = NHCl) with N-chlorosuccinamide was followed by dehydrohalogenation with alkali. The resulting imine (**50a**, R_1 = OH, R_2 = NH) was hydrolyzed to the ketone (**50a**, R_1 = OH, R_2 = O), which on treatment with diazomethane and chromatography of the reaction mixture afforded 7-oxo-deacetamidocolchicine (**50a**, R_1 = OCH_3, R_2 = O) and the corresponding iso derivative.

In view of the fact that the β-lumi derivative of 7-oxodeacetamidocolchicine is known as "lumicolchicone," 7-oxodeacetamidocolchicine will hereafter be referrred to as "colchicone." Interestingly, although lumicolchicone has been isolated from a natural source and characterized (Section III,A,3,a), colchicone itself has not been found in nature (Canonica *et al.*, 1969b).

Colchicone may serve as the starting point for many interesting colchicine derivatives and the method used by Canonica *et al.* (1969a) to prepare the lumicolchicone derivatives (ninhydrin oxidation of the corresponding *N*-deacetyllumicolchicine) may provide a more convenient method for the preparation of colchicone, starting from *N*-deacetylcolchicine (**20**). The yield of lumicolchicone from deacetyllumicolchicine is 22%.

Zeitler and Niemer (1969) have reported the conversion of colchicine directly to colchicone by the bacterium *Arthrobacter colchovorum* when this organism is grown on a nitrogen-free medium (except for the added colchicine). Although the yield of product is not given, this method may find application in the preparation of colchicone.

The amide function of colchicine has been recognized for over 80 years, yet only recently have haloacetyl derivatives of colchicine been reported (Lettré *et al.*, 1972). These compounds [**50b**, $R_1 = OCH_3, N(CH_3)_2$, or SCH_3; $R_2 = NHCOCH_2X$, where X = F, Cl, Br, or I] are prepared by treating deacetylcolchicine (**20** or **50b**, $R_1 = OCH_3$, $R_2 = NH_2$) with the appropriate haloacetyl halide. Reaction of the bromo derivative with NaI affords the iodo compound. Some of these compounds are of greater antimitotic activity than colchicine itself, and some possess promising antitumor activity.

The simplest derivative of colchicine known to possess microtubule protein binding activity (Section III,B,1) is a bicyclic compound (**13**, $R_1 =$ 2,3,4-trimethoxyphenyl, $R_2 = H$) (Fitzgerald, 1973). This compound has been prepared in 15% yield by treatment of a solution of 5-aminotropolone (**13**, $R_1 = NH_2$, $R_2 = H$) and trifluoroacetic acid in 2,3-dimethoxyphenol with isoamyl nitrite and copper followed by treatment with diazomethane.

B. Biology of Colchicine

The most significant biological properties of colchicine are its ability to inhibit mitosis in metaphase and its effectiveness in alleviating acute attacks of gout. In recent years it has become increasingly evident that both these actions of colchicine derive from a more fundamental property of the drug, i.e., its interaction with microtubule protein, the subunit of microtubules. Therefore a discussion of microtubules, the role of microtubules in mitosis, and the nature of the colchicine–microtubule protein interaction is presented as a prelude to the section on colchicine's antigout effects (Section III,B,2).

1. MICROTUBULES AND THE ANTIMITOTIC ACTION OF COLCHICINE

The potent and specific antimitotic action of colchicine was first observed by Pernice (1889) but remained generally unknown until its rediscovery by Lits (1934) and Dustin *et al.* (1937). These findings kindled the interest of many workers and it soon became apparent that colchicine inhibited cell division in metaphase by halting the formation of spindles as well as by causing the dissolution of preformed spindles. Despite considerable research effort, the mechanism of colchicine's antimitotic action remained elusive until a few years ago.

Comprehensive monographs on the early work with colchicine (Eigsti and Dustin, 1955) and on the physiology of cell division (Mazia, 1961) are available.

An essential prelude to understanding this action of colchicine was a knowledge of the nature of the mitotic apparatus. This entity includes the spindle fibers, the chromosomes, and the amorphous material in which these structures are embedded (Mazia, 1961). Isolation of the intact mitotic apparatus was first accomplished by Mazia and Dan (1952), who also determined that disulfide linkages played a significant role in the assembly of the proteins into a mitotic apparatus. Microtubules were subsequently identified as the major element of the spindle fibers (DeHarven and Bernhard, 1956). It was originally believed that microtubules consisted largely of a single protein (Weisenberg *et al.*, 1968) but more recent investigations (Bryan and Wilson, 1971; Bryan, 1972a; Everhart, 1971) showed that the structural unit of microtubules is actually a heterodimer composed of two very similar proteins (designated α and β). The proteins have molecular weights between 55,000 and 60,000 and exhibit very similar amino acid compositions. Microtubule protein is also characterized by a strong tendency to aggregate, by association with bound guanine nucleotide, and by precipitation by calcium ion and vinblastine. In addition, the known metaphase-specific mitotic poisons, viz., colchicine, podophyllotoxin, vinblastine, and vincristine, all bind to microtubule protein.

Using the colchicine-binding activity as an indicator, a number of workers have found that microtubule disappearance from specimens of isolated mitotic apparatus, as determined by electron microscopy, parallels the appearance in extracts of the specimens of a colchicine-binding protein (Kiefer *et al.*, 1966; Borisy and Taylor, 1967b; Taylor, 1965; Bibring and Baxandall, 1971).

The colchicine-binding species is the heterodimer (110,000 M.W.) consisting of an α and a β chain and binds 1 mole of colchicine per mole of dimer. This species also binds 2 moles of guanosine triphosphate (GTP), one of which is exchangeable and the other not. Podophyllotoxin, an antimitotic agent similar in action to colchicine, also binds to microtubule protein (Wilson and Friedkin, 1967). Wilson (1970) has shown that podophyllotoxin blocks colchicine binding but that it stabilizes the colchicine–protein complex once it has been formed, and he suggests that podophyllotoxin may bind at a site different from the colchicine binding site. However, Bryan (1972b) has incubated colchicine and podophyllotoxin together with suspensions of vinblastine-induced crystals of microtubule protein from sea urchin eggs (Wilson used chick embryo brain) and has obtained results indicating that the inhibition observed with podophyllotoxin is competitive and that the two drugs compete for the same site on the dimer. He also confirms that 1 mole of colchicine is bound per mole of dimer and calculated thermodynamic values for the binding process: $\Delta F^0 = -6.7$ kcal/mole, $\Delta H^0 = 16$ kcal/mole, $\Delta S^0 = 80$ e.u. (at 13°C). These values are consistent with the idea that colchicine binds in a hydrophobic or nonpolar pocket on the protein. It has also been reported that iodoacetic acid, N-ethylmaleimide, and 5-nitro-2-methoxytropone have no effect on colchicine binding even when these substances are present in very large excess. Additional information on microtubule protein and its interaction with colchicine has been obtained using the technique of circular dichroism (CD) (Ventilla *et al.*, 1972). Using the 6S protein subunit (this corresponds to the 110,000 M.W. dimer) from porcine brain these workers have determined that at 4°C and pH 6.5 (conditions of maximum protein stability) the subunit consists of 22% α helix, 30% β structure (a pleated-sheet conformation), and 48% random coil. At 37°C (a temperature of low protein stability but maximum colchicine binding activity) and pH 6.5 the subunit shows 0% α helix, 56% β structure, and 44% random coil. Colchicine, vinblastine, and various guanosine nucleotides protect the protein against denaturation as observed by CD measurements at 220 nm. The authors believe their results are consistent with the idea that colchicine binding activity is highly dependent on protein conformation and that the conformation to which colchicine binds is probably an energetically unfavorable one.

The other well-known antimitotic agent, vinblastine, appears to bind to a different species (perhaps a higher molecular weight aggregate) of the protein (Wilson and Friedkin, 1967; Weisenberg and Timasheff, 1970). Lumicolchicine, which has no antimitotic activity, neither binds to microtubule protein nor inhibits nor enhances colchicine binding (the particular isomer or mixture of lumicolchicine isomers was not specified) (Wilson and Friedkin, 1967).

Microtubules and microtubule subunit protein are not limited in their distribution to spindle fibers but occur in many different tissues and non-dividing cells (Borisy and Taylor, 1967a). Evidence suggesting their participation in various cell functions has accumulated. Thus, in addition to their role in mitosis, microtubules may also be involved in platelet aggregation (White, 1969), degranulation and secretion (Gillespie *et al*., 1968; Lacy *et al*., 1968; Levy and Carlton, 1969; Malawista and Bodel, 1967; Poisner and Bernstein, 1971; Williams and Wolff, 1970), chemotaxis (Caner, 1965), axonal flow (Dahlström, 1968), and phagocytosis (Journey, 1964).

At the present time colchicine's antimitotic activity is believed to be a function of its ability to bind to a protein subunit of microtubules. If microtubules (in nondividing cells as well as in the mitotic spindle) were in dynamic equilibrium with smaller protein subunits in surrounding cytoplasm (Inoué, 1964) the binding of colchicine to a smaller subunit (such as the sub-unit protein dimer) would inhibit their further aggregation (Weisenberg *et al*., 1968) and would shift the equilibrium towards dissociation of the microtubules. Various factors that affect formation of the colchicine–protein complex have been described and may be of significance in microtubule function. It has been shown that GTP; the vinca alkaloids, vinblastine and vincristine; and high concentrations of glucose, NaCl, or sodium glutamate stabilize the colchicine–protein complex. The binding of colchicine to the protein is apparently irreversible but on deactivation of the colchicine–protein complex colchicine is released (Wilson, 1970). Therefore, colchicine is not covalently bound to the protein. What relation these *in vitro* observations have to actual conditions in a viable cell is not known.

The association of cyclic AMP and calcium with cell processes (Jost and Rickenberg, 1971) led to the question of whether the functions of microtubules also involved interaction with these agents. Goodman *et al*. (1970) suggest that the secretory process in the neurotubule–vesicle system might involve cyclic AMP-dependent phosphorylation of microtubules followed by activation of the phosphorylated protein by calcium ion in analogy to the role of these two intracellular messengers in the activation of the phosphorylase systems in cardiac muscle. Colchicine did not inhibit the cyclic AMP-mediated phosphorylation of microtubules observed by these workers. Purified rat brain microtubule protein was phosphorylated by a cyclic AMP-dependent kinase from hog brain (Murray and Froscio, 1971). These workers found that incubation of the phosphorylated microtubule protein with rat brain extract resulted in loss of ability of the phosphorylated microtubule protein to absorb to DEAE Sephadex. They speculated that this was related to microtubule assembly. Evidence that the soluble component in rat brain extract was a protein was obtained and the protein was shown to be insensitive to colchicine treatment. Cyclic AMP and its $N^6,O^{2'}$-dibutyryl derivative

altered cell shape and growth characteristics (Hsie and Puck, 1971; Johnson
et al., 1971). That these changes involved microtubule protein was suggested
by the fact that colchicine, demecolcin (Colcemid), and vinblastine were
inhibitory at low concentrations. Gillespie (1971) studied the effect of cyclic
AMP and calcium on colchicine in tissue slices. In order to explain the
biphasic response of colchicine binding activity observed with variation of
cyclic AMP concentrations the following scheme was proposed.

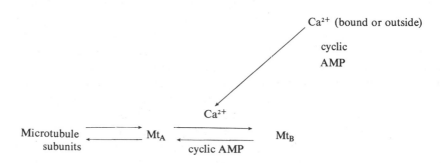

This proposal assumes that there are two forms of microtubules, Mt_A and
Mt_B, which represent any difference in a microtubule, a portion thereof, or
a subunit. Also, it is assumed that only one of the forms breaks down into
subunits and that calcium and cyclic AMP regulate the equilibrium between
Mt_A and Mt_B. Thus, either calcium or cyclic AMP can stimulate or inhibit
microtubule function.

An integrated picture of the control mechanisms for regulation of subunit–microtubule equilibria essential to the formation and dissociation of
microtubules, as well as the mechanisms involved in the various functions of
microtubules, has yet to emerge. However, a beginning is being made.
Several studies on the role of guanosine nucleotide in phophorylation reactions have appeared, although no general hypothesis has been formulated
(Berry *et al.*, 1971; Bryan, 1971; Soifer, 1971). Weisenberg and Timasheff
(1970) have examined certain aspects of the aggregation dynamics of microtubule protein that may be of significance in the association and dissociation
of microtubules. They find that magnesium or calcium induces reversible
aggregation of microtubule protein, that colchicine increases the divalent
ion-induced aggregation, and that vinblastine induces aggregation and alters
the effect of divalent ions. Roth *et al.* (1970) have challenged the assumption
that microtubules of different stability possess subunits of different structure
and suggest that microtubules are all derived from identical subunits and that
allosteric effects and regulatory molecules are responsible for differences in
stability and function of microtubules.

Two reviews that discuss the nature of microtubules and the interaction of colchicine with microtubule protein have appeared (Margulis, 1973; Olmsted and Borisy, 1973).

2. ANTIGOUT ACTIVITY OF COLCHICINE

The ability of *Colchicum* extracts to relieve attacks of gout was first recognized about 14 centuries ago (Eigsti and Dustin, 1955; Hartung, 1954). The isolation of colchicine from the *Colchicum* plant made available the pure compound for medicinal use. Colchicine's notable lack of influence on urate excretion, urate blood levels, or any aspect of urate metabolism, as well as its failure to exhibit analgesic properties posed a riddle concerning its mechanism that only recently began to become disentangled. The discovery of colchicine's antimitotic properties was of little assistance in understanding its antigout effect. Nevertheless, even after many investigators had failed to find a relationship between these two activities of colchicine it was a concept difficult to abandon; indeed, for lack of experimental evidence the law of parsimony was invoked (Goodman and Gilman, 1955).

Events of the past decade have changed all this, and at the present time it is believed that the antimitotic and antigout activities of colchicine may indeed share a common mechanism. As developed by Malawista (1968) this hypothesis suggests that the sol–gel transformations associated with the properties and function of the mitotic spindle are related to the sol–gel transformations responsible for such cellular properties as shape and movement. Colchicine may interfere with the organization of protoplasmic gels by virtue of its effect on microtubules, which are likely candidates for mediating such sol–gel transformations.

The PMN, because of its central role in acute gout (Section II,B,3), has been regarded as the possible locus of colchicine's action, and, therefore, the effect of colchicine on various functions of PMN's has been the subject of numerous investigations. Initially the phagocytic activity of PMN's was considered as a possible target of colchicine's activity (Seegmiller *et al.*, 1962). By inhibiting phagocytosis, it was suggested, colchicine interrupted the cycle of events (Section II,B,3) leading to inflammation. Subsequent investigation showed that microtubules in PMN's were no longer seen in cells after incubation with colchicine (Malawista and Bensch, 1967) but that the cells nevertheless continued to phagocytize α-streptococci. Instead, colchicine was found to inhibit the increased metabolism associated with phagocytosis and the subsequent fusion of lysosomes with the vacuoles (Malawista and Bodel, 1967). Although these observations would seem to cast doubt on inhibition of phagocytosis as a site of action for colchicine, other workers presented evidence that colchicine did indeed suppress phagocytosis. Chang

(1968), for instance, found a differential inhibition of phagocytosis by colchicine in PMN's depending on the nature of the particle offered to the cells. Colchicine ($1 \times 10^{-4} M$) was able to suppress phagocytosis of *Pseudomonas aeruginosa* or starch granules but even at a concentration of $25 \times 10^{-3} M$ colchicine did not affect phagocytosis of *Staphlococcus aureus*. Wallingford and McCarty (1971) showed that colchicine ($1 \times 10^{-4} M$) inhibited uptake of starch or monosodium urate crystals by human PMN's. A good correlation between decreased oxygen consumption and inhibition of uptake of polystyrene particles in PMN's was observed when the cells were incubated with colchicine (2.9×10^{-3} to $11.1 \times 10^{-3} M$), although the concentration of drug was rather high (Kvarstein and Stormorken, 1971). Much lower concentrations of colchicine ($10^{-6} M$) were observed to reduce Zymosan particle uptake in murine macrophages (Weissmann *et al.*, 1971) and to decrease phagocytosis of urate crystals by human PMN's (Phelps, 1970). Somewhat earlier, Goldfinger *et al.* (1965) noted a suppression of phagocytosis of urate crystals by human leukocytes as a result of colchicine ($2 \times 10^{-6} M$) treatment.

Fusion of lysosomes with the phagocytic vacuole containing a urate crystal, and subsequent events, may be the basis of acute gouty inflammation (Section II,B,3), and the fusion process is considered a possible site of action for colchicine. It has been shown that colchicine interferes with lysosomal degranulation and formation of the phagolysosome in human PMN's (Malawista and Bodel, 1967). This prevents eventual cell rupture and spillage of the lysosomal enzymes and other potential inflammatory mediators into the joint space. Microtubules may well be involved in guiding the lysosome to the phagocytic vacuole. Because colchicine does not stabilize isolated lysosomes (Weissmann, 1966) its action in preventing lysosomal degranulation may be mediated through its ability to cause disruption of microtubules.

Phelps (1969a) found that random motility of PMN's induced by dissolved urate could be inhibited by colchicine at low ($10^{-8} M$) concentrations. It was subsequently established (Phelps, 1969b) that PMN's released a chemotactic factor following phagocytosis of urate crystals. Colchicine interferred with the generation of this factor at concentrations as low as $10^{-10} M$. Suppression of chemotactic factor generation by colchicine was greater than could be accounted for by colchicine's ability to diminish phagocytosis of urate crystals. Wallace and Ertel (1969) pointed out that the concentration of colchicine in the blood after a therapeutic dose (2 mg, i.v.) of colchicine in humans was in the same range as those concentrations of colchicine which suppressed both the urate-induced random motility of PMN's and the generation of chemotactic activity. Inhibition of other PMN functions, such as phagocytosis or lysosomal degranulation, required much higher concentrations of the drug.

Although the exact site or sites of colchicine's antigout activity have yet to be rigorously established it seems likely that the drug interferes in some way with PMN function and thereby diminishes the contribution of this cell to the inflammatory process. Furthermore, it is also likely that colchicine's effects on PMN functions reflect its ability to bind to microtubule protein and thereby disrupt microtubules, which seem to be involved in a number of cellular functions. The combined action of colchicine on motility, chemotactic activity generation, phagocytosis, and lysosomal degranulation may be more significant than its effect on any of these processes alone. It is possible, of course, that colchicine's antigout activity reflects its interaction at other points in the inflammatory process that have yet to be uncovered.

3. STRUCTURE–ACTIVITY RELATIONSHIPS OF COLCHICINE'S ANTIGOUT ACTIVITY

Although the relationship between colchicine's molecular structure and its antimitotic activity has been the subject of intensive study (Černoch et al., 1954; Deysson, 1968; Lettré, 1951; Schindler, 1965) the structure–activity relationship of colchicine's antigout activity has been little investigated. (Colchicine derivatives tested for antiinflammatory activity are presented in Table II.) This is not surprising when one considers that animal models of gout have only recently become available following the establishement of microcrystalline sodium urate as the etiologic agent. In fact, lack of experimental models of gout and the necessity of using human subjects have probably had a deterrent effect on studies concerning structural aspects of colchicine's antigout activity. Nevertheless, Wallace (1959) has investigated five colchicine derivatives for their effect against acute gout. Although demecolcin (26) and deacetylthiocolchicine (51) exhibit antigout activity equivalent to that of colchicine and produce less gastrointestinal disturbance than colchicine, routine use of these agents is discouraged because of their tendency to produce agranulocytosis. Colchicoside (52) is less active than colchicine, and colchiceine (17) is completely ineffective. Deacetylcolchiceine (19) is as effective as colchicine with respect to antigout activity but does not produce gastrointestinal distress and it does not appear to elicit the hematologic toxicity that accompanies demecolcin (26) and deacetylchiocolchicine (51).

Phelps and McCarty (1969) compared the effects of colchicine (11), deacetylcolchiceine (19), colchiceine (17), and colchicoside (52) on the random motility of PMN's stimulated either by urate crystals or by killed bacteria. Inhibition of urate-stimulated random motility followed the order: colchicine > deacetylcolchiceine > colchicoside > colchiceine; colchiceine possessed some effectiveness. The same order of activity for

TABLE II

Comparison of Antiinflammatory and Antimitotic Activities among Colchicine Derivatives and Related Compounds

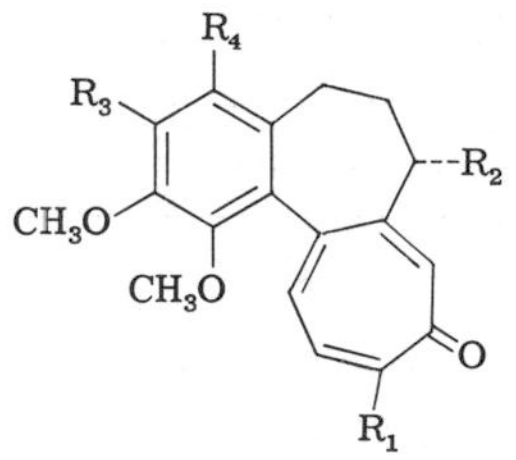

Compound	R_1	R_2	R_3	R_4	Antiinflammatory activity[a,b]	Antimitotic activity[a]
Colchicine (11)	OCH_3	$NHCOCH_3$	OCH_3	H	++(h,m,r)	++
Colchiceine (17)	OH	$NHCOCH_3$	OCH_3	H	0(h,m) +(r)	+
Deacetylcolchiceine (TMCA, 19)	OH	NH_2	OCH_3	H	++(h) 0(m,r)	0
Deacetylcolchicine (20)	OCH_3	NH_2	OCH_3	H	++(m,r)	++
N-Deacetyl-N-methylcolchicine (demecolcin, Colcemid, 26)	OCH_3	$NHCH_3$	OCH_3	H	++(h,r)	++
Deacetamidocolchicine (37, R = OCH_3)	OCH_3	H	OCH_3	H	0(m)	+++
4-Cyanocolchicine (49, R = CN)	OCH_3	$NHCOCH_3$	OCH_3	CN	+(m)	?
Deacetylthiocolchicine (51)	SCH_3	NH_2	OCH_3	H	++(h,r)	++
Colchicoside (52)	OCH_3	$NHCOCH_3$	$OC_6H_{11}O_5$ (glucose)	H	+(h) 0(r)	+
Colchicinamide (Section VI)	NH_2	$NHCOCH_3$	OCH_3	H	++(r)	++
TMCA ethyl ether (Section VI)	OCH_2CH_3	$NHCOCH_3$	OCH_3	H	++(r)	++
Colchicosamide (Section VI)	NH_2	$NHCOCH_3$	$OC_6H_{11}O_5$ (glucose)	H	0(r)	0
N-Benzoyl-TMCA (Section VI)	OH	$NHCOC_6H_5$	OCH_3	H	0(r)	0

332

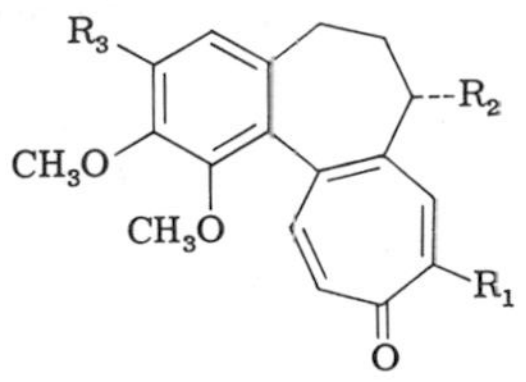

Compound	R_1	R_2	R_3	Antiinflammatory activity[a,b]	Antimitotic activity[a]
Isocolchicine (**18**)	OCH_3	$NHCOCH_3$	OCH_3	0(m,r)	+
Isocolchiceinamide (Section VI)	NH_2	$NHCOCH_3$	OCH_3	0(r)	0
Deacetylisocolchicine (Section VI)	OCH_3	NH_2	OCH_3	0(r)	0

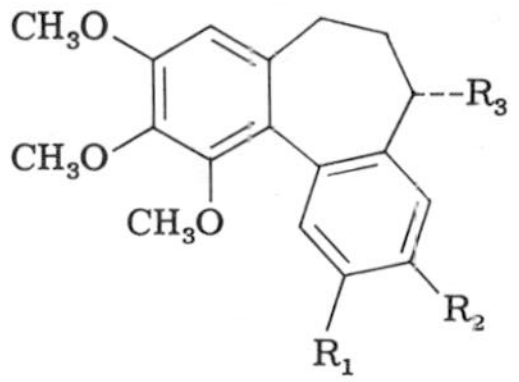

Compound	R_1	R_2	R_3	Antiinflammatory activity[a,b]	Antimitotic activity[a]
N-Acetylcolchinol (Section VI)	H	OH	$NHCOCH_3$	++(r)	+
Colchinol (**28** and Section VI)	H	OH	NH_2	0(r)	+
N-Acetyliodocolchinol (Section VI)	I	OH	$NHCOCH_3$	+(r)	+
Allocolchiceine (colchinoic acid, Section VI)	H	COOH	$NHCOCH_3$	0(r)	0

Table II (*continued*)

Compound	Antiinflammatory activity[a,b]	Antimitotic activity[a]
Tropolone (**12**) R = H	0(m)	0
2-Methoxytropone (**13**) R = CH₃	0(m)	0
1,2,3-Trimethoxybenzene (**53**)	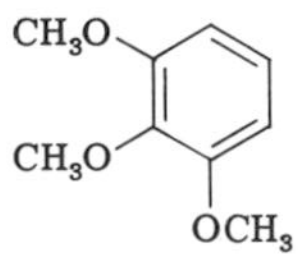 0(m)	?

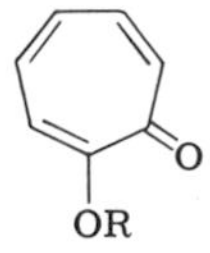

[a] + +, more active than colchicine; + +, activity equal to colchicine; +, less active than colchicine; 0, no activity; ?, not tested.
[b] h, human gout (Wallace, 1959); m, urate-induced paw swelling in mice (Fitzgerald et al., 1971a); r, urate-induced paw swelling in rats: colchicine (Denko and Whitehouse, 1970); demecolcin (Trnavský and Kopecký, 1966). In addition to colchicine and demecolcin, all other compounds indicated by "r" were reported by Zweig et al. (1972).

these compounds was observed in the case of killed bacteria-stimulated chemotactic motility from some individuals but when PMN's from other individuals were employed colchiceine was more effective than colchicoside. The authors point out that the suppressive effects of colchiceine and colchicoside differ depending on the stimulus.

Urate-induced paw swelling in mice has also been used to examine structure–activity relationships of colchicine's antiinflammatory action (Fitzgerald et al., 1971a). A number of compounds representing portions of the skeletal structure of colchicine or retaining the basic carbon skeleton but possessing modified functional groups (Table II) has been examined for their ability to suppress sodium urate-induced paw swelling. Tropolone (1 2), 2-methoxytropone (13), and 1,2,3-trimethoxybenzene (53) are ineffective in doses of 50, 50, and 150 mg/kg, respectively. In contrast, colchicine at a dose of 2 mg/kg almost completely abolishes paw swelling. Colchiceine (17) at 10 mg/kg and isocolchicine (18) at 50 mg/kg are ineffective. Deacetylcolchicine (20) as the tartrate (15 mg/kg) and 4-cyanocolchicine (49) at 10 mg/kg are able to reduce the urate-induced paw swelling but are completely ineffective at 2 mg/kg. Neither deacetylcolchiceine (19) nor deacetamidocolchicine (37, R = OCH_3) suppresses paw swelling at doses of 2 mg/kg and they are only effective when administered at a dose of 100 mg/kg. These results suggest that both the nitrogen function and the methoxytropone system are necessary for activity in the mouse paw swelling model. According to Malawista (1968) the antiinflammatory and antimitotic actions of colchicine share a common mechanism based on the drug's ability to interact with microtubule protein. Therefore, the low activity exhibited by deacetamidocolchicine is surprising because this substance is a more potent antimitotic agent than colchicine itself. Lack of activity with isocolchicine is taken to indicate that the position of the methoxy group on the tropone ring is critical.

Using rat brain microtubule protein, Zweig and Chignell (1973) examined the influence of a series of colchicine derivatives on [^{3}H] colchicine binding by protein. It was found that demecolcin (26) and deacetylthiocolchicine (51) were effective displacers of colchicine, whereas colchiceine (17) was a poor displacer. These results were in accordance with the antigout activity found for these compounds in humans (Wallace, 1959). However, deacetylcolchiceine (TMCA, 19) exhibited poor displacing ability, in contrast to its effective antigout activity in humans (Wallace, 1961). This observation, in conjunction with the low activity of this compound in the mouse paw model, suggests that whatever antiinflammatory activity this substance might possess, it would function by a mechanism different than that of colchicine. The nature of the antiinflammatory action of deacetylcolchiceine (19) deserves further examination.

Hibino (1971) compared the activities of colchicine, colchicoside (52), and thiocolchicoside (52, R_1 = SCH_3) on a variety of experimental inflammatory states. None of the inflammations were induced with microcrystalline sodium urate. Rat paw edema induced with mustard was inhibited by nontoxic doses of colchicoside and thiocolchicoside, as were cotten pellet granuloma and adjuvant arthritis. In general, the author recommended thiocolchicoside over colchicine for the treatment of chronic inflammation.

[3H]Lumicolchicine, prepared by irradiating colchicine tritiated in the acetyl group, did not bind to microtubule protein and had no antimitotic activity (Wilson and Friedkin, 1967). This suggests that the tropone ring is necessary for binding activity at the colchicine binding site.

Further evidence on this point was presented by Aronson and Inoué (1970). They demonstrated that demecolcin (N-deacetyl-N-methylcolchicine, 26) induced mitotic inhibition could be reversed by irradiation of the culture with long-wave ultraviolet light (366 nm). Demecolcin was known to undergo a photoisomerization analogous to colchicine to give lumi derivatives of the type shown (54). Dissociation of this product from the demecolcin receptor was probably responsible for the observed reversal of the mitotic inhibition. Borisy (1971) demonstrated that colchicine inhibition of porcine brain microtubule protein aggregation could also be reversed by ultraviolet irradiation. Several lines of evidence were presented to show that the effect of the radiation was indeed on the bound colchicine and that the microtubule protein was not affected in any way.

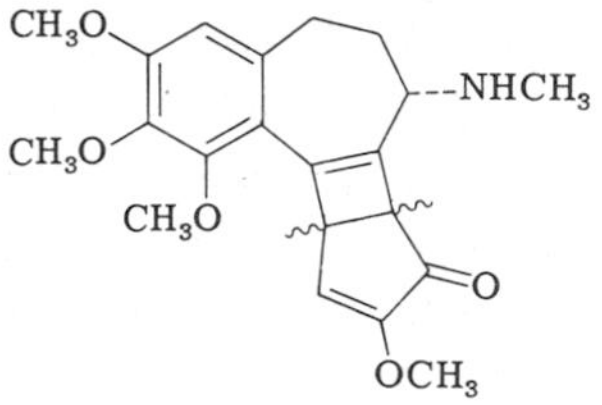

54

Sagorin et al. (1972) irradiated an alcoholic solution of colchicine until no residual colchicine was left, as determined by thin-layer chromatography. The photorearrangement product prepared in this way was examined for antimitotic activity in human lymphocytes in tissue culture. At a concentration of 10^{-6} M this preparation of lumicolchicine was without antimitotic action, whereas colchicine was highly active even at a concentration of 10^{-7} M. The authors suggested that these and other findings of lack of antimitotic effects of lumicolchicines might have clinical relevance because they found large concentrations of lumicolchicines in batches of colchicine for intravenous injection packaged in clear glass vials.

Although lumicolchicines appear to be without effect on mitosis and microtubule protein, these substances (or at least one of them) have recently been observed to block nucleoside transport in a number of mammalian cell lines, as does colchicine itself (Mizel and Wilson, 1972). This activity is discussed more fully in Section III,B,4.

Malawista *et al.* (1972) reported that colchicine reversed the passive Arthus reaction in rats but that lumicolchicines (a mixture of isomers) lacked colchicine's antiinflammatory activity in this system.

Continued investigation of various colchicine derivatives in animal models of gout is important not only because it can reveal the molecular features of the colchicine molecule that are involved in antiinflammatory activity but also because such studies are essential for elucidating the mechanisms by which these agents work and may lead to the introduction of more effective and less toxic agents. Also, through comparative studies of these derivatives using models in various species of animals, important clues to the nature of the inflammation itself are likely to be uncovered.

4. OTHER BIOCHEMICAL AND PHARMACOLOGICAL ASPECTS OF COLCHICINE

Several reports in the literature that colchicine-binding activity had been observed in association with structures other than microtubules led Stadler and Franke (1972) to examine this possibility in detail. These authors found that although the supernatant of rat brain homogenate possessed 100% of the colchicine-binding activity, the supernatant of rat liver homogenate exhibited only 2% of the colchicine-binding activity. In fact, the highest colchicine-binding activity of the liver extracts was found among those fractions representing nuclei and membranes. The authors proposed that proteins similar to microtubule protein were associated with chromatin and membranes and functioned as nuclei for the growth of microtubule crossbridges or microtubules themselves. Alternatively, these microtubulelike proteins might serve as stores of microtubule protein when bound to chromatin or membranes.

In an investigation of earlier reports on the inhibition of DNA and RNA synthesis by colchicine, Mizel and Wilson (1972) found that although colchicine had no effect on incorporation of nucleosides into DNA and RNA, colchicine did inhibit nucleoside uptake in a number of mammalian cell lines. This effect appeared to be independent of colchicine's interaction with microtubules and was about two orders of magnitude less sensitive to colchicine than was disruption of microtubules. Podophyllotoxin was more effective than colchicine, whereas demecolcin (*N*-deacetyl-*N*-methyl-colchicine, **26**) was about equipotent. Lumicolchicine (a mixture of isomers) was slightly more effective than colchicine, whereas isocolchicine (**18**) was about tenfold less active. Deacetylcolchiceine (TMCA, **19**), which neither inhibits mitosis nor interacts with microtubule protein, did not inhibit nucleoside transport. Deacetylcolchiceine (**19**) was reported to be as effective as colchicine in treating gout, however (Wallace, 1961). This compound was inactive against urate-induced paw swelling in mice (Fitzgerald *et al.*, 1971a). The colchicine-inhibited transport of adenine, guanosine, uridine, and thymidine appeared to be competitive and was incompletely reversible.

A number of other actions of colchicine have been reported and may have some bearing on colchicine's antigout activity and/or toxicity. DeChatelet *et al.* (1971) observed colchicine-mediated inhibition of the hexose monophosphate shunt without bacteriocidal activity of human leukocytes' being altered. Colchicine was found to increase collagenase activity in cultures of rheumatoid synovium (Harris and Krane, 1971). Successful treatment with colchicine of the periarticular inflammation associated with sarcoidosis was reported by Harris and Millis (1971). Rosenbloom and Ferguson (1968) observed generalized fatty changes in organs of rats treated with colchicine (0.5 mg/kg). Colchicine in obese humans induced marked increases in fecal sterol and bile acids and at the same time lowered serum cholesterol (Rubulis *et al.*, 1970). It was suggested that colchicine lowered the serum cholesterol level by interfering with the enterohepatic cycle of bile acids and neutral sterols. In isolated cat papillary muscles colchicine was found to enhance contractile force, decrease excitability, and distort the electrogram (Fink and Ferguson, 1968). Cohen and McNamara (1970) studied the effect of colchicine on guinea pig intestinal enzyme activity and suggested that colchicine was probably only toxic to the disaccharidase system of the intestinal mucosa and not to the entire mucosal cell population. When the effect of colchicine on various intestinal disaccharidases in rats was examined by Herbst *et al.* (1970), it was observed that a significant depression of lactase, invertase, and alkaline phosphatase occurred. It was concluded that colchicine depressed these enzymes by a direct effect on the differentiated cells of the villus and not by decreasing cellular renewal. Finally, a reappraisal of colchicine intoxication appeared in which tissue changes were correlated with clinical manifestations (Stemmermann and Hayashi, 1971).

5. METABOLISM OF COLCHICINE

Studies on the metabolism of colchicine began long before the structure of the compound was known. In 1890 Jacobj suggested that colchicine was oxidized in the body to a product, oxydicolchicine, he believed to be composed of two molecules of colchicine connected by an oxygen atom. This material, which he found to be more toxic to frogs than colchicine itself, was obtained by treating colchicine with ozone or by perfusing colchicine-containing blood through porcine kidney.

Somewhat later,' the interesting observation was made that hibernating bats, with lower body temperature, were not affected by colchicine in doses that were lethal in awake and warmer bats (Hausmann, 1906). Fühner (1920) subsequently demonstrated that colchicine was several hundredfold more toxic to frogs at 30°–32°C than at 15°–20°C. At the higher temperature the toxicity (s.c.) of colchicine to frogs (LD_{50}, 3.3 mg/kg) was similar to that of warm blooded animals (LD_{50} in mice, 1.9 mg/kg) (Kocsis et al., 1958). These observations suggested that colchicine was metabolized at the higher temperature to a more toxic substance. Alternative explanations might relate to the rate of metabolism or rate of a toxic reaction. Recently, Wilson (1970) observed that colchicine binding to microtubule protein was affected by temperature. He found that at 0°C colchicine did not bind to microtubule protein. However, once the colchicine was bound at 37°C the colchicine–protein complex was stable at 0°C. Whether there is a relationship between these observations and the effects of temperature on colchicine toxicity in frogs has not been determined.

Early attempts to study distribution (Brues, 1942) and excretion (Lettré and Lutze, 1944) of colchicine were hampered by lack of sensitivity (for the former) or selectivity (for the latter) in the methods used for detection. With the advent of radioactive colchicine (Walaszek et al., 1952) these difficulties were overcome. Back and Walaszek (1953), using randomly labeled [^{14}C] colchicine prepared by the biosynthetic method, studied the distribution of the drug in normal and tumor-bearing mice. All animals were sacrificed 4 hours after administration of colchicine. In normal animals colchicine was distributed among the intestines (18–23%), kidney (23–29%), liver (7–15%), and spleen (39–47%). No radioactive material was found in the heart, brain, or muscle. In tumor-bearing mice, however, the spleen contained no detectable radioactivity, whereas the level in the intestines was about double the amount in normal animals. Similar results were obtained in normal mice that had been injected with tumor homogenates 24 hours before administration of colchicine. The authors suggested that this phenomenon might be caused by some substance produced by the tumor. This interesting suggestion does not seem to have been followed up experimentally.

In 1952 Orsini and Pansky reported a remarkable resistance to the toxic effects of colchicine by the golden hamster compared to other animals. The LD_{50} (i.p.) for colchicine in the hamster is 470 mg/kg; in the mouse, 3.5 mg/kg (Fleischmann et al., 1962); and in the rat, 4 mg/kg (Barnes and Eltherington,

1966); in rabbits the minimum lethal dose is 7.5 mg/kg, s.c. (Barnes and Eltherington, 1966). A lethal dose of colchicine in dogs is reported as 0.57 mg/kg, s.c. (Barnes and Eltherington, 1966). Kocsis *et al.* (1958) suggested that the liver and/or the gut was important in detoxifying colchicine in the hamster because this animal resisted such large doses of the drug given orally or intraperitoneally.

Other investigators also attempted to ascertain the nature of the hamster's resistance to colchicine. Using both heterologous and homologous tissues grafted in the hamster as well as human and hamster cells grown *in vitro*, Midgley *et al.* (1959) demonstrated that the hamster had a cellular resistance to colchicine as revealed by the much higher doses of colchicine (100-fold) necessary to inhibit mitosis in hamster cells and tissues. It has not yet been determined whether colchicine is unable to enter the cell or whether hamster microtubules are resistant to colchicine.

Fleischmann *et al.* (1968) have established that the urine and bile are the major pathways for the excretion of colchicine by the golden hamster.

The excretion of radioactive colchicine in humans and a number of animal species was studied by Walaszek *et al.* (1960). Colchicine randomly labeled with ^{14}C by the biosynthetic method and colchicine labeled with ^{14}C in the carbonyl carbon of the acetyl group were used. A number of findings emerged from these studies. It was observed that normal mice and humans excreted more unchanged colchicine than did tumor-bearing mice or tumor-bearing humans. The amount of unchanged colchicine excreted by two patients with gout was similar to that of six cancer patients but the gout patients excreted a much higher percentage of metabolites. In one patient with gout 4% of the administered dose of acetyl-labeled colchicine was detected in expired CO_2 in 67 minutes. A patient with prostatic carcinoma was also given acetyl-labeled colchicine; 39% of the administered radioactivity was recovered as urea. When randomly labeled colchicine was employed in the former patient no radioactive CO_2 was detected. No radioactivity was detected in urea from the latter patient when randomly labeled colchicine was used. From the results obtained with the acetyl-labeled colchicine it appeared that deacetylation might be a major route of metabolism and therefore deacetylcolchicine (20) might be a metabolite of colchicine.

Metabolism of colchicine by microorganisms has also been reported. Zeitler and Niemer (1969) have discovered a soil bacteria, *Arthobacter colchovorum*, that when cultivated in a colchicine-containing medium converts the colchicine to deacetylcolchicine (20) along with traces of colchicone (50a, R_1 = OCH_3, R_2 = O). If the growth medium contains no inorganic nitrogen, colchicine is converted mainly to colchicone whereas only small amounts of deacetylcolchicine (20) are formed. When glucose and inorganic nitrogen are deleted from the medium colchicone is formed to the near exclusion of deacetylcolchicine (20).

Plasma levels of [^{14}C](tropone methoxy)colchicine were studied in humans by Wallace et al. (1970). It was found that colchicine very rapidly left the blood and became distributed in a volume in excess of extracellular water, suggesting a rapid entry of the drug into cells. This also led the authors to suggest that little if any significant binding by colchicine to plasma protein occurs. The mean 15-minute plasma level, after a 2-mg dose (i.v.) of colchicine was 1.14 ± 0.85 μg per 100 ml; the mean extrapolated zero time concentration was 1.92 ± 0.88 μg per 100 ml. These levels correspond to the concentrations of colchicine that interfere with random motility and chemotactic-induced motility (Section III,B,2) and are far below those concentrations which affect other PMN activities. It is suggested by the authors that this information supports interference with PMN motility as the mechanism of colchicine's antigout activity.

Schönhartung et al. (1973) subjected colchicine to a modified form of the Udenfriend system, which is an artificially constructed redox system considered to simulate, in many respects, the reactions of the microsomal enzyme system. These workers isolated and characterized four products from this mixture. One of the products was colchiceine (17). Two of the other products were 2- and 3-demethylcolchicine (i.e., replacement of either the 2- or 3-methoxy group on the benzene ring with a hydroxy group). A rearranged tropone ring of colchicine in the form of an o-hydroxybenzaldehyde structure constituted the fourth product and was designated "colchinal."

An extensive investigation of the biliary excretion and metabolism of colchicine in rats, dogs, rabbits, and golden hamsters was reported (Hunter, 1973). In bile collected from rats 52% of an administered dose of ^{3}H-(tropone methoxy)colchicine was excreted in 2 hours. Of this, 53% was unchanged colchicine, 15% demethylated (benzene ring) metabolite(s), and 32% represented polar (i.e., water-soluble) metabolites. Deacetylcolchicine (20) was ruled out as a possible metabolite by thin-layer chromatography. The studies in hamsters showed that neither increased biliary excretion nor increased biotransformation of colchicine were responsible for the high tolerance of the golden hamster to the toxic effects of colchicine.

A recent finding by Vesell et al. (1970) that allopurinol alters the metabolism of certain drugs (Section IV,C) demands an investigation of the metabolic interactions of allopurinol as concerns both acute and chronic toxicity of colchicine and the antigout activity of colchicine.

IV. ALLOPURINOL

A. Allopurinol in Gout

Allopurinol (pyrazolo[3,4-d] pyrimidine-4-ol, **55**) was originally prepared as a potential antitumor agent (Robins, 1956) because it represented an isomeric purine molecule. The original synthetic scheme is shown here; however, other pathways have since been developed, particularly for preparation of substituted derivatives (Hildick and Shaw, 1971; Baker and Kozma, 1968, and references therein). This compound and several others synthesized in the same series are inhibitors of xanthine oxidase, the enzyme responsible for

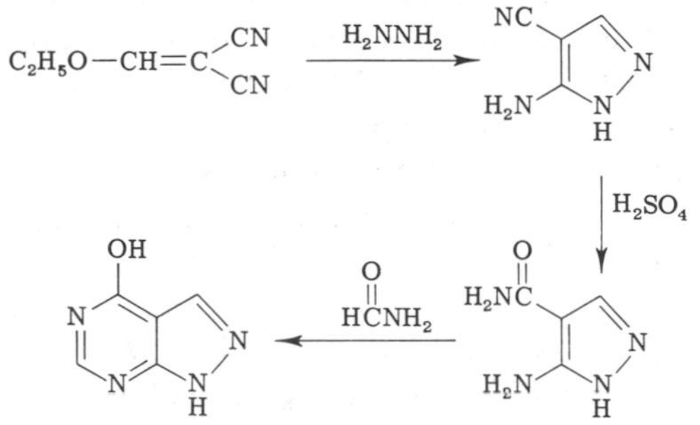

$$C_2H_5O-CH=C\underset{CN}{\overset{CN}{\big\langle}} \xrightarrow{\;H_2NNH_2\;}$$

(pyrazole intermediate, via H_2SO_4)

55

conversion of hypoxanthine (**4**) and xanthine (**5**) to uric acid (**6**) (Feigelson *et al.*, 1957). In an effort to increase the activity of 6-mercaptopurine (**56**), which is converted to the inactive 6-thiouric acid (**57**) by xanthine oxidase, Elion *et al.* (1963) have studied the activity of allopurinol. This compound, which appears to be otherwise biologically inert, exhibits a potent inhibition of xanthine oxidase and increases the antitumor activity of 6-mercaptopurine severalfold. Allopurinol has been recommended for use in the treatment of gout (Rundles *et al.*, 1963) and has since enjoyed wide application in gout therapy (Rundles *et al.*, 1969). Sales of this drug, marketed as Zyloprim, have rapidly increased in the years since it was first introduced into therapy. The large sales volume reflects the ready acceptance of allopurinol by physicians.

Administration of allopurinol to gouty patients (orally, 200–800 mg/day) for 3–5 days effectively lowers serum urate to normal levels (6 mg per 100 ml) or less. There is a corresponding drop in urinary excretion of urate but the increase in urinary oxypurines, hypoxanthine and xanthine, is not as great as expected. This is believed to be because of reutilization of hypoxanthine and xanthine in *de novo* biosynthesis of nucleic acids and because of feedback inhibition in purine biosynthesis resulting from the accumulation of purine intermediates. Although hypoxanthine is more soluble in serum than sodium urate, xanthine is about equally soluble.* Nevertheless, no problems arising from crystallization of these compounds in gouty patients have been encountered. This is because of the more efficient renal clearance of hypoxanthine and xanthine as compared to urate. Furthermore, there is an overall lowering of total purine output for reasons just mentioned. Thus, the serum levels of hypoxanthine and xanthine, as well as levels of urate, remain below the limits of solubility of these substances.

	R_1	R_2	R_3
4	OH	H	H
5	OH	OH	H
6	OH	OH	OH
56	SH	H	H
57	SH	OH	OH

B. Mechanism of Action

1. XANTHINE OXIDASE

This enzyme is widely distributed in nature, occurring in microorganisms (*Escherichia coli*) as well as man. Although it is found in several tissues, the highest xanthine oxidase activity in man is found in the liver. Bovine milk is a rich source of the enzyme and most of the xanthine oxidase used experimentally is from this source. Rat liver xanthine oxidase is occasionally employed experimentally also.

Xanthine oxidase is a complex enzyme and, although its ability to oxidize hypoxanthine and xanthine to uric acid has been known since 1904 its catalytic mechanism is only recently coming to light (DeRenzo, 1956; Mahler and Cordes, 1966). The enzyme was first obtained in crystalline form in 1955 (Avis *et al.*, 1955), and, more recently, it has been ascertained that the oxidative mechanism involves enzyme-bound molybdenum, flavin adenine nucleotide (FAD), and nonheme iron associated with labile sulfide in the ratio 2:2:8:8 per molecule of enzyme (Massey *et al.*, 1969). Xanthine oxidase is an enzyme of rather low specificity with regard to substrate and

---

*According to the Merck Index (Stecher, 1968) the solubility of monosodium urate in water is 830 mg/liter, that of xanthine 70 mg/liter, and that of hypoxanthine 700 mg/liter. In serum, however, the high sodium level lowers the solubility of sodium urate through the common ion effect. Thus, the calculated solubility of monosodium urate in serum is 64 mg/liter (Seegmiller, 1967). Because hypoxanthine and xanthine are not appreciably ionized at physiological pH (7.4), their solubilities in serum are not affected.

electron acceptors. Oxidation of purines other than xanthine and hypoxanthine, as well as of pyrimidines, pterins, aldehydes, and DPNH, is catalyzed
by this enzyme. The overall oxidation of xanthine can be illustrated as shown
in Scheme I. At the present time it cannot be stated with certainty whether
dehydrogenation of the hydrated substrate is the actual initial event or
whether introduction of the hydroxyl group takes place after dehydrogenation. A number of substances can function as electron acceptors for this
enzyme among which are, including the natural acceptor, O_2, artificial dyes,
ferricyanide, and cytochrome c.

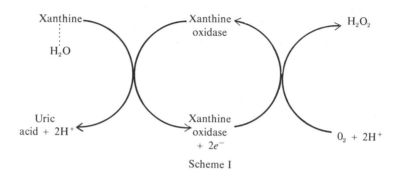

Scheme I

Reduction of the enzyme, as measured by absorbance at 450 nm, by
various substrates is biphasic. A rapid phase, in which the absorbance is
brought to 52–58% of the original, is followed by a slower phase bringing
the absorbance to 34–41% of the original. If dithionite is then added the
absorbance is lowered to 28%. In the fast phase four electrons, representing
2 moles of substrate, are taken up per equivalent of enzyme-bound FAD.
Two of these electrons are used in reducing FAD through its neutral semi-
quinone (FADH) to $FADH_2$. A third electron is involved in reducing Mo(VI)
to Mo(V), and the fourth appears to be taken up by the nonheme iron. The
fate of the three electrons taken up in the slow phase is not clear. One
electron may be accepted by the nonheme iron system. Two electrons may be
involved in reducing Mo(V) to Mo(III) and the eighth (dithionite) electron
may reduce the molybdenum to the Mo(II) state. Alternatively, the slow
phase may involve reduction of disulfide instead of molybdenum. In this
case the dithionite electron reduces Mo(V) to Mo(IV). The reduced enzyme
is rapidly reoxidized to its catalytic state by molecular oxygen.

The flow of electrons in this reaction was thought to be: substrate $\longrightarrow$
Mo $\longrightarrow$ FAD $\longrightarrow$ Fe–S $\longrightarrow O_2$. However, dissociation of the FAD by
treating the enzyme with high concentrations of calcium or manganese ions
resulted in loss of xanthine oxygen reductase activity without affecting the
ability of the molybdenum or iron to be oxidized by other electron acceptors

(Komai *et al.*, 1969). This suggested that it was the flavin that reacted with oxygen rather than the nonheme iron.

Incubation of the enzyme with xanthine under anaerobic conditions results in a biphasic reduction of the enzyme. The first phase is rapid and the second phase, which reduces the enzyme nearly to the level produced by dithionite, is much slower. Admission of air to the system reoxidizes the enzyme to its catalytic state. Allopurinol under these conditions gives the rapid phase of reduction followed by only a small change; no further changes corresponding to the slow second phase seen with xanthine occur even after long periods of incubation (Massey *et al.*, 1970). Admitting air to the system causes the visible spectrum to change to one only slightly modified from that of the original enzyme. This reoxidized enzyme is not reduceable by either xanthine or allopurinol under anaerobic conditions. Alloxanthine (**58**), the oxidation product of allopurinol, is unable

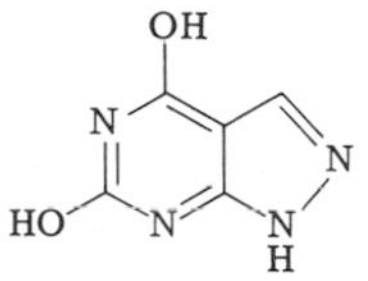

58

to reduce xanthine oxidase under conditions favorable to reduction by allopurinol or xanthine. However, this compound is able to inactivate xanthine oxidase when incubated in the presence of xanthine under both anaerobic and aerobic conditions. Under anaerobic conditions, in the presence of xanthine, a rapid reduction phase occurs followed by a slight spectral modification similar to that seen with allopurinol. Reoxidation of the alloxanthine-modified enzyme gives a spectrum identical with that obtained on reoxidation of the allopurinol-reduced enzyme, and, as with allopurinol, enzyme activity is abolished. These observations suggest that alloxanthine may be the agent responsible for allopurinol inactivation of xanthine oxidase. Removal of unreacted allopurinol and unbound alloxanthine from [^{14}C] allopurinol-inactivated xanthine oxidase followed by heat denaturation of the complex demonstrates the presence of [^{14}C] alloxanthine.

The nature of the allopurinol inactivation of xanthine oxidase was considered by the same authors in more detail. It was found that both the flavin and nonheme iron–sulfur chromophores of the enzyme were reduced by allopurinol. Each of the two different iron–sulfur chromophores can accept one electron and the flavin moiety can accept a third. This would account for 2 of the 3 moles of product formed by each mole of enzyme. Reduction of Mo(VI) to Mo(IV) could account for the third mole of product.

Ferricyanide titrations and electron paramagnetic resonance studies of alloxanthine-inactivated xanthine oxidase suggested that combining alloxanthine with reduced enzyme prevented further electron flow to molybdenum. The alloxanthine might be complexed with molybdenum trapped in the Mo(IV) oxidation state. However, studies on the interaction of alloxanthine-inhibited xanthine oxidase with dichlorophenolindophenol led Gurtoo and Johns (1971) to conclude that the molybdenum in the complex existed as Mo(V) rather than Mo(IV).

2. STRUCTURE–ACTIVITY RELATIONSHIPS OF XANTHINE OXIDASE INHIBITORS

Early studies with purine derivatives made it apparent that there were multiple binding modes on xanthine oxidase. Bergmann *et al.* (1958) showed that whereas 8-hydroxypurine and hypoxanthine (6-hydroxypurine, **4**) were oxidized at the 2 position, 2-hydroxypurine was oxidized at the 8 position.

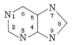

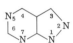

Purine   Pyrazolo[3, 4-*d*]pyrimidine
numbering system   numbering system

Adenine (6-aminopurine), however, was oxidized at the 8 position, whereas the 2-amino and 8-amino derivatives were oxidized at the 6 position. Results obtained with *N*-methylated purines further indicated that more than one route of purine oxidation was available on xanthine oxidase. Whereas 2-amino and 2-methylaminopurines were oxidized at the 6 position, oxidation of the 2-dimethylamino compound occurred at the 8 position. Most of these substances were at best only poor substrates for the enzyme, and the hydroxylated dimethylamino derivatives did not function as substrates at all. The latter group of compounds, however, might have been bound to the enzyme, but no estimation of their inhibitory ability was made. Leonard *et al.* (1962) studied a series of 2-hydroxy-6-substituted purines for their inhibitory activity on the dehydrogenase and oxidase activities of xanthine oxidase using xanthine as substrate. The former activity was determined by using the dye dichlorophenolindophenol (DCI) as the electron acceptor and measuring the decrease in optical density at 600 nm. Oxidase activity was assayed by measuring increase in optical density at 290 nm (λ_{max} of uric acid). The findings that some derivatives were more inhibitory toward dehydrogenase activity than toward oxidase activity although the reverse was true with other derivatives and that both competitive and noncompetitive inhibition was observed among the compounds as well as in a single compound at different concentrations led these workers to suggest the presence of more than one binding site for purines on xanthine oxidase.

Pyrazolopyrimidine derivatives were first examined by Feigelson *et al.* (1957) for their ability to inhibit xanthine oxidase. Although these authors presumably had allopurinol (4-hydoxypyrazolo[3,4-*d*]pyrimidine, **55**) at their disposal it was not included in this study. However, of the substances tested, 4-amino-6-hydroxypyrazolo[3,4-*d*]pyrimidine (**61**) was shown to be a potent competitive inhibitor with 50% inhibition at 10^{-6} *M*. In these studies the dehydrogenase activity of the enzyme was measured using DCI.

Massey *et al.* (1970) showed that, like alloxanthine(**58**), other 6-substituted pyrazolo[3,4-*d*]pyrimidines were unable to reduce xanthine oxidase in the absence of xanthine. However, these compounds were able to reduce the enzyme on addition of xanthine, and all compounds produced the same reduced [i.e., complexed to Mo(IV)] complex as discerned by spectral evidence. However there was a considerable difference among the complexes formed by the various compounds when compared to the native enzyme. The complexes of inactivated enzyme and inhibitor eventually dissociated on exposure to air. The enzyme, thus recovered, possessed full catalytic activity. Only the complex of (**62**) exhibited a half-life (1220 minutes) greater than that of the alloxanthine complex (300 minutes) leading the authors to suggest that the former's effects might be longer *in vivo* than those of alloxanthine (**58**).

	R_1	R_2
58	OH	OH
59	SH	OH
60	SH	SH
61	NH$_2$	OH
62	OH	SH

Among structure–activity relationship studies of xanthine oxidase inhibitors the most extensive were carried out by Baker and co-workers. These studies were initiated with the objective of constructing a selective irreversible inhibitor of xanthine oxidase in tumor cells, which inhibitor would have little or no effect on the enzyme in normal cells. Such an inhibitor would find use in chemotherapy of cancer as an adjunct to the use of 6-mercaptopurine, which is inactivated by the action of xanthine oxidase. Inhibition of xanthine oxidase by the various derivatives was determined by measuring the increase in absorption at 290 nm. The enzyme employed in these studies was derived from bovine milk, and hypoxanthine was employed as the substrate.

In order to design such an active-site-directed, irreversible inhibitor (Baker, 1967) it was first necessary to determine the structural features involved in reversible binding of the substrate to the enzyme in order to achieve good binding properties. The next step was to determine where on the substrate molecule large or bulky groups could be placed without interfering with the binding process (bulk tolerance). Covalent bond-forming groups could then be placed on the bulky substituent for irreversible binding to the enzyme.

The initial investigations of Baker's group (Baker and Hendrickson, 1967) revealed certain features relating to reversible binding efficiency.

1. If no hydroxyl, thiol, or amino group was present in the purine, binding was poor.
2. A thiol group often gave better binding than a hydroxyl group.
3. More than one OH could be detrimental to the binding process.

The enzyme was able to accommodate large groups in both the 2 and the 8 position of hypoxanthine, as illustrated by the 11-fold and threefold increases in binding of (63) and (64), respectively, over hypoxanthine. Such compounds as substituted pyrimidines and 5-aminoimidazole-4-carboxamide, representing fragments of the hypoxanthine and xanthine molecules, were not particularly good inhibitors of xanthine oxidase.

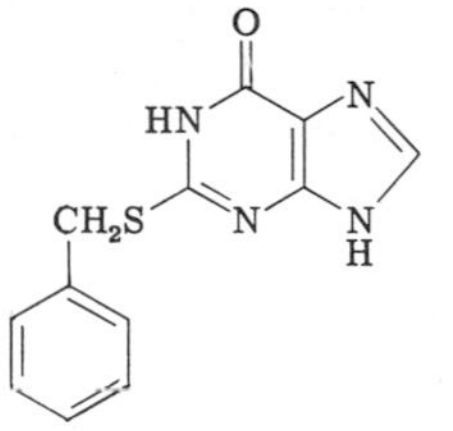

63

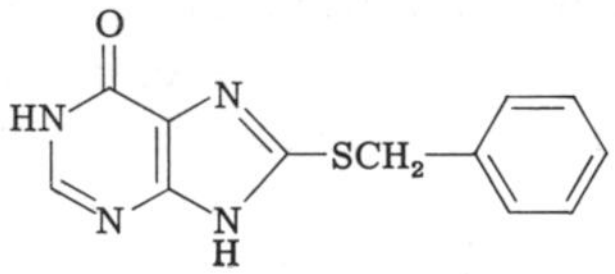

64

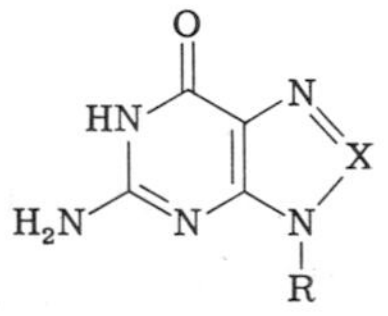

65   R = [phenyl]   , X = CH

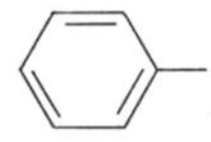

66   R = Cl—[phenyl]—   , X = N

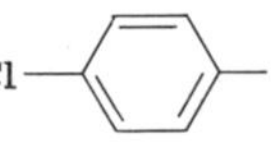

Among the best reversible inhibitors of xanthine oxidase were 9-phenylguanine (65) and 9-(p-chlorophenyl)-8-azaguanine (66). Preparation and testing of a large number of 9-phenylguanine derivatives led Baker and Wood (1967) to propose that a hydrophobic region at the binding site on xanthine oxidase exists in the area enclosed by the dotted line in structure (67).

Further studies (Baker and Wood, 1968) with substituted 9-phenylguanine derivatives, including irreversible binding compounds, allowed a detailed map of the hydrophobic bonding site adjacent to the purine binding site to be drawn (68). In addition, it was concluded that the phenyl ring should be coplanar to the purine ring for optimum binding. With this information in hand it was possible to devise potential irreversible inhibitors of xanthine

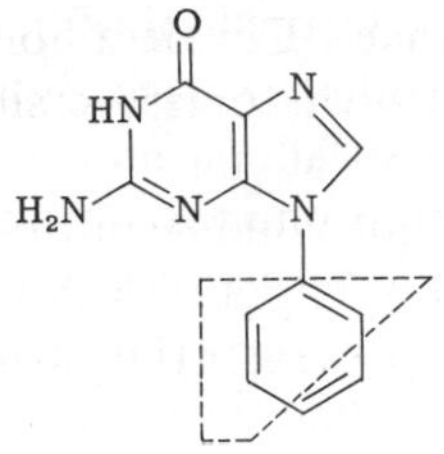

67

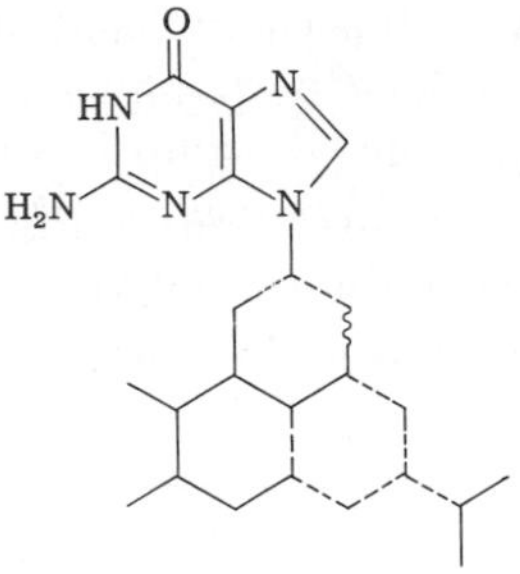

68

— Hydrophobic

--- Not hydrophobic

∿ Unknown

oxidase. Among the most potent irreversible agents prepared was **69**, inactivating 50% of the enzyme activity in 1 minute or less at a concentration of 2.8×10^{-7} *M*; although (**70**) exhibited a very high degree of reversible binding, it did not inactivate the enzyme (Baker and Wood, 1969).

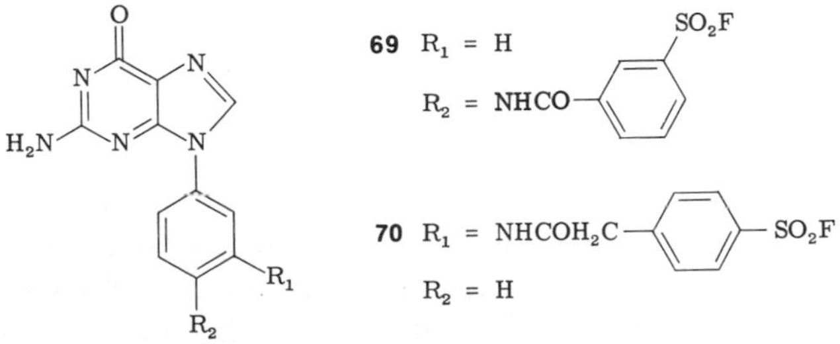

A number of 8-phenyladenines (**71**) was found to possess high reversible inhibitory activity, being complexed with xanthine oxidase up to 400-fold better than the substrate, hypoxanthine. Although the development of irreversible inhibitors from the 8-phenyladenine derivatives was pursued, none of the candidate inhibitors showed particularly good enzyme inactivation (Baker and Kozma, 1968).

In additional studies by these workers (Baker *et al.*, 1968) the nature of the allopurinol (**55**) binding site was probed using several derivatives of

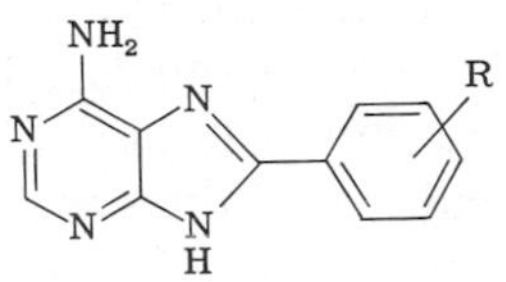

71

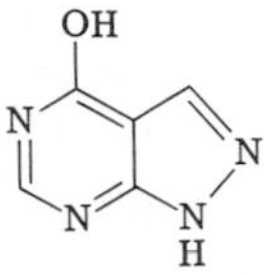

55

this compound. It became clear that multiple modes of binding of the purines and pyrazolo[3,4-*d*]pyrimidines to xanthine oxidase existed. For instance, introducing a phenyl group in the 1 position of allopurinol resulted in a 300-fold loss in binding wheras 9-phenylhypoxanthine was bound nearly as well as hypoxanthine. Therefore, these phenyl derivatives of allopurinol and hypoxanthine could not have been binding in the same way. That the mode of binding was also dependent on the nature of the polar substituents was evident from results obtained with candidate irreversible derivatives of allopurinol (72) and (73). Whereas (72) inactivated xanthine oxidase, (73) did not. The two compounds must, therefore, bind differently to the enzyme. Both substances showed good reversible binding, (73) being complexed sixfold better than (72).

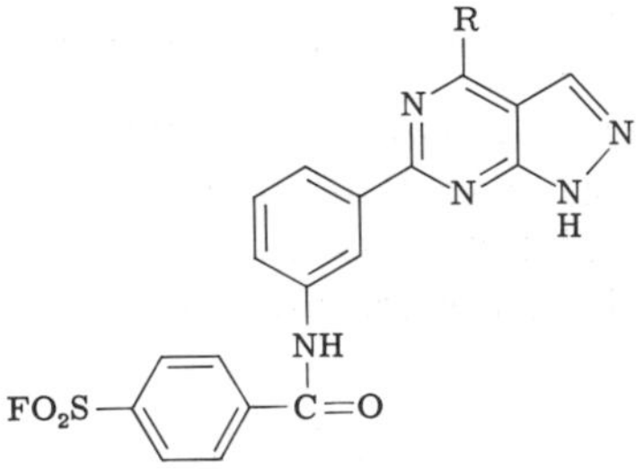

72 R = OH
73 R = NH$_2$

Taking a cue from the work of Baker's group, Parmar *et al.* (1972) prepared some 3-hydroxy-1-nitrophenyl-1*H*-pyrazolo[4,3-*c*] pyridines. These compounds were inhibitory toward xanthine oxidase but did not inhibit adenosine deaminase, guanosine deaminase, or guanine deaminase. The inhibitory activity of these compounds on xanthine oxidase isolated from rat liver was determined at 290 nm using hypoxanthine as substrate. The 2′,4′-dinitrophenyl derivative (74) was the most potent inhibitor of the enzyme, producing 50% inhibition at 5×10^{-5} *M*. These results suggest that the nitrogen at the 7 position of allopurinol is not required for the binding process.

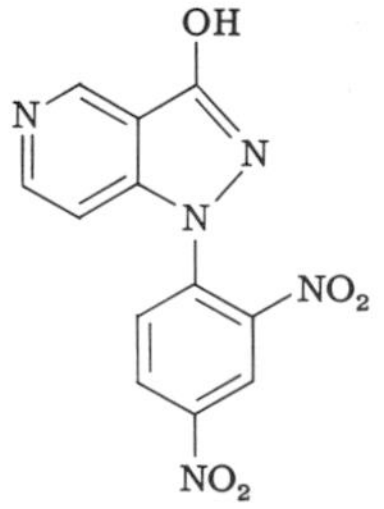

74

Few, if any, of the compounds prepared by the various groups of workers mentioned in this section have been evaluated for toxicity or for xanthine oxidase inhibitory activity in animals or in man. None of the compounds appears to have been evaluated for usefulness in gout therapy.

C. Other Effects of Allopurinol

Although allopurinol has been considered to be a specific inhibitor of xanthine oxidase, there have been a number of reports in recent years concerning the ability of this drug to interact with other systems. These interactions may have significant consequences, influencing the use of allopurinol in the treatment of gout.

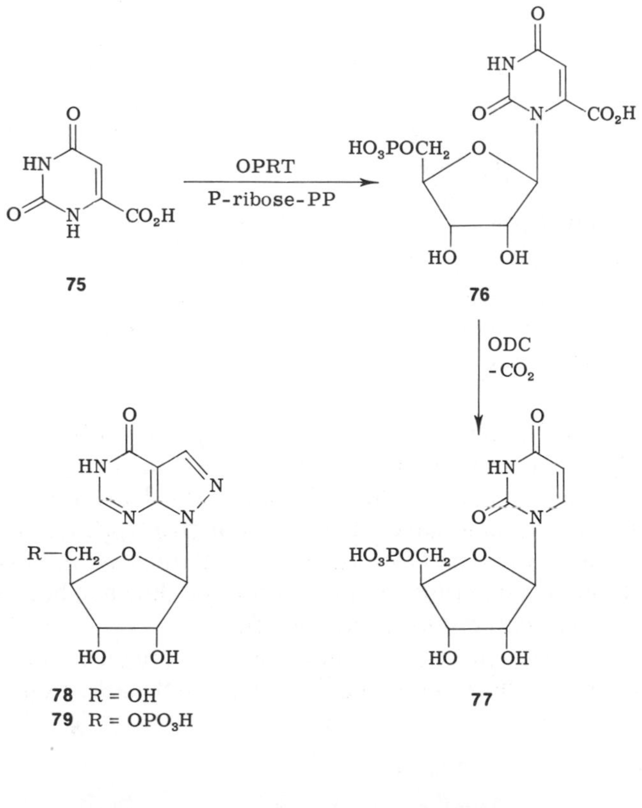

The administration of allopurinol or alloxanthine was found to result in an increased urinary secretion of orotic acid (75) and orotidine (76), suggesting that these drugs might interfere with pyrimidine biosynthesis. Using cultured human fibroblasts Kelley et al. (1971) determined that allopurinol and alloxanthine were indeed able to inhibit pyrimidine biosynthesis at one of the two steps in the conversion of orotic acid (75) to uridine 5′-monophosphate (77). Alloxanthine is much more potent than allopurinol in this respect. Allopurinol, alloxanthine, allopurinol ribonucleoside (78), allopurinol ribinucleotide (79), hypoxanthine (4), and xanthine (5) had no effect on orotate phosphoribosyltransferase (OPRT). Of these substances only allopurinol ribonucleotide (79) inhibited orotodine decarboxylase (ODC). Because alloxanthine could not be converted to allopurinol ribonucleotide, its *in vivo* inhibitory action was left unexplained. Subsequently, Beardmore and Kelley (1971) conducted studies in gouty humans and observed the effect of allopurinol and alloxanthine on the metabolism of [7-^{14}C]orotic acid. Expired $^{14}CO_2$ and urinary ^{14}C metabolites were measured. In addition, the effects of allopurinol and alloxanthine on hemolyzates lacking hypoxanthine–guanine phosphoribosyltransferase (HGPRT) activity and hemolyzates lacking OPRT activity were studied. HGPRT is the enzyme necessary for the conversion of allopurinol to allopurinol ribonucleotide (79). From the results of their studies these investigators concluded that the 1- and 7-alloxanthine ribonucleotides (80 and 81, respectively) in addition to allopurinol ribonucleotide (79) and xanthosine monophosphate (previously shown to inhibit ODC) were responsible for the inhibition of pyrimidine biosynthesis *in vivo*. The 1-ribonucleotide of alloxanthine (80) appeared to be formed by the action of HGPRT, whereas the 7-ribonucleotide (81) was apparently a product of OPRT.

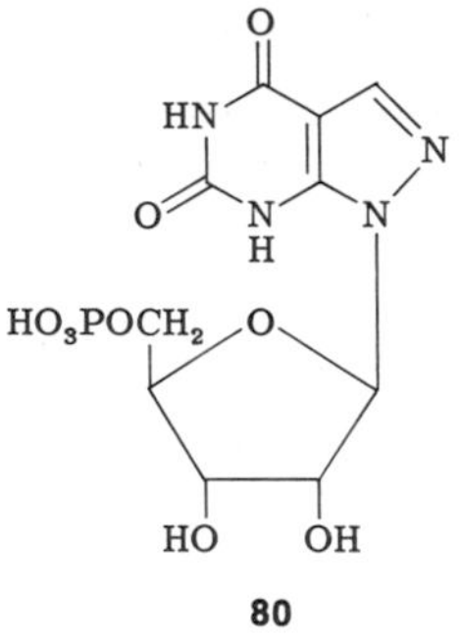

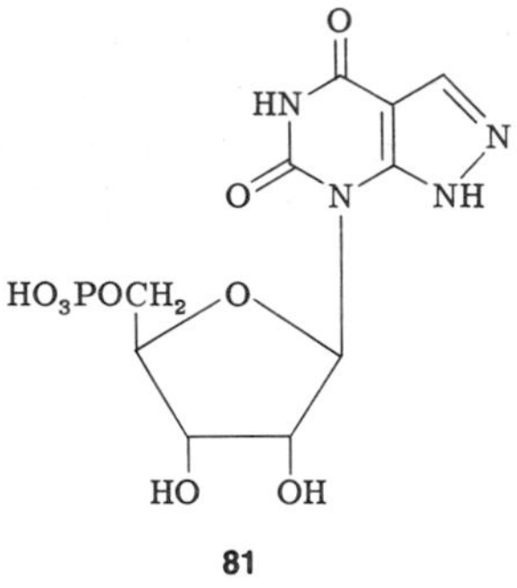

Goldfinger (1971) has pointed out that allopurinol ribonucleotide can theoretically be incorporated into nucleic acids; the same possibility exists for the metabolites of alloxanthine. Although this has not been shown to occur, it does not seem to have ruled out. Perhaps a 1-phenyl-1*H*-pyrazolo-[4,3-*c*]pyridine of the type (74) presented by Parmar *et al.* (1972) can be substituted, should allopurinol or alloxanthine be shown to be incorporated into nucleic acids with resulting adverse effects.

Vesell *et al.* (1970) observed an impairment of drug metabolism by allopurinol. In these studies it was found that allopurinol markedly increased the plasma half-life of antipyrine and bishydroxycoumarin in normal humans. Using rats treated with allopurinol these authors observed a decrease in the activity of hepatic microsomal drug metabolizing enzymes and a slightly lowered level of cytochrome P-450. It was suggested that the reduced activity of the microsomal components was the result of reduced microsomal protein. In light of these findings it would be of interest to determine the effects of allopurinol and its metabolites on the toxicity and antigout activity of colchicine and other antiinflammatory agents and uricosuric agents used in the treatment of gout.

In addition to its ability to lower urate formation through its inhibitory action on xanthine oxidase, allopurinol may have other beneficial effects when used in the treatment of gout. An antiinflammatory action of allopurinol has been claimed (Riesterer and Jaques, 1969) as well as an antinociceptive activity (Jaques and Helfer, 1971). The drug was found to be effective (10–30 mg/kg) in reducing the 24-hour volume of turpentine-induced pleural exudate but was less active against kaolin-induced paw swelling in rats. Essentially no activity against the paw swelling of adjuvant-induced arthritis was observed.

Low doses (3 mg/kg) were found effective in preventing the writhing syndrome in mice induced by either arachidonic acid peroxide or phenyl-*p*-benzoquinone. Xanthine had a similar but less marked effect and hypoxanthine and uric acid were inactive. Xanthine and allopurinol were also effective in reducing peritoneal leakage induced by the writhing agents, as measured by peritoneal concentration of an intravenously administered dye. The authors suggested that the beneficial effects of allopurinol in gout might also result from the increased levels of xanthine.

V. APPENDIX

Uricosuric Agents

The rationale for using uricosuric agents in gout is based on the ability of these drugs to enhance renal excretion of uric acid and thereby lower serum urate levels. Most widely employed in therapy are probenecid (Benemid; **82**, R = H) and sulfinpyrazone (Anturane, **83**). The common feature of uricosuric agents is that they are all organic acids. An exception to this, however, is zoxazolamine (**84**), which is a weak organic base. This substance is no longer used because of its association with severe hepatotoxicity. An extensive review of uricosuric agents, their mechanism of action, and their structure–activity relationships has appeared (Gutman, 1966).

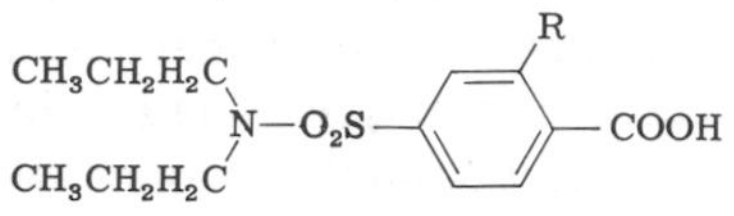

As mentioned in Section II,A, the uricosuric action of probenecid and sulfinpyrazone results from inhibition by these drugs of tubular reabsorption of urate. Tubular reabsorption of urate in man is believed to be an active transport process with limited but large capacity. Uricosuric drugs apparently compete with urate for this transport mechanism, and their ability to limit interaction of urate with the transport mechanism is related to their relative affinities for the organic acid transport system.

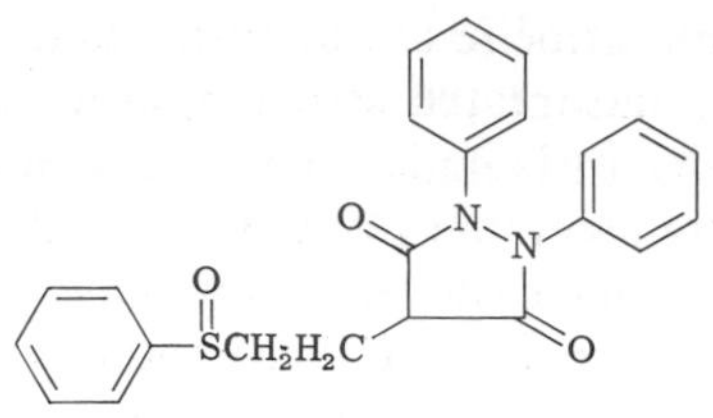

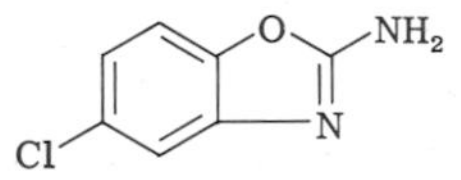

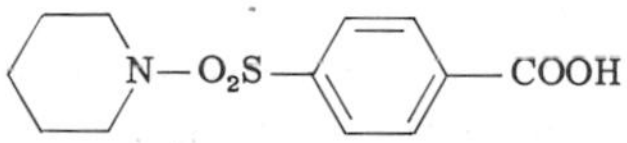

Zoxazolamine, in contrast to probenecid and sufinpyrazone, is a weak organic base. The mechanism of its uricosuric action is not known.

Structure–activity relationship studies of uricosuric agents have been carried out. Among various N,N-dialkyl analogs of probenecid (which is the N,N-dipropyl compound), lipid solubility correlates with clearance of the drugs in dogs (Weiner et al., 1960). More recently an evaluation of the uricosuric activity of 2-substituted probenecid analogs (**82**, R = Cl, OH, or NO_2) in Cebus monkeys has revealed that these derivatives are more potent than probenecid (Blanchard et al., 1972). Israili et al. (1972) have studied the uricosuric activity of several metabolites of probenecid in dogs and concluded that these metabolites may contribute to the action of probenecid. The piperidyl analog (**85**) is included in these studies and is similar to probenecid in its uricosuric activity.

A large number of sulfinpyrazone derivatives and related compounds has been investigated, and the results are summarized by Gutman (1966). In this series of agents, uricosuric activity is related only to acidity (pK_a). No relationship with lipid solubility has been discerned.

In addition to increasing urinary excretion of uric acid, probenecid and sulfinpyrazone also increase excretion of allopurinol. Nevertheless, uricosuric agents are often used in conjuction with allopurinol to lower serum urate levels (Seegmiller, 1969).

In addition to the uricosuric agents described so far, there are two others, benziodarone (**86**, R = I) and benzbromarone (**86**, R = Br), that have been used extensively in Europe in the treatment of gout (Ryckewaert and Kuntz, 1968; Famaey and Vandenabeele, 1970). Both agents are phenols and, despite the presence of electronegative substituents in the ortho position, are less acidic than probenecid and sulfinpyrazone. Nevertheless, benziodarone and benzbromarone appear to be more potent uricosurics than probenecid and sulfinpyrazone. Their mechanism of action is not known.

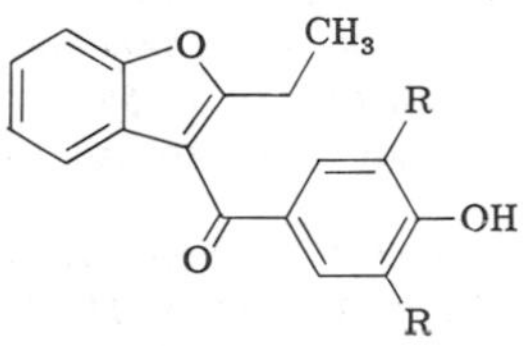

CH_3
R
OH
R

86

VI. ADDENDUM

Zweig *et al.* (1972) have recently reported on the ability of colchicine and of 17 colchicine derivatives to inhibit urate-induced paw swelling in rats. The results of this investigation are included in Table II for comparison with data obtained by other workers. Paw swelling in this case is evaluated by weighing the amputated paw 6 hours after administering urate. In general it has been found that those compounds most closely related to colchicine in molecular structure are able to inhibit paw swelling with a potency similar to colchicine's. Podophyllotoxin and vinblastine are also active in suppressing paw swelling. This is in contrast to the lack of activity with podophyllotoxin observed by Denko and Whitehouse (1970) in a similar animal system. *N*-Acetylcolchicinol, which possesses a benzenoid ring in place of the tropone system, shows good activity, suggesting that the tropone moiety of colchicine may not be necessary for antiinflammatory activity in this system. Deacetylcolchiceine (TMCA, **19**) was inactive in this system, paralleling the observation of Fitzgerald *et al.* (1971a) that this substance is also inactive against urate-induced paw swelling in mice. Deacetylcolchiceine (TMCA, **19**) is of interest because it has been found by Wallace (1961) to be as effective as colchicine in the treatment of gout.

Antiinflammatory activity as expressed by suppression of paw swelling was well correlated with the antimitotic activity of the various compounds tested. This correlation was offered as support by these workers for the hypothesis (Malawista, 1968) that the antimitotic and antiinflammatory activity of colchicine shared a common mechanism of action based on the drug's ability to disrupt microtubules. It was suggested that certain analogs of colchicine, such as colchiceinamide, deacetylcolchicine, and TMCA ethyl ether, might be useful in the treatment of gout in view of their action on paw swelling and their lower toxicity compared to colchicine.

REFERENCES

Aronson, J., and Inoué, S. (1970). *J. Cell. Biol.* **45**, 470.
Avis, P. G., Bergel, F., and Bray, R. C. (1955). *J. Chem. Soc., London* p. 1100.
Back, A., and Walaszek, E. J. (1953). *Cancer Res.* **13**, 552.
Baker, B. R. (1967). "Design of Active-Site-Directed Irreversible Enzyme Inhibitors," p. 156. Wiley, New York.
Baker, B. R., and Hendrickson, J. L. (1967). *J. Pharm. Sci.* **56**, 955.
Baker, B. R., and Kozma, J. A. (1968). *J. Med. Chem.* **11**, 657.
Baker, B. R., and Wood, W. F. (1967). *J. Med. Chem.* **10**, 1101.
Baker, B. R., and Wood, W. F. (1968). *J. Med. Chem.* **11**, 644.
Baker, B. R., and Wood, W. F. (1969). *J. Med. Chem.* **12**, 214.
Baker, B. R., Wood, W. F., and Kozma, J. A. (1968). *J. Med. Chem.* **11**, 661.
Barnes, C. D., and Eltherington, L. G. (1966). "Drug Dosage in Laboratory Animals. A Handbook," p. 73. Univ. of California Press, Berkeley.
Beardmore, T. D., and Kelley, W. N. (1971). *J. Lab. Clin. Med.* **78**, 696.
Bergmann, F., Levin, G., Kwietny-Govrin, H., and Ungar, H. (1958). *Biochim. Biophys. Acta* **47**, 1.
Berry, R. W., Ventilla, M., Cantor, C., and Shelanski, M. L. (1971). *Abstr., 11th Annu. Meet. Amer. Soc. Cell Biol.* p. 29.
Bertelli, D. J., and Andrews, T. G. (1969). *J. Amer. Chem. Soc.* **91**, 5280.
Bertelli, D. J., Andrews, T. G., and Crews, P. O. (1969). *J. Amer. Chem. Soc.* **91**, 5286.
Bibring, T., and Baxandall, J. (1971). *J. Cell Biol.* **48**, 324.
Blade-Font, A., and Muller, G. (1964). French Patent 1,359,637; *Chem. Abstr.* **61**, 13362f (1964).
Blade-Font, A., and Muller, G. (1968). French Patent 1,512,320; *Chem Abstr.* **70**, 78217 (1969).
Blanchard, K. C., Maroske, D., May, D. G., and Weiner, I. M. (1972). *J. Pharmacol. Exp. Ther.* **180**, 397.
Bluhm, G. B., Riddle, J. M., and Barnhart, M. I. (1969). *Arthritis Rheum.* **12**, 283.
Borisy, G. G. (1971). *Abstr. 11th Annu. Meet. Amer. Soc. Cell Biol.* p. 35.
Borisy, G. G., and Taylor, E. W. (1967a). *J. Cell Biol.* **34**, 525.
Borisy, G. G., and Taylor, E. W. (1967b). *J. Cell Biol.* **34**, 535.
Briseid, K., Arntzen, C., and Dyrud, O. (1971). *Acta Pharmacol. Toxicol.* **29**, 265.
Brues, A. M. (1942). *J. Clin. Invest.* **21**, 646.
Bryan, J. (1971). *Abstr. 11th Annu. Meet. Amer. Soc. Cell Biol.* p. 38.
Bryan, J. (1972a). *J. Mol. Biol.* **66**, 157.
Bryan, J. (1972b). *Biochemistry* **11**, 2611.
Bryan, J., and Wilson, L. (1971). *Proc. Nat. Acad. Sci. U.S.* **8**, 1792.
Buchanan, G. L., McKillop, A., Porte, A. L., and Sutherland, J. K. (1964). *Tetrahedron* **20**, 1449.
Caner, J. (1965). *Arthritis Rheum.* **8**, 752.

Canonica, L., Danieli, B., Manitto, P., Russo, G., and Bombardelli, E. (1967). *Chim. Ind. (Milan)* **49**, 1304.

Canonica, L., Danieli, B., Manitto, P., and Russo, G. (1969a). *Tetrahedron Lett.* p. 607.

Canonica, L., Danieli, B., Manitto, P., Russo, G., Bonati, A., and Bombardelli, E. (1969b). *Gazz. Chim. Ital.* **99**, 1059.

Černoch, M., Malinský, J., Tělupilová, O., and Šantavý, F. (1954). *Arch. Int. Pharmacodyn. Ther.* **99**, 141.

Chang, Y.-H. (1968). *Arthritis Rheum.* **11**, 473.

Chapman, O. L., Smith, H. G., and King, R. W. (1963a). *J. Amer. Chem. Soc.* **85**, 103.

Chapman, O. L., Smith, H. G., and King, R. W. (1963b). *J. Amer. Chem. Soc.* **85**, 806.

Chapman, O. L., Smith, H. G., and Barks, P. A. (1963c). *J. Amer. Chem. Soc.* **85**, 3171.

Cohen, M. I., and McNamara, H. (1970). *Amer. J. Dig. Dis.* [N.S.] **15**, 247.

Cook, J. W., Gibb, A. R., Raphael, R. A., and Somerville, A. R. (1950). *Chem. Ind. (London)* p. 427.

Corrodi, H., and Hardegger, E. (1955). *Helv. Chim. Acta* **38**, 2030.

Corrodi, H., and Hardegger, E. (1957). *Helv. Chim. Acta* **40**, 193.

Coyne, W. E. (1970). *In* "Medicinal Chemistry" (A. Burger, ed.), 3rd ed., Vol. 2, pp. 953–975. Wiley (Interscience), New York.

Crunkhorn, P., and Meacock, S. C. R. (1971). *Brit. J. Pharmacol.* **42**, 392.

Dahlström, A. (1968). *Eur. J. Pharmacol.* **5**, 111.

Dauben, W. G., and Cox, D. A. (1963). *J. Amer. Chem. Soc.* **85**, 2130.

DeChatelet, L. R., Cooper, M. R., and McCall, C. E. (1971). *Infec. Immunity* **3**, 66.

DeHarven, E., and Bernhard, W. (1956). *Z. Zellforsch. Mikrosk. Anat.* **45**, 378.

Denko, C. W., and Whitehouse, M. W. (1970). *Pharmacology* **3**, 229.

DeRenzo, E. C. (1956). *Advan. Enzymol.* **17**, 293.

Dewar, M. J. S. (1945). *Nature (London)* **155**, 141.

Dewar, M. J. S., and Trinajstic, N. (1970). *Croat. Chem. Acta* **42**, 1.

Deysson, G. (1968). *Int. Rev. Cytol.* **24**, 99.

Dustin, A., Havas, L., and Lits, F. (1937). *C. R. Ass. Anat.* **32**, 170.

Eigsti, O. J., and Dustin, P., Jr. (1955). "Colchicine—in Agriculture, Medicine Biology and Chemistry." Iowa State Coll. Press, Ames.

Elion, G. B., Callahan, S., Nathan, H., Bieber, S., Rundles, R. W., and Hitchings, G. H. (1963). *Biochem. Pharmacol.* **12**, 85.

Ertel, N. H., and Wallace, S. L. (1970). *Biochem. Med.* **4**, 181.

Ertel, N. H., Omokoku, B. A., and Wallace, S. L. (1967). *Excerpta Med. Found. Int. Congr. Ser.* **143**, 14.

Everhart, L. P. (1971). *J. Mol. Biol.* **61**, 745.

Faires, J. S., and McCarty, D. J., Jr. (1962). *Lancet* **2**, 282.

Famaey, J. P., and Vandenabeel, G. (1970). *J. Belge Rhumatol. Med. Phys.* **25**, 5.

Fanelli, G. M., Bohn, D. L., and Reilly, S. S. (1970). *J. Pharmacol. Exp. Ther.* **175**, 259.

Fanelli, G. M., Bohn, D. L., and Reilly, S. S. (1971). *J. Pharmacol. Exp. Ther.* **177**, 591.

Fanelli, G. M., Bohn, D. L., Reilly, S. S., and Baer, J. E. (1972). *J. Pharmacol. Exp. Ther.* **180**, 377.

Feigelson, P., Davidson, J., and Robins, R. (1957). *J. Biol. Chem.* **226**, 993.

Fink, J., and Ferguson, F. C. (1968). *Arch. Int. Pharmacodyn. Ther.* **174**, 451.

Fitzgerald, T. J. (1973). *Pharmacologist.* **15**, 204.

Fitzgerald, T. J., Williams, B., and Uyeki, E. M. (1971a). *Proc. Soc. Exp. Biol. Med.* **136**, 115.

Fitzgerald, T. J., Williams, B., and Uyeki, E. M. (1971b). *Pharmacology* **6**, 265.

Fleischmann, W., Russell, O. Q., and Fleischmann, S. K. (1962). *Med. Exp.* **6**, 101.

Fleischmann, W., Price, H. G., and Fleischmann, S. K. (1968). *Pharmacology* **1**, 48.

358   THOMAS J. FITZGERALD

Floersheim, G. L., Brune, K., and Seiler, K. (1973a). *Agents and Actions.* 3, 20.
Floersheim, G. L., Brune, K., and Seiler, K. (1973b). *Agents and Actions.* 3, 24.
Forbes, E. J. (1955). *J. Chem. Soc., London* p. 3864.
Freudweiler, M. (1901). *Deut. Arch. Klin. Med.* 69, 105.
Fühner, H. (1920). In "Handbuch der experimentellen Pharmakologie" (A. Heffter, ed.) Vol. 2, p. 493. Springer, Berlin.
Gillespie, E. (1971). *J. Cell Biol.* 50, 544.
Gillespie, E., Levine, R. J., and Malawista, S. E. (1968). *J. Pharmacol. Exp. Ther.* 164, 158.
Goldfinger, S. E. (1971). *N. Engl. J. Med.* 285, 1303.
Goldfinger, S. E., Howell, R. R., and Seegmiller, J. E. (1965). *Arthritis Rheum.* 8, 1112.
Goodman, D. B. P., Rasmussen, H., DiBella, R., and Guthrow, C. E., Jr. (1970). *Proc. Nat. Acad. Sci. U.S.* 67, 652.
Goodman, L., and Gilman, A., eds. (1955). "The Pharmacological Basis of Therapeutics," 2nd ed., p. 305. Macmillan, New York.
Grewe, R., and Wulf, W. (1951). *Chem. Ber.* 84, 621.
Gurtoo, H. L., and Johns, D. G. (1971). *J. Biol. Chem.* 246, 286.
Gutman, A. B. (1966). *Advan. Pharmacol.* 4, 91.
Gutman, A. B. (1973). *Arthritis Rheum.* 16, 431.
Hahn, E. F. (1971). *Diss. Abstr. B* 31, No. 2, Part 1, 7184B.
Harris, E. D., and Krane, S. M. (1971). *Arthritis Rheum.* 14, 669.
Harris, E. D., and Millis, M. (1971). *Arthritis Rheum.* 14, 130.
Hartung, E. F. (1954). *Ann. Rheum. Dis.* 13, 190.
Hausmann, W. (1906). *Arch. Gesamte Physiol. Menschen Tiere* 113, 317.
Herbst, J. J., Hurwitz, R., Sunshine, P., and Kretchmer, N. (1970). *J. Clin. Invest.* 49, 530.
Hibino, R. (1971). *Gifu Daigaku Igakubu Kiyo* 19, 739; *Chem. Abstr.* 77, 14112 (1972).
Hildick, B. G., and Shaw, G. (1971). *J. Chem. Soc., C* p. 1610.
His, W., Jr. (1900). *Deut. Arch. Klin. Med.* 76, 81.
Hrbek, J., Jr., Jennings, J. P., Klyne, W., and Šantavý F. (1964). *Collect. Czech. Chem. Commun.* 29, 2822.
Hsie, A. W., and Puck, T. T. (1971). *Proc. Nat. Acad. Sci. U.S.* 68, 358.
Hunter, A. (1973). "Biliary Excretion of Colchicine by Rats, Dogs, Rabbits, and Hamsters". Doctoral Dissertation. University of Kansas Medical Center, Kansas City, Kansas.
Inoué, S. (1964). In "Primitive Motile Systems in Cell Biology" (R. D. Allen and N. Kamiya, eds.), p. 549. Academic Press, New York.
Israili, Z. H., Perel, J. M., Cunningham, R. F., Dayton, P. G., Yü, T. F., Gutman, A. B., Long, K. R., Long, R. C., and Goldstein, J. H. (1972). *J. Med. Chem.* 15, 709.
Jacobj, C. (1890). *Arch. Exp. Pathol. Pharmakol.* 27, 119.
Jaques, R., and Helfer, H. (1971). *Pharmacology* 5, 49.
Johnson, G. S., Friedman, R. M., and Pastan, I. (1971). *Proc. Nat. Acad. Sci. U.S.* 68, 425.
Johnson, W. J., Stavric, B., and Chartrand, A. (1969). *Proc. Soc. Exp. Biol. Med.* 131, 8.
Jost, J.-P., and Rickenberg, H. V. (1971). *Annu. Rev. Biochem.* 40, 741.
Journey, L. J. (1964). *Cancer Res.* 24, 1393.
Kaneko, S., and Matsui, M. (1968). *Agr. Biol. Chem.* 32, 995.
Kelley, W. N., Beardmore, T. D., Fox, I. H., and Meade, J. C. (1971). *Biochem. Pharmacol.* 20, 1471.
Kelley, W., Green, M., Rosenbloom, F., Henderson, J., and Seegmiller, J. (1969). *Ann. Intern. Med.* 70, 155.
Kiefer, B., Sakai, H., Solari, A., and Mazia, D. (1966). *J. Mol. Biol.* 20, 75.
King, M., DeVries, J., and Pepinsky, R. (1952). *Acta Crystallogr.* 5, 437.
Kocsis, R., Balek, W., and Walaszek, E. J. (1958). *J. Pharmacol. Exp. Ther.* 122, 39A.

Komai, H., Massey, V., and Palmer, G. (1969). *J. Biol. Chem.* **244**, 1692.
Kreppel, E. (1959). *Med. Exp.* **1**, 285.
Kvarstein, B., and Stormorken, H. (1971). *Biochem. Pharmacol.* **20**, 119.
Lacy, P. E., Howell, S. L., Young, D. A., and Fink, C. J. (1968). *Nature (London)* **219**, 1177.
Leonard, E. O., Orme-Johnson, W. H., McMurtray, R. R., Skinner, C. G., and Shive, W. (1962). *Arch. Biochem. Biophys.* **99**, 16.
Lettré, H. (1951). *Angew. Chem.* **63**, 421.
Lettré, H., and Lutze, M. (1944). *Hoppe-Seyler's Z. Physiol. Chem.* **281**, 58.
Lettré, H., Dönges, K.-H., Barthold, K., and Fitzgerald, T. (1972). *Justus Liebigs Ann. Chem.* **758**, 185.
Levy, D. A., and Carlton, J. A. (1969). *Proc. Soc. Exp. Biol. Med.* **130**, 1333.
Levy, L. (1969). *Life Sci.* **8**, 601.
Lits, F. (1934). *C. R. Soc. Biol.* **115**, 1421.
McCarty, D. J., Jr. (1970). *Annu. Rev. Med.* **21**, 357.
McCarty, D. J., Jr., and Hollander, J. L. (1961). *Ann. Intern. Med.* **54**, 452.
McCarty, D. J., Jr., Phelps, P., and Pyenson, J. (1966). *J. Exp. Med.* **124**, 99.
McKracken J., Owen, P., and Pratt, J. (1946). *J. Amer. Med. Ass.* **131**, 367.
McLaughlin, G. E., McCarty, D. J., Jr., and Prescott, D. J. (1970). *Top. Med. Chem.* **3**, 263.
Magid, R. M., Grayson, C. R., and Cowsar, D. (1968). *Tetrahedron Lett.* p. 4819.
Mahler, H., and Cordes, E. (1966). "Biological Chemistry," p. 579. Harper, New York.
Malawista, S. E. (1968). *Arthritis Rheum.* **11**, Part 1, 191.
Malawista, S. E., and Bensch, K. G. (1967). *Science* **156**, 521.
Malawista, S. E., and Bodel, P. (1967). *J. Clin. Invest.* **46**, 786.
Malawista, S. E., Chang, Y.-H., and Wilson, L. (1972). *Arthritis Rheum.* **15**, 641.
Margulis, L. (1973). *Int. Rev. Cytol.* **34**, 333.
Margulis, L., Banerjee, S., and White, T. (1969). *Science* **164**, 1178.
Martel, J., Toromanoff, E., and Haynh, C. (1965). *J. Org. Chem.* **30**, 1752.
Massey, V., Brumby, P., and Komai, H. (1969). *J. Biol. Chem.* **244**, 1682.
Massey, V., Komai, H., Palmer, G., and Ellion, G. (1970). *J. Biol. Chem.* **245**, 2837.
Mazia, D. (1961). In "The Cell" (J. Brachet and A. E. Mirsky, eds.), Vol. 3 pp. 77–412. Academic Press, New York.
Mazia, D., and Dan, K. (1952). *Proc. Nat. Acad. Sci. U.S.* **38**, 826.
Midgley A. R., Pierce, B., and Dixon, F. J. (1959). *Science* **130**, 40.
Mizel, B., and Wilson, L. (1972). *Biochemistry* **11**, 2573.
Muller, G. (1963). French Patent 1,344,474; *Chem. Abstr.* **60**, 15928 (1964).
Muller, G., and Poittevin, A. (1964). French Patent 1,375,049; *Chem. Abstr.* **62**, 5312b (1965).
Muller, G., Blade-Font, A., and Bordoneschi, R. (1963). *Justus Liebigs Ann. Chem.* **662**, 105.
Murray, A. W., and Froscio, M. (1971). *Biochem. Biophys. Res. Commun.* **44**, 1089.
Nakamura, T. (1962). *Chem. Pharm. Bull.* **10**, 299.
Nakamura, T., Murase, Y., Hayasi, R., and Endo, Y. (1962). *Chem. Pharm. Bull.* **10**, 281.
Nozoe, T. (1959). In "Non-Benzenoid Aromatic Compounds" (D. Ginsburg, ed.), pp. 339–463. Wiley (Interscience), New York.
Olmsted, J. B., and Borisy, G. G. (1973). *Annu. Rev. Biochem.* **42**, 507.
Orsini, M., and Pansky, B. (1952). *Science* **115**, 88.
Pagliara, A. S., and Goodman, A. D. (1969). *N. Engl. J. Med.* **281**, 767.
Parmar, S., Dwivedi, C., and Basheer, A. (1972). *J. Pharm. Sci.* **61**, 179.
Pernice, B. (1889). *Sicil. Med.* **1**, 265.
Phelps, P. (1969a). *Arthritis Rheum.* **12**, 189.
Phelps, P. (1969b). *Arthritis Rheum.* **12**, 197.
Phelps, P. (1970). *Arthritis Rheum.* **13**, 1.

Phelps, P., and McCarty, D. J., Jr. (1966). *J. Exp. Med.* **124**, 115.
Phelps, P., and McCarty, D. J., Jr. (1967). *J. Pharmacol. Exp. Ther.* **158**, 546.
Phelps, P., and McCarty, D. J., Jr. (1969). *Postgrad. Med.* **45**, 87.
Phelps, P., Prockop. D. J., and McCarty, D. J., Jr. (1966). *J. Lab. Clin. Med.* **68**, 433.
Poisner, A. M., and Bernstein, J. (1971). *J. Pharmacol. Exp. Ther.* **177**, 102.
Potěšilová, H., Wiedermannová, J., and Šantavý, F. (1969). *Collect. Czech. Chem. Commun.* **34**, 3642.
Raffauf, R., Farren, A., and Ullyot, G. (1953). *J. Amer. Chem. Soc.* **75**, 2576.
Rapoport, H., and Lavigne, J. B. (1955). *J. Amer. Chem. Soc.* **77**, 667.
Rapoport, H., and Lavigne, J. B. (1956). *J. Amer. Chem. Soc.* **78**, 2455.
Riesterer, L., and Jaques, R. (1969). *Pharmacology* **2**, 288.
Robins, R. K. (1956). *J. Amer. Chem. Soc.* **78**, 784.
Rosenbloom, S. J., and Ferguson, F. C. (1968). *Toxicol. Appl. Pharmacol.* **13**, 50.
Rosenthale, M. E., Kassarich, J., and Schneider, F., Jr. (1966). *Proc. Soc. Exp. Biol. Med.* **122**, 693.
Roth, L. E., Pihlaja, D. J., and Shigenaka, Y. (1970). *J. Ultrastruct. Res.* **30**, 7.
Rubulis, A., Rubert M., and Faloon, W. W. (1970). *Amer. J. Clin. Nutr.* **23**, 1251.
Rundles, R. W., Wyngaarden, J., Hitchings, G., Elion, G., and Silberman, H. (1963). *Trans. Ass. Amer. Physicians* **76**, 126.
Rundles, R. W., Wyngaarden, J., Hitchings, G., and Elion, G. (1969). *Annu. Rev. Pharmacol.* **9**, 345.
Ryckewaert, A., and Kuntz, D. (1968). *Actual. Rheumatol.* **5**, 125.
Sagorin, C., Ertel, N. H., and Wallace, S. L. (1972). *Arthritis Rheum.* **15**, 213.
Schindler, R. (1962). *Nature (London)* **196**, 73.
Schindler, R. (1965). *J. Pharmacol. Exp. Ther.* **149**, 409.
Schönhartung, M., Pfaender, P., Reiker, A., and Siebert, G. (1973). *Hoppe-Seyler's Z. Physiol. Chem.* **354**, 421.
Schreiber, J., Leimgruber, W., Pesaro, M., Schudel, P., and Eschenmoser, A. (1959). *Angew. Chem.* **71**, 637.
Schreiber, J., Leimgruber, W., Pesaro, M., Schudel, P., Threlfall, T., and Eschenmoser, A. (1961). *Helv. Chim. Acta* **44**, 540.
Scott, A. I., McCapra, F., Buchanan, R. L., Day, A. C., and Young, D. W. (1965). *Tetrahedron* **21**, 3605.
Seegmiller, J. E. (1967). *In* "Gout" (J. H. Talbott, ed.), 3rd ed., pp. 38–55. Grune & Stratton, New York.
Seegmiller, J. E. (1969). *Postgrad. Med.* **45**, 99.
Seegmiller, J. E., Howell, R. R., and Malawista, S. E. (1962). *J. Amer. Med. Ass.* **180**, 469.
Shimanouchi, H., and Sasada, Y. (1970). *Tetrahedron Lett.* p. 2421.
Skeith, M. D., and Healey, L. A. (1968). *Amer. J. Physiol.* **214**, 582.
Soifer, D. (1971). *Abstr. 11th Ann. Meet. Soc. Cell Biol.* p. 283.
Spilberg, I., and Osterland, C. K. (1970). *J. Lab. Clin. Med.* **76**, 472.
Stadler, J., and Franke, W. W. (1972). *Nature (London), New Biol.* **237**, 237.
Stecher, P. G., ed. (1968). "Merck Index," 8th ed. pp. 559, 968, and 1119. Merck and Co., Inc., Rahway, New Jersey.
Stemmermann, G. N. and Hayashi, T. (1971). *Hum. Pathol.* **2**, 321.
Sunagawa, G., Nakamura, T., and Nakazawa, J. (1962). *Chem. Pharm. Bull.* **10**, 291.
Talbott, J. H., ed. (1967). "Gout," 3rd ed. Grune & Stratton, New York.
Taylor, E. W. (1965). *J. Cell Biol.* **25**, 145.
Trnavský, K., and Kopecký, Š. (1966). *Med. Exp.* **15**, 322.
Tse, R. L., and Phelps, P. (1970). *J. Lab. Clin. Med.* **76**, 403.

Tse, R. L., and Phelps, P. (1971). *Arthritis Rheum.* **14**, 418.

Uyeki, E. M., Klassen, R. S., and Llacer, V. (1969). *Proc. Soc. Exp. Biol. Med.* **132**, 1140.

van Tamelen, E. E., Spencer, T. A., Jr., Allen, D. S., Jr., and Orvis, R. L. (1959). *J. Amer. Chem. Soc.* **81**, 6341.

van Tamelen, E. E., Spencer, T. A., Jr., Allen, D. S., Jr., and Orvis, R. L. (1961). *Tetrahedron* **14**, 8.

Vesell, E. S., Passananti, G. T., and Green, F. E. (1970). *N. Engl. J. Med.* **283**, 1484.

Ventilla, M., Cantor, C. R., and Shelanski, M. (1972). *Biochemistry* **11**, 1554.

von E. Doering, W., and Detert, F. L. (1951). *J. Amer. Chem. Soc.* **73**, 876.

Walaszek, E. J., Kelsey, F. E., and Geiling, E. M. K. (1952). *Science* **116**, 225.

Walaszek, E. J., Kocsis, J. J., Leroy, G. V., and Geiling, E. M. K. (1960). *Arch. Int. Pharmacodyn. Ther.* **125**, 371.

Wallace, S. L. (1959). *Arthritis Rheum.* **2**, 389.

Wallace, S. L. (1961). *Ann. Intern. Med.* **54**, 274.

Wallace, S. L., and Ertel, N. H. (1969). *Bull. Rheum. Dis.* **20**, 582.

Wallace, S. L., Omokoku, B., and Ertel, N. H. (1970). *Amer. J. Med.* **48**, 443.

Wallingford, W. R., and McCarty, D. J. (1971). *Arthritis Rheum.* **14**, 189.

Weiner, I. M., Washington, J. A., and Mudge, G. H. (1960). *Bull. Johns Hopkins Hosp.* **106**, 333.

Weiner, M., and Piliero, S. J. (1970). *Annu. Rev. Pharmacol.* **10**, 171.

Weisenberg, R. C., and Timasheff, S. C. (1970). *Biochemistry* **9**, 4110.

Weisenberg, R. C., Borisy, G. G., and Taylor, E. W. (1968). *Biochemistry* **7**, 4466.

Weissmann, G. (1966). *Arthritis Rheum.* **9**, 834.

Weissmann, G. (1971). *Hosp. Pract.* **6**, 43.

Weissmann, G. Dukor, P., and Zurier, R.-B. (1971). *Nature (London), New Biol.* **231**, 131.

White, J. G. (1969). *Amer. J. Pathol.* **54**, 467.

Williams, J. A., and Wolff, J. (1970). *Proc. Nat. Acad. Sci. U.S.* **67**, 1901.

Willis, A. L. (1970). *Pharmacol. Res. Commun.* **2**, 297.

Wilson, L. (1970). *Biochemistry* **9**, 4999.

Wilson, L., and Friedkin, M. (1967). *Biochemistry* **6**, 3126.

Winter, C. A., Risley, E. A., and Nuss, G. W. (1963). *Proc. Soc. Exp. Biol. Med.* **111**, 544.

Woodward, R. B. (1965). *Harvey Lect.* **59**, 31.

Zeitler, H.-J., and Niemer, H. (1969). *Hoppe-Seyler's Z. Physiol. Chem.* **350**, 366.

Zweig, M. H., and Chignell. C. F. (1973). *Biochem. Pharmacol.* **22**, 2141.

Zweig, M. H., Maling, H. M., and Webster, M. E. (1972). *J. Pharmacol. Exp. Ther.* **182**, 344.

Chapter 11

Antiinflammatory Proteins and Peptides

J. D. FISHER

Biochemistry Research Department
Armour Pharmaceutical Co.
Kankakee, Illinois

I. INTRODUCTION

Normal healthy animals respond to a noxious insult by several means: some involve physical responses, such as avoidance of further exposure; some involve biological responses to isolate the insult; and some involve chemical responses that reinforce both the physical and biological responses and may assist in terminating or minimizing the injury to the host.

The generation of endogenous modulators of inflammation is part of a healthy inflammatory response. When these modulators are deficient, as in adrenalectomized animals, which cannot respond to ACTH liberated by stressful situations, or in human subjects with emphysema, who lack anti-proteases, the severity of inflammation is increased. In recent years there has been a modest revival of interest in elucidating the physiology of inflammation from the viewpoint of understanding the mechanisms by which the host is cushioned or "buffered" from extensive autoinjury, extending beyond the original site of the inflammagenic insult. Some of these studies point the way to manipulating the host's response to increase the titer of natural antiinflammatory or inflammalytic agents and raise the possibility of adding replacement therapy to the other therapeutic modes presently available to combat chronic inflammatory disease.

II. ADRENOCORTICOTROPIC HORMONES (ACTH'S)

The anterior pituitaries of all mammals studied secrete a 39-amino acid polypeptide that stimulates the adrenal cortex, without species specificity, to secrete glucocorticoids. There is evidence that an ACTH may in addition stimulate the secretion of mineral corticoids (i.e., aldosterone) by human and dog adrenals and exhibit a range of hormonal effects on extraadrenal tissues, e.g., influencing fat metabolism, pigmentation in melanocytes (Engel and Lebovitz, 1966), or relaxing human bronchial muscle (Svedmayr et al., 1970). The relationship of these extraadrenal activities of ACTH to its antiinflammatory activity is still uncertain. There is repeated testimony but as yet little scientific evidence that the therapeutic activity of ACTH in treating inflammatory diseases is not exactly reproduced by substituting synthetic corticosteroids for the ACTH.

A. Composition and Assay

Analysis of amino acid content and sequences have been completed for the human, porcine, bovine, and ovine species (Fig. 1), which are of prime interest in medicine. The structures of all these four ACTH's have been recently revised. The porcine and human sequences were revised by Graf et al. (1971) and these revisions have been independently confirmed and extended (Riniker et al., 1972). The bovine and ovine sequences have been corrected by Li (1972). A sequence for human ACTH described by Lee et al. (1965) is of some importance as it is the foundation for early synthetic work to provide adequate amounts of "human" material for extensive clinical

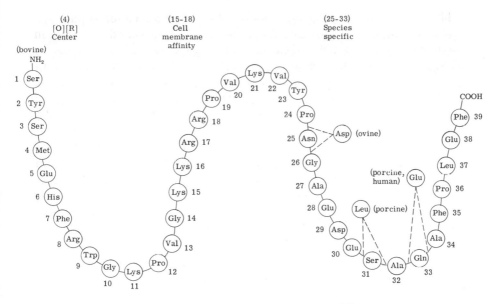

Fig. 1 Revised bovine, ovine, porcine, and human ACTH structures.

evaluation (Szporny *et al.*, 1968; Laszlo *et al.*, 1970; El-Shaboury, 1970; Yamashiro and Li, 1973).

Natural ACTH (monomer) can form dimers and trimers (Li, 1962). The full 1–39 ACTH sequence has the form of a random coil with no secondary or tertiary structures (Li, 1962). A possible conformation of the partial ACTH sequence 1–24 at its receptor site has been described (Seelig *et al.*, 1971). A reversible oxidation–reduction center (methionine sulfur) exists (Hofmann and Yajima, 1962) that is critical for biological activity (Fig. 1).

Fractionation of human plasma via the Cohn methods has indicated ACTH activity associated with fractions II and III and occasionally fractions IV_1 and IV_4 (Bethune *et al.*, 1958). Yalow and Berson (1971) have presented evidence for the existence in plasma and extracts of human pituitary glands of immunoreactive components closely resembling ACTH but of larger molecular size than ACTH 1–39 (as well as of components resembling ACTH). The larger molecular weight fraction is represented as ACTH bound in covalent linkage to a larger peptide.

The whole sequence of 39 amino acids is not essential for adrenocorticotropic activity. The first 24 amino acids from the N-terminal serine are common to the ACTH's from all mammals, and the first 20 amino acids are essential for the manifestation of full biological activity (Hofmann *et al.*, 1962). The synthesis of this 1–24 sequence (Kappeler and Schwyzer, 1961; Schwyzer and Kappeler, 1963) has been rapidly followed by clinical trials and its introduction as a therapeutic agent in both short-acting and long-acting formulations. The structure–action relationship for the various partial sequences is still under active investigation, using a variety of biological assays. The following are two principle methods of assay for standardization and detection of ACTH's in plasma.

1. *In vivo* methods that determine depletion of adrenal ascorbate (in rat only) and/or rise in circulating C-21 oxysteroids (all species) after administration of an ACTH preparation.

2. *In vitro* methods in which an ACTH sample is incubated with isolated adrenal tissue slices (Saffran and Schally, 1955) or isolated cells (Schwyzer *et al.*, 1971; Richardson and Schulster, 1970) and the tissue response is measured by steroid output, reduction of reducing capacity (Daly *et al.*, 1972; Chaven *et al.*, 1972), or displacement of radio-labeled ACTH from receptor (Lefkowitz *et al.*, 1970; Wolfsen *et al.*, 1972, Finn *et al.*, 1972; Besser, 1973).

Low quantities of ACTH given to rats may raise steroid output without affecting the adrenal ascorbic acid content, indicating that different threshold doses should be associated with different effects even within the same target tissue (Fisher, 1962; Evans *et al.*, 1966).

Radioimmune assays using specific antibodies are used to detect and quantify circulating ACTH and to permit distinction between sequences within the whole ACTH molecule that vary with the animal source. A pitfall in quantitating ACTH preparations is that their relative efficacy may change with the mode of administration, whether intramuscular, intravenous, or subcutaneous. *In vitro* assays agree more closely with *in vivo* results following intravenous administration, although it must be recognized that in therapeutic use these preparations are nearly always given intramuscularly. Assays of potency are generally reported on a weight basis (i.e., units per milligram). When expressed on a molar basis the partial peptide sequences of ACTH are generally less active than the intact 1–39 sequence.

B. Biological Effects

ACTH is as a rule administered by injection. The literature describes attempts to give modified peptides by buccal or nasal routes (Felber *et al.*, 1969; Keenan and Chamberlain, 1969).

In general the spectrum of responses to an ACTH parallel those to the prime corticosteroid secreted by that animal's adrenal cortex (corticosterone in the rat, cortisol in man). However, the peptide itself also has a pharmacology that is distinct from that of the elicited steroid in terms of affecting separate receptors, although it is sometimes extremely difficult to disentangle the effect of the peptide from the steroid in some extra-adrenal tissues. For example, ACTH inhibits steroid inactivation in isolated fibroblasts (Berliner, 1964) and slows the conjugation of cortisol with glucuronic acid (Kornel and Meador, 1964). In these instances ACTH exhibits a bifunctional control of steroid metabolism—both stimulating production in one organ and retarding degradation in another. Some ACTH fragments (partial sequences) may show kinin activity, inducing changes in vascular permeability (J. D. Fisher, unpublished, 1968) that are in fact antagonized by the steroids.

Compounds having androgenic, estrogenic, and progestational activities are secreted by the normal adrenal in small amounts. After ACTH stimulation their plasma titers usually increase. How much of a role these noncorticoid hormonal steroids play in the spectrum of responses attributed to ACTH administration is not well known.

Aldosterone secretion is stimulated in man far more extensively by the synthetic 1–24 sequence than by the whole 39-amino acid sequence (Arguelles et al., 1964). This raises the question of whether degraded fragments of ACTH, which have been found to be present in sera by using specific antibodies (Besser, 1973; Matsuyama et al., 1972b), do not in turn exhibit further pharmacological activities over and above that of the intact ACTH molecule (or the steroids formed in response to intact ACTH). It is also clear that as more of the synthetic peptide sequences, "mini ACTH's" are fully evaluated in laboratory animals and hopefully in man (Schröder and Lübke, 1966), we shall have to revise our concepts of what even the intact, or "maxi," ACTH may be capable of (Rittel, 1971).

The half-life in man of exogenous ACTH varies depending on the detection assay methods employed; biological in vivo assays give 4–18 minutes and radioimmune assays give 10–25 minutes for the half-life of the whole 1–39 sequence (Matsuyama et al., 1972a).

The various active peptides stimulate adrenal steroidogenesis through a mechanism involving the synthesis of a protein with a rapid rate of turnover. The level of this protein then determines the rate of steroidogenesis (Garren et al., 1971) by controlling the conversion of cholesterol to pregnenolone, the rate-limiting step under hormonal control (Gill, 1972). Cyclic AMP serves as the mediator of ACTH action within the cell. The mechanism of action of ACTH has been fully reviewed elsewhere (Ferguson, 1972; Gill, 1972).

The intact 1–39 sequence contains a number of antigenic determinants. These determinants are sited in the 25–39 portion of the amino acid sequence. Antibodies directed toward the whole 1–39 sequence demonstrate occasional cross-responses with the partial sequence 1–24 (Forssman and Mulder, 1971). However, the tetracosapeptide (1–24) is also immunogenic and the antibody produced to it appears to be directed mainly against the C-terminal of this polypeptide (Gelzer, 1968). Circulating antibodies directed toward natural porcine ACTH, administered over short- (5 weeks) and long-term schedules (200 weeks), have been demonstrated (Landon *et al*., 1967). The antibody that is evoked is generally of low titer and appears in most cases to have had no adverse clinical effects in that there is no demonstrable reduction in responsiveness to further administrations of exogenous hormone, and endogenous levels of ACTH from the subjects own pituitary are not evidently suppressed (Fleischer *et al*., 1967). There is evidence that resistance and allergic responses can occur occasionally following the administration of either the natural porcine ACTH or the partial sequences, such as the tetracosapeptide (1–24) (Glass *et al*., 1971).

A negative feedback loop exists in most, if not all, hormonal systems, i.e., the product(s) of the stimulated organ can inhibit the other organ, from which the stimulator originates, to shut down further release of excessive stimulator in order to maintain a homeostatic balance. Thus, there exists a hypothalamus–pituitary–adrenal cortex closed loop. Excess or prolonged use of corticosteroids inhibits the release of endogenous ACTH, on exposure to stress, from the pituitary and thereby suppresses normal adrenal function. Long-term use of ACTH has also been demonstrated to suppress the pituitary but to a lesser degree. It has been concluded (Daly and Glass, 1971) that because of the possible adrenal hypertrophy following long-term use of ACTH, levels of plasma corticosteroid (adrenal origin) are reduced to a lower degree than that demonstrated after withdrawal of treatment with an exogenous steroid.

C. Clinical Use

For clinical use in man the following formulations are currently employed (Malone and Strong, 1972).

1. Natural porcine material, in a rather concentrated form, that contains a mixture of the parent ACTH with its deamino derivative and other altered forms, either artifacts of isolation or truly endogenous products representing naturally synthesized variants (Dixon, 1964; Lerner *et al*., 1968). It is available in lyophilized form for resolubilization in saline or in a depot form, admixed with either 16% degraded gelatin or a zinc phosphate suspension or carboxymethylcellulose. (This last formulation is not available in the United States.)

2. Synthetic 1–24 sequence (Synacthen, Cortrosyn): 1 mg is equivalent to approximately 80 units of the international standard ACTH preparation. This synthetic material is formulated either in aqueous solution or with a

zinc phosphate suspension. A dose of 0.25 mg will give maximum stimulation of the human adrenal for diagnostic purposes.

For acute allergic disorders and asthma, 10–25 units of porcine ACTH may be given in a continuous intravenous infusion over an 8-hour period. For dermatological and rheumatoid diseases, ACTH is usually given as 40–80 units in a repository form (H.P. Acthar Gel, Cortrotropin-zinc) intramuscularly or subcutaneously every 24–72 hours or in 25–40-unit doses three times daily. The synthetic partial peptide (1–24 sequence) has a shorter half-life and gives a shorter duration of response. For therapeutic purposes it must be administered in the long-acting repository form.

III. ENZYMES AS THERAPY FOR INFLAMMATION

Approximately one third of the agents available in the United States and listed as having clinical antiinflammatory activity in recent editions of the "Physicians Desk Reference" have been enzymes. Although not employed widely to treat established inflammatory states, they seem to have an especial value as prophylactic agents (especially when administered pretrauma) in preventing the normal inflammatory response from running its full course. Therefore, they have been frequently used for minimizing the postoperative trauma after dental surgery or for "preventing" physical incapacitation following athletic injuries.

Before the use of proteases (and nucleases) for treating inflammation are considered, some major drawbacks to their use must be discussed.

1. The general uncertainty as to how they may act.

2. Incredulity that such large molecules could be absorbed through cells and across phase boundaries by mechanisms that have nothing to do with intrinsic lipophilic character, the chief of these being pinocytosis (Leake, 1972); i.e. physical incorporation into the cell of a portion of the extracellular, drug-containing, medium. By such a mechanism, insulin may perhaps truly affect intracellular receptors and enzymes.

3. The small number of well-controlled clinical studies of the agents.

4. The much larger, relatively unscientific, literature devoted to these agents, which can best be described as "testimonials."

5. The inflammagenic activity of many proteolytic enzymes.

It should be noted that the first four difficulties cited above have not prevented gold preparations from being accepted as possible therapies of choice in certain well-defined stages of rheumatoid arthritis because of the purely pragmatic observation that these gold preparations may afford more real benefit to the patient than alternative available therapies. The fifth point is dealt with in Section III,A.

A. Endogenous Enzymes in Inflammation

The basic symptomatic features of inflammation are heat, redness, pain, swelling, and consequent reduction in function (Houck, 1968). Inflammation is preceded by cell and tissue injury (Movat, 1971). Subsequent to these injuries, vascular changes take place that are related to the severity of injury. Dilation of the arterial portion of the terminal vascular bed and hyperemia of the entire bed occurs in the immediate area of injury. Slowing of blood flow and eventual blood stasis may follow this hyperemia, depending on the severity of injury. Stasis may be caused by (a) loss of plasma into the tissues because of changes in vascular permeability, (b) emigration of leukocytes, hemorrhage, and thrombosis, and (c) release of tissue breakdown products into blood. Proteolytic enzymes and vasoactive peptides, e.g., kinins, contribute to both thrombus formation and hemorrhage. Proteolytic enzymes are released at the time of injury from lysosomes of monocytes, and from fibroblasts, mast cells, platelets, and lymphocytes. Most if not all these enzymes may participate in the propagation of both injury and the subsequent counterinjury (inflammalytic) phase (Foster, 1972; Janoff, 1972). Some of these relationships are indicated in Fig. 2.

Different irritants produce inflammation via different pathways and the mechanism of induction is often characteristic of the irritants. The migration of cells into, and away from, an injury site is characteristic of the time of observation postinjury and the intensity of injury and is related to the nature of the irritant. The type of (a) tissue involved and (b) cell migration elicited can both contribute to a characteristic milieu as demonstrated by the events

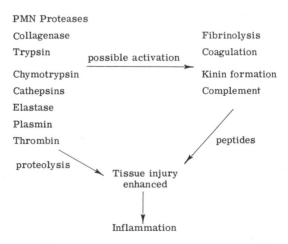

Fig. 2 Trauma. Redrawn from suggestions of R. C. Talamo (1971).

following a burn insult (Sevitt, 1964). The appearance of different proteases (Bertelli, 1972) at the site of inflammation is related to tissue type, severity of the inflammagenic stimulus, and time. In the first phase (i.e., within only a few hours after injury) chymotryptic-like enzymes appear followed by other catheptic enzymes. Aminopeptidase and carboxypeptidase can be found in tissues several weeks after the initiation of the inflammatory state.

The types of intra- and extracellular enzymes that can participate in different phases of the inflammatory process are collagenases (collagenase or collagenolytic cathepsins); trypsin; chymotrypsin; cathepsins A, B, and C; aminopeptidase; carboxypeptidase; plasmin; elastase; ribonuclease; SH-dependent proteases; and plasma kallikrein (Janoff, 1972; Bazin and Delaunay, 1972).

B. Exogenous Enzymes and Inflammation

A variety of proteolytic enzymes of animal, vegetable, bacterial, and fungal origin (see Tables I and II) have been administered orally and by injection into both experimental animals and man with demonstration of varying degrees of antiinflammatory activity.

Although local enzymes of tissue and cell origin apparently contribute to the excitation of the inflammatory process, injected proteolytic enzymes, of exogenous origin, inhibit experimentally induced inflammation initiated by an earlier trauma.

The injected enzyme is also an irritant, and this property may or may not depend on the enzyme's activity as an inflammagen. The antiinflammatory effects produced following the administration of a second irritant (counter-irritant) are probably mediated via systemic processes and have been generally regarded as nonspecific. Atkinson (1971) compared the systemic antiinflammatory activity of three different irritants in the rat. He concluded that the inflammatory affect of each counterirritant was mediated by a different mechanism. One possible mechanism that he proposed was competition of two inflammatory sites for precursors of inflammatory mediators (e.g., bradykinogen). Edema produced by an agent is more likely to be inhibited if the counterirritant is the same as the initiating agent; for example, carrageenan versus carrageenan, dextran versus dextran. By extension of this argument, an exogenous enzyme may be considered as being particularly appropriate for bringing about the inhibition of inflammation elicited by endogenous enzymes.

Keller and Schauwecker (1972) reported that tissue mast cells and their constituents, including various hydrolytic enzymes, contributed to the immediate (in contrast to delayed) inflammatory response. This conclusion

TABLE I

Activities and Substrates for Some Antiinflammatory Proteases[a]

Enzyme	Activity	Convenient substrate for assay
Trypsin	Esterase	(BAEE) benzoyl-L-arginineethyl ester
		(TAME) P-toluenesulfonyl-L-argininemethyl ester
	Proteolytic	Casein or hemoglobin
	Amidase	Benzoyl-L-Argininamide
		Benzoyl-DL-arginine P-nitroanilide (BANA)
Chymotrypsin	Esterase	(ATEE) N-acetyl-L-tyrosineethyl ester
		(BTEE) N-benzoyl-L-tyrosineethyl ester
		(ZTNE) N-benzyloxycarbonyl-L-tyrosine-p-nitrophenyl ester
Papain	Proteolytic	Casein
	Esterase	(BAEE)
		(CTNP)-p-nitrophenylcarbobenzoxytyrosine
Ficin	Proteolytic	Casein
		(p-NPZG) p-nitrophenylcarbobenzoylglycinate
Bromelain	Proteolytic	Casein or hemoglobin
	Esterolytic	(BAEE)
	Amidase	(BAA) n-benzoyl-L-arginine amide
Pronase	Proteolytic	Casein
	Esterolytic	(BAEE)
	Aminopeptidase	L-leucylglycine
	Carboxypeptidase	Carbobenzoxyglycl-L-leucine
Streptokinase (SK)	Proteases	Lysis of standard fibrin clot; through activation of plasminogen to plasmin; clot formed from a standard Fibrinogen (containing, human plasminogen) SK + human plasminogen; assaying the rate of hydrolysis of lysinemethyl ester (LMe).
Collagenase	Proteases	Collagen, Gelatin Z-gly-pro-gly-gly-pro-ala-OH

[a] Perlman and Lorand (1970) .

stemmed from experimental systems wherein depletion of the mast cells (rat) reduced the acute (immediate) inflammatory signs. Horakova and Muratova (1965) parenterally administered trypsin and demonstrated an inhibition of rat paw edema caused by local injection of trypsin. Intraperitoneal administration of chymotrypsin alone (rabbits) induced a leukocytic response reflected in an approximately 50% depletion of neutrophil cells (Seneca, 1965). Parenteral administration of mediators of some phases of inflammation, e.g., histamine, serotonin, and bradykinin, diminished the local reaction induced by the identical inflammagenic agent (Bertelli, 1972).

TABLE II

Type and Origin of Enzymes Evaluated Both as Inflammagens and as Antiinflammatory Agents

Oral enzyme	Derivation	Approximate molecular weight
Trypsin	Pancreas	24,000
Chymotrypsin	Pancreas	25,000
Elastase	Pancreas	25,000
Papain	Papaya latex	21,000
Ficin	Latex of fig tree	26,000
Bromelain	Stem of pineapple	35,000
Pronase	*Streptomyces griseus*	Mixture
Alcolase	*Bacillus subtilis*	28,000
Maxatase	*Bacillus subtilis*	28,000
Streptokinase (SK) Streptodornase	Streptococci	48,000 (SK)
Collagenase	*Clostridium histolyticum*	50,000–100,000

When different inflammagenic agents were used to institute edema in the rat paw (Table III) and varying types of proteases (animal, vegetable, bacteria) were administered orally, these enzymes were found to have significant type-specific actions on the edema generated. Pancreatic enzymes and the plant enzymes ficin and bromelain each demonstrated significant antiedemic activity in most edema states, whereas papain, another enzyme of plant origin, and the bacterial enzymes displayed little or no effect. These differences again indicated a type-specific inflammation and the need to utilize a variety of different experimental assay systems for characterization of each agent (Winter *et al.*, 1964).

TABLE III

Some Animal Models Used for Studying the Antiinflammatory Effect of Enzymes

Animal	Assay condition	Inflammagenic agent or procedure
Rat	Rat paw edema	Serotonin creatinine sulfate, egg white, dextran, brewers yeast, carrageenan (Netti *et al.*, 1972)
Rat	Granuloma pouch	Croton oil (Hakim *et al.*, 1964) Carbon tetrachloride (Innerfield *et al.*, 1966)
Rabbit	Scab size	UV light (Seneca, 1965)
	Burn-dry	Dry ice (Seneca, 1965)
	Burn	Steam
	Edema (Paw)	Crushed, controlled
Monkey	Edema (Head-Forearm)	Crushed (Seneca, 1965)

Netti *et al.* (1972) also found that a threshold dose might be required to affect these particular assay systems. At low doses a certain percentage of rats responded, and as the dose was increased, an increasing percentage of animals responded favorably. Thus, an all-or-none, rather than a dose–response, relationship was apparent. In any given population of animals (man?) the experimental results might indeed reflect this threshold difference.

At least five different natural (plasma protein) protease inhibitors have been identified. These proteins may regulate the activity of intracellular proteases and those proteases involved in the blood clotting processes. The two major inhibitors have been identified as α_1-antitrypsin (AT) and α_2-macroglobulin. The former represents approximately 90% of the inhibitory titer in plasma. Because complexes formed between α_1-antitrypsin and trypsin of either bovine pancreatic or human origin are enzymatically inactive (Travis and Coan, 1972), their pathophysiological role is believed to be that of modulating excessive proteolysis. AT has a wide spectrum of inhibitory activity, as demonstrated by its ability to complex with at least six animal proteases, namely trypsin, chymotrypsin, elastase, collagenase, thrombin, and plasmin. This antiprotease, the titer of which may be changed on injury, may play a systemic role in affecting the antiinflammatory activity of exogenously administered enzyme (Whitehouse, 1969; Margetts *et al.*, 1972). A number of possible explanations have been suggested as plausible mechanisms by which orally administered enzymes can intercede in an inflammatory process. One of these proposals suggests that there is a restoration of microcirculation (reduction of edema) by augmenting fibrin resolution. Augmentation of fibrinolysis, according to this theory, may take place by saturation of the normal serum antiproteases with the absorbed enzyme, which indirectly enhances plasmin activity and fibrinolysis (DeN'Yeurt, 1972). Chakrabarti *et al.* (1969) reported that a significant rise in serum enzyme inhibitors occurs during an episode of fibrinolytic shutdown which may minimize the antiinflammatory action of endogenous fibrinolytic enzymes. These changes can result in a restriction of microcirculation and lead to the localized edema.

An excellent description of the possible physiological role of α_2-macroglobulin has been recently given (Rinderknecht and Geokas, 1973). Unlike the trypsin complex with α_1-antitrypsin, the enzyme complex formed with α_2-macroglobulin, although retaining little proteolytic activity, still retains 80–90% of the original esterolytic activity (equivalent to free trypsin) against low molecular weight substrate.

Although there is clinical evidence that exogenous enzymes may alter the titer of α_1-antitrypsin (Margetts *et al.*, 1972; Fisher *et al.*, 1974), the effective concentration of circulating α_2-macroglobulin does not seem to be changed after administering these same enzymes. The augmented anti-inflammatory counterirritant effects of a variety of agents may alter the ratio of free α_2-globulin to globulin complexed with enzymes. Ambrus and his colleagues (1962) indicate that the complex formed by union of plasmin with antiplasmin is effective in lyzing fibrin clots. Ganrot (1967) suggested that the retention of peptidase activity by this complex may indicate that it still has a role in detoxifying peptides, whereas the other functions of plasmin are considerably diminished. Rinderknecht and Geokas (1973) reported that the α_2-macroglobulin–trypsin complex is still able to destroy both angiotensin and vasopressin. Thus, one possible systemic effect of exogenous enzyme may be to contribute to the formation of a circulating α_2-macroglobulin complex that functions to somehow reduce some phase of the inflammatory process. Whether this simply involves some form of complement depletion (away from the site of irritation) is quite uncertain at the present time.

Utilizing varying clinical criteria, evidence for the effectiveness of oral enzymes has been reported by a number of investigators (Cirelli, 1962; Lie et al., 1967; Shaw, 1969; Tsomides and Goldberg, 1969; Schwinger, 1970; Rathgeber, 1971; DeN'Yeurt, 1972, DeFiebre et al., 1967). Proof of oral absorption has been reported for trypsin and chymotrypsin (Ambrus et al., 1967; Martin et al., 1957; Moriya et al., 1967; Kobacoff et al; 1963; Avakian, 1964; Miller, 1968; Seneca, 1965) when either increases in serum esterase levels or radioactive tracers incorporated into the enzymes are used. Similar demonstrations of bromelain absorption by both animals and man (Bodi, 1965; Miller, 1965; Martin, 1965; Bogner and Snyder, 1962; Seneca, 1965) have been reported.

The evidence for clinical effectiveness has been challenged for a variety of reasons (Korlof et al., 1969; Calnan et al., 1963; Council on Drugs, 1964), including (a) the fact that all enzymes do not necessarily act in an equivalent manner and (b) the lack of specific objective measurable evidence to parallel the subjective criteria of effectiveness.

Oral enzyme preparations currently being utilized clinically in the United States and western Europe are:

1. Bromelain: Available as 50,000 and 100,000 unit tablets. The unit is derived from an assay involving the proteolysis of casein. The dose recommended initially is 100,000 units q.i.d. and for maintenance, 100,000 units b.i.d. or 50,000 units q.i.d.

2. Trypsin and chymotrypsin combinations, e.g. (a) Trypsin and chymotrypsin in a ratio of 6:1. Available as 50,000- or 100,000-unit tablets. The unit is derived from an assay involving the proteolysis of hemoglobin (Anson procedure). The dose schedule recommended is 50,000–100,000 q.i.d. The recommended time of administration is before meals and as soon as possible after trauma. (b) Trypsin and chymotrypsin in a ratio of 35,000-units (14 mg

crystalline) trypsin to 15,000-units (15 mg crystalline) chymotrypsin. Available as 50,000 unit tablets. The unit is derived from an assay involving the proteolysis of hemoglobulin (Anson Procedure). The dose schedule recommended is 100,000 units 4 times a day initially and a maintenance dose of 50,000 units 3 or 4 times per day.

3. Papain: Available as 100,000-unit tablets. The unit is derived from the use of a milk clotting assay. The prophylactic schedule recommended (dose may be administered either orally or via buccal route) is two tablets 1 or 2 hours before surgery (episeotomy). Therapeutic dose recommended is two tablets q.i.d. for 5 days.

IV. OTHER ANTIINFLAMMATORY PROTEINS

The literature contains many reports of the existence of such proteins, usually detected by their ability to suppress a subsequent inflammation when injected into naive rats. Some of these may in effect be crude animal proteases; others may be the antiproteases, or other protective proteins, formed as part of a response to previous inflammation. Yet others may be counterirritants, in turn causing a release of endogenous proteases and production of endogenous modulators of inflammation, e.g., complement inhibitors. Some recent references can be found in a short review by Paulus and Whitehouse (1973). If these are truly protective, then it should be a responsibility of experimental pharmacologists to find out whether a drug being considered for clinical trial has any deleterious effect on the formation of these natural antiinflammatory materials.

V. CHALONES: NATURAL ANTIPROLIFERATIVE AGENTS

The previous sections of this chapter have discussed some large molecules, present in blood or the inflamed tissues of animals, that may augment such natural antiinflammatory hormones as the corticoids secreted by the adrenal. As sections II and III have shown, these large molecules may be supplemented or simulated by exogenous antiinflammatory agents prepared from readily available animal sources.

This section is concerned with certain other high molecular weight materials that may be the natural analogs of the cytotoxic–antiproliferative–immunosuppressant drugs that are increasingly being used to augment antiinflammatory drugs in severe crippling or life-threatening inflammatory diseases (see Paulus, Chapter 1 in this volume). A complete listing of all the natural analogs of such immunosuppressant agents must include such diverse agents as the corticosteroids, on the one hand, and immunoregulatory globulins, on the other. As the title of this section indicates, this discussion is primarily devoted to considering a few agents the mechanisms of action of which have at least been fairly well defined, even if not yet understood, at the cellular level. They have in common the potential for regulating cellular proliferation, associated with both the immunological and the nonimmunological events, that ensues following invasion of a tissue by a foreign component.

A. Background

Events involved in the restoration of tissue integrity, i.e., healing, have been extensively covered in the excellent review by Schilling (1968). The following events, occuring both concurrently and sequentially, are the changes that take place following a noxious insult: platelet aggregation and blood clotting, formation of fibrin, cellular injury and necrotic tissue formation, alterations in the ground substance, endothelial and capillary proliferation, fibroblast proliferation and collagen production, epithelial proliferation and surface covering, variable regeneration of certain cell types, and restructuring of the affected tissue. Until there is adequate restructuring and restoration of function, healing is not complete.

When a tissue is damaged, enhanced cellular mitotic activity occurs that results in an increase of the specific cells to replace those damaged, in order to restore and maintain the structural integrity of the tissue. When a sufficient number of new cells has been produced to restructure the damaged tissue, mitotic activity subsides. The functional integrity of a tissue or organ is also dependent on cellular multiplication, which occurs when cells are lost during an aging process. Thus, an equilibrium or dynamic balance appears to exist between the number of aged and functional cells and the creation of new cells.

At least two possible mechanisms have been defined to insure regulatory control over enhanced mitotic activity. One proposes that a wound hormone, or mitotic stimulator (Pashkis, 1958), is released from damaged cells to initiate mitosis. A second and contrasting postulate suggests that inhibitory or repressor substances exist, that when depleted, enhance mitotic activity (Bullough, 1968). Furthermore, when restoration of cell production and functional integrity is achieved, it appears there is a slowing down or cessation of mitotic activity because of an increase in these inhibitory substance(s). Thus, a negative feedback control is instituted. Weiss and Kavanau (1957) speculating on the basis of mathematical models defining the features of a typical sigmoidal growth curve, have suggested that a self-limiting expression (inhibitor) of growth must exist for each cell type, that there are as many inhibitors as there are cell types, and that each is specific for its own type. Bullough and Laurence have designated the inhibitor(s) as "chalone(s)," i.e., an internal secretion produced by a tissue to control, by inhibition, the rate of cell production in that tissue. Basing their hypothesis on some early observations with mouse epidermal tissue, Bullough and Laurence (1960) postulated that the chalone is tissue specific. After extracting and purifying the mitotic inhibitor from both mouse and other mammalian epidermal tissue, as well as from codfish, they have been able to demonstrate that chalone from cod epidermis tissue inhibits mitosis in mouse epidermis. This leads to the important conclusion that chalones are tissue specific but not species specific and raises the prospect that chalones of animal origin may be of real service in medicine.

B. Properties of Some Chalones

In general, the chalones have been characterized (Bullough, 1969) as being produced in the cells in which they act and as being tissue specific in their antimitotic activity. Their action is readily reversible and certain of the stress hormones (adrenalin, glucocorticoids) act as cofactors (Bullough and Laurence, 1964, 1968). Halprin and Taylor (1971) have reported on a factor from human epidermal tissue that has the characteristics of a chalone, is tissue specific and species nonspecific, but that does not require adrenalin as a cofactor.

A variety of chalones has been isolated and their mode of action studied (Elgjc et al., 1971, 1972; Voorhess and Duell, 1971; Laurence et al., 1972). Epidermal chalone was the first to be thus evaluated (Bullough et al., 1967; Boldingh and Laurence, 1968; Marrs and Voorhess, 1971a,b). Chalones from other tissues and cell populations that have been evaluated include the blood erythrocyte (Kivilaakso and Rytomaa, 1971), the granulocyte (Paukovits, 1972), and the lymphocyte (Garcia-Giralt et al., 1970; Houck et al., 1971). Spleen, thymus, liver (Verly et al., 1971), and melanocytes of skin have been utilized as source materials.

A diurnal or circadian cycle of mitotic activity in the epidermis and other tissues has been observed for many years. The proposed role of the adrenal hormones in mitotic inhibition is tied to the circadian incidence of low steroid titer with high mitotic state, and conversely, of high steroid titer with low mitotic activity. The specific role of the 11-oxycorticosteroids in the enhancement of mitotic rate is not clear. The corticoids in general have been shown to alter the rate of RNA and protein synthesis. Depending on dose or concentration (*in vivo* and *in vitro*, respectively), the steroids affect both increased synthesis of hepatic RNA, possibly messenger RNA and its associated protein, and RNA polymerase in the liver, and decreased RNA polymerase in the thymus. Proteins that specifically bind corticoids have been found in many cell types. Only the liver and lymphoid system appear to be organ specific for the corticoids. A number of hepatic steroid-binding proteins have been characterized (Snart *et al.*, 1972) and are postulated to play a role in the control of protein synthesis both at the transcriptional and at the translational level (e.g., an acid cytonuclear receptor that may play a role as a derepressor and a basic receptor protein that may act as a repressor in the hormonal stimulation of protein synthesis).

Nucleohistones are examples of inhibitor proteins that may be considered a prototype of the chalones. The histones appear to be gene inhibitors, suppressing activity according to cell type and contributing to gene specificity and cellular individuality (Butler, 1964; Busch *et al.*, 1964). They function by virtue of their adherence to the surface of DNA and only with their removal can the DNA serve as a template for RNA synthesis. Further evidence for the functional similarity of histone and chalone is that liver regeneration is inhibited in rats after the intraperitioneal administration of a histone (Sluyser, 1967). This analogy of the chalone with the histone may be quite misleading, however. Whereas the histones certainly act within the nucleus, where they are synthesized *de novo*, there is yet no evidence that the chalones are taken up by their target cells and penetrate into the cell nucleus.

The epidermal chalone isolated by Bullough and Laurence has been classified as a simple protein or glycoprotein with a molecular weight of between 30,000 and 50,000 Daltons. This preparation is further characterized by the fact that it is degraded by trypsin but not by pepsin. Houck and co-workers (1971) have isolated a lymphoid chalone from the spleen of the pig, cow, and rat. This preparation is characterized as being thermolabile and trypsin degradable, with M. W. between 30,000 and 50,000. Rytomaa and Paukovits (1972) have isolated a granulocyte chalone from rat marrow that inhibits DNA synthesis in cultured granulocytes. This preparation has been characterized as being a dialyzable polypeptide with M. W. well under 10,000. These protein substances have been demonstrated to specifically inhibit DNA synthesis in the receptor tissue or cells for which they are chalones, i.e., from which they were isolated.

Schilling (1968) has further suggested the possibility that because tryptic degradation of histones reduces their DNA inhibitory capacity, the trypsin-like activities associated with inflammatory exudates and mast cells may be of some importance in degrading endogenous histones, "DNA inhibitors," thus allowing RNA synthesis and cellular regeneration. The proteolytic

events accompanying an inflammatory process may therefore be essential for
instituting the reparative or wound-healing phase.

C. Natural Mitotic Stimulants

In contrast to the inhibitory chalones described in Sections V,A and V,B
Byyny *et al.* (1972) have reported an epidermal growth factor (EGF) from
mouse submaxillary glands that can cause generalized epithelia growth in
mouse and that is also active in stimulating a variety of epithelial tissues from
several animal species. Epidermal growth factor is a heat-stable, nondialyz-
able polypeptide with approximately 6400 M.W. It contains all of the common amino acids, except phenylalanine, alanine, and lysine, and has a
C-terminal arginine residue. Crude extracts apparently are complexed with
a binding protein of approximately 29,000 M.W., which is an arginine
esterase. Two molecules of EGF and two of the arginine esterase form a
complex of molecular weight of approximately 74,000. EGF has been reported to increase mouse mammary gland epithelium in organ culture and
concurrently to increase DNA synthesis. The activity of EGF also appears
to be hormone and cofactor dependent. Testosterone has been identified
as the specific cofactor.

D. Conclusion

The potential therapeutic value of tissue-specific chalones is manifold.
For example, because lymphocytes are involved in the inflammatory processes accompanying rheumatoid arthritis and the rejection of transplants,
a lymphocyte-specific chalone is potentially of considerable value in the
treatment of these disease states. With the development of more suitable
assays to facilitate quality control, it ought to be feasible to obtain fairly
large quantities of these remarkable tissue regulators from slaughterhouse
materials and, after rigorous purification, to initiate therapeutic trials in
man.

REFERENCES

Ambrus, C. M., Black, N., and Ambrus, J. L. (1962). *Circ. Res.* **10**, 161.
Ambrus, J. L., Lassman, H. B., and De Marchi, J. J. (1967). *Clin. Pharmacol. Ther.* **8**, 362.
Arguelles, A. E., Chekherdemian, M., Ricca, A., and Cardinali, D. P. (1964). *J. Clin. Endocrinol. Metab.* **24**, 1277.
Atkinson, D. C. (1971). *Arch. Int. Pharmacodyn. Ther.* **193**, 391.
Avakian, S. (1964). *Clin. Pharmacol. Ther.* **5**, 712.
Bazin, S., and Delaunay, A. (1972). *J. Dent. Res.* **51**, No. 2 Part 1, 244.

Berliner, D. L. (1964). *Ann. N. Y. Acad. Sci.* **116**, 1078.

Bertelli, A. (1972). *J. Dent. Res.* **51**, No. 2 Part 1, 235.

Besser, G. M. (1973). *In* "Immunological Methods in Endocrinology" (K. Fedulin, E. N. Hales, and J. Kracht, eds.). Suppl. Ser. No. 3, pp. 78–81. Academic Press, New York.

Bethune, J. E., Despointes, R. H., Antoniades, H. N., and Nelson, D. H. (1958). *Proc. Soc. Exp. Biol. Med.* **97**, 69.

Bodi, T. (1965). *Exp. Med. Surg., Suppl. Issue* p. 51.

Bogner, R. L., and Snyder, C. C. (1962). *J. Int. Coll. Surg.* **3**, 280.

Boldingh, W. H., and Laurence, E. B. (1968). *Eur. J. Biochem.* **5**, 191.

Bullough, W. S. (1968). *Biol. Basis Med.* **1**, 311–332.

Bullough, W. S. (1969). *Sci. J.* (April), 71.

Bullough, W. S., and Laurence, E. B. (1964). *Exp. Cell. Res.* **33**, 176.

Bullough, W. S., and Laurence, E. B. (1968). *Cell Tissue Kinet.* **1**, 5.

Bullough, W. S., Laurence, E. B., Iversen, O. H., and Elgjc, K. (1967). *Nature (London)* **214**, 578.

Busch, H., Steele, W. J., Hnilica, L. S., and Taylor, C. (1964). *In* "The Nucleohistones" (J. Bonner and P. O. P. Ts'o, eds.), pp. 242–245. Holden-Day, San Francisco, California.

Butler, J. A. V. (1964). *In* "The Nucleohistones" (J. Bonner and P. O. P. Ts'o, eds.), pp. 36–45. Holden-Day, San Francisco, California.

Byyny, R. L., North, D., and Cohen, S. (1972). *Endocrinology* **90**, 1261.

Calnan, J., Kulatilake, A. E., and Saad, M. N. (1963). *Brit. J. Surg.* **3**, 743.

Chakrabarti, H., Hocking, E. D., and Fernly, G. R. (1969). *J. Med. Pathol.* **22**, 659.

Chayen, J., Loveridge, N., and Daly, J. R. (1972). *Clin. Endocrinol.* **1**, 219.

Cirelli, M. G. (1962). *Del. Med. J.* **34**, 159.

Council on Drugs. (1964). *J. Amer. Med. Ass.* **188**, 857.

Daly, J. R., and Glass, D. (1971). *Lancet* **1**, 476.

Daly, J. R., Loveridge,N., Bitensky, L., and Chaven, J. (1972). *Ann. Clin. Biochem.* **9**, 81.

DeFiebre, C. W., Ramsay, A. G., Goldberg, R. I., and Schuman, F. I. (1967). *In* "Drugs of Animal Origin." (A. Leonardi and J. Walsh, eds.), pp. 103–110. Ferro Edizioni, Milan.

DeN'Yeurt, A. (1972). *J. Roy. Coll. Gen. Pract.* **22**, 633.

Dixon, H. B. F. (1964). *In* "The Hormones" (G. Pincus, K. V. Thimann, and E. B. Astwood, eds.), Vol. 5, pp. 1–59. Academic Press, New York.

Elgjc, K., Laerum, O. D., and Edgehill, W. (1971). *Virchows Arch., B* **8**, 277.

Elgjc, K., Laerum, O. D., and Edgehill, W. (1972). *Virchows Arch., B* **10**, 299.

El-Shaboury, A. H. (1970). *Acta Allergol.* **25**, 451.

Engel, F. L., and Lebovitz, H. F. (1966). *In* "The Pituitary Gland" (G. W. Harris and B. T. Donovan, eds.), Vol. 2, p. 563. Univ. of California Press, Berkeley.

Evans, H. B., Sparks, L. L., and Dixon, J. S. (1966). *In* "The Pituitary Gland" (G. W. Harris and B. T. Donovan, eds.), Vol. 1, pp. 318–352. Univ. of California Press, Berkeley.

Felber, J. P., Aubert, M. L., and Debuillaume, R. (1969). *Experientia* **24**, 119w.

Ferguson, J. J., Jr. (1972). *In* "Biochemical Actions of Hormones (G. Litwack, ed.), Vol. 2, pp. 317–335. Academic Press, New York.

Finn, F. B., Widnell, C. C., and Hofmann, K. (1972). *J. Biol. Chem.* **247**, 5695.

Fisher, J. D. (1962). *Methods Horm. Res.* **1**, 641–666.

Fisher, J. D., Weeks, R. L., Curry, W. M., Rosen, L. L., and Hrinda, M. E. (1974). *J. Med.* To be published.

Fleischer, N., Abe, K., Liddle, G. W., Orth, D. N., and Nicholson, W. E. (1967). *J. Clin. Invest.* **46**, 196.

Forssman, O., and Mulder, J. (1971). *Lancet* **1**, 1024.

Foster, J. (1972). *J. Dent. Res.* **51**, No. 1, Part. 1, 257.

Ganrot, K. (1973). *Biochim. Biophys. Acta* **295**, 245–251.

Garcia-Giralt, E., Lasalvia, E., Florentin, I., and Mathé, G. (1970). *Eur. J. Clin. Biol. Res.* **15**, 1012.

Garren, L. D., Gill, G. N., Masui, H., and Walton, G. M. (1971). *Recent Progr. Horm. Res.* **27**, 433.

Gelzer, J. (1968). *Immunochemistry* **5**, 23–31.

Gill, G. N. (1972). *Metab. Clin. Exp.* **21**, 571.

Glass, D., Morley, D. J., Williams, T. J., and Daly, J. R. (1971). *Lancet* **1**, 547.

Graf, L., Bajusz, S., Patthy, A., Barat, E., and Cseh, G. (1971). *Acta Biochim. Biophys.* **6**, 415.

Hakim, A. A., Dailey, V. P., and Lesh, J. B. (1964). *Excerpta Med. Found. Int. Congr. Ser. n82*, p. 265.

Halprin, K. M., and Taylor, J. K. (1971). *Advan. Clin. Chem.* **14**, 319.

Hofmann, K., and Yajima, H. (1962). *Recent Progr. Horm. Res.* **18**, 41.

Hofmann, K., Liu, T., Yajima, H., Yanaihara, N., Yanaihara, C., and Humes, J. L. (1962). *J. Amer. Chem. Soc.* **84**, 4481.

Horáková, Z, and Muratová, J. (1965). *Int. Symp, Non-Steroidal Anti-Inflammatory Drugs, Proc. 1964* pp. 237–244.

Houck, J. C. (1968). *In* "Chemical Biology of Inflammation," (B. F. Forscher, ed.), pp. 1–3. Pergamon, Oxford.

Houck, J. C., Inranusquin, H., and Leikin, S. (1971). *Science* **173**, 1139.

Innerfield, I., Cohen, H., and Zweil, T. (1966). *Proc. Soc. Exp. Biol. Med.* **123**, 871.

Janoff, A. (1972). *Annu. Rev. Med.* **23**, 177–190.

Kappeler, H., and Schwyzer, R. (1961). *Helv. Chim. Acta* **44**, 1136.

Keenan, J., and Chamberlain, M. A. (1969). *Brit. Med. J.* **4**, 407.

Keller, R., and Schauwecker, H. H. (1972). *J. Dent. Res.* **51**, No. 2, Part 1, 228.

Kivilaakso, E., and Rytomaa, T. (1971). *Cell Tissue Kinet.* **4**, 1.

Kobacoff, B. L., Wholman, A., Umhey, M., and Avakian, S. (1963). *Nature* (*London*) **199**, 815.

Korlof, B., Ponten, B., and Ugland, O. (1969). *Scand. J. Plast. Reconst. Surg.* **3**, 27.

Kornel, L., and Meador, C.K. (1964). *Abstr., Endocrine Soc., 1964*

Landon, J., Friedman, M., and Greenwood, F. R. (1967). *Lancet* **1**, 652.

Laszlo, F. A., Kovacs, K., Faredin, I., Czako, L., Durszt, F., Sziggi, I., Toth, I., Biro, A., and Julesz, M. (1970). *Acta Med.* (*Budapest*) **27**, 223.

Laurence, E. G., Randers-Hansen, E., Christophers, E., and Rytomaa, T. (1972). *Rev. Eur. Etud. Clin. Biol.* **17**, 133.

Leake, C. D. (1972). *Proc. West. Pharmacol. Soc.* **15**, 227.

Lee, T. H., Lerner, A. B., and Buettner-Janusch, V. (1965). *J. Biol. Chem.* **236**, 2970.

Lefkowitz, R. J. (1970). *Science* **170**, 633.

Lefkowitz, R. J., Roth, J., Pricer, W., and Pastan, I. (1970). *Proc. Nat. Acad. Sci. U.S.* **65**, 745.

Lerner, A. B., Upton, G. V., and Lande, S. (1968). *Advan. Exp. Biol. Med.* **2**, 203–212.

Li, C. H. (1962). *Recent Progr. Horm. Res.* **18**, 1.

Li, C. H. (1972). *Biochem. Biophys. Res. Commun.* **49**, 835.

Lie, K. K., Larsen, R. D., and Posch, J. L. (1967). *Surg., Gynecol. Obstet.* **125**, 595.

Malone, D. N. S., and Strong, J. A. (1972). *Practitioner* **208**, 329.

Margetts, G., Barber, K., Christie, R. B., Jones, W. E., and Bowder, W. T. (1972). *Brit. J. Clin. Pract.* **26**, 293.

Marrs, J. M., and Voorhess, J. J. (1971a). *J. Invest. Dermatol.* **56**, 174.

Marrs, J. M., and Voorhess, J. J. (1971b). *J. Invest. Dermatol.* **56**, 353.

Martin, G. J. (1965). *Int. Symp. Non-Steroidal Anti-Inflammatory Drugs, 1964* p. 90.

Martin, G. J., Bogner, R. L., and Edeman, A. (1957). *Amer. J. Pharm.* **129**, 386.
Matsuyama, H., Harada, G., Rhumann-Wennhold, A., Nelson, D. H., and West, C. D. (1972a). *J. Clin. Endocrinol. Metab.* **34**, 713.
Matsuyama, H., Rhumman-Wennhold, A., Johnson, L. R., and Nelson, D. H. (1972b). *Metab., Clin. Exp.* **21**, 30.
Miller, J. M. (1965). *Exp. Med. Surg., Suppl.* p. 26.
Miller, J. M. (1968). *Clin. Med.* **75**(10), 35.
Moriya, H., Moriwaki, C., Akomoto, S., Yamaguchi, K., and Iwadare, M. (1967). *Chem. Phar. Bull.* **15**, 1662.
Movat, H. Z. (1971). "Inflammation, Immunity and Hypersensitivity," pp. 2–129. Harper, New York.
Netti, C., Bandi, G. L., and Pecile, A. (1972). *Farmaco, Ed. Prat.* **27**, 453.
Pashkis, K. E. (1958). *Cancer Res.* **18**, 981.
Paukovits, W. R. (1972). *Cell Tissue Kinet.* **4**, 539.
Paulus, H. E., and Whitehouse, M. W. (1973). *Annu. Rev. Pharmacol* **13**, 118.
Perlman, G., and Lorand, L., eds. (1970). "Methods in Enzymology" Vol. 19. Academic Press, New York.
Rathgeber, W. F. (1971). *S. Afr. Med. J.* **45**, 181.
Rees, L. H., Ratcliffe, J. G., Besser, G. M., Kramer, R., and Landon, J. (1973). *Nature (London) New Biol.*, **241**, 84.
Richardson, M. C., and Schulster, D. (1970). *Biochem. J.*, **120**, 25.
Rinderknecht, H., and Geokas, M. C. (1973). *Biochim. Biophys. Acta* **295**, 233.
Riniker, B., Sieber, P., and Rittel, W. (1972). *Nature (London) New Biol.* **235**, 114.
Rittel, W. (1971). *Biochem. J.* **25**, 56.
Rytomaa, T., and Paukovits, W. R. (1972). *Int. Chalone Conf. 1st, 1972* Reported in *Chem. Eng. News* June, 23 (1972).
Saffran, M., and Schally, A. V. (1955). *Endocrinology* **56**, 523.
Schilling, J. A. (1968). *Physiol. Rev.* **48**, 374.
Schröder, E., and Lübke, K. (1966). "The Peptides," Vol. 2, pp. 194–251. Academic Press, New York.
Schwinger, U. (1970). *Wien. Med. Wochensch.* **36**, 1.
Schwyzer, R., and Kappeler, H. (1963). *Helv. Chim. Acta* **46**, 1550.
Schwyzer, R., Schiller, P., Seelig, S., and Sayers, G. (1971). *FEBS Lett.* **19**, 229.
Seelig, S., Sayers, G., Schwyzer, R., and Schiller, P. (1971). *FEBS Lett.* **19**, 232.
Seneca, H. (1965). *Exp. Med. Surg., Suppl.*, p. 63.
Sevitt, S. (1964). "Injury, Inflammation, and Immunity," pp. 183–209. Williams & Williams, Baltimore, Maryland.
Shaw, P. C. (1969). *Brit. J. Clin. Pract.* **23**, 25.
Sluyser, M. (1967). *In* "Regulation of Nucleic Acid and Protein Biosynthesis" (V. V. Koningsberger and L. Bosch, eds.), pp. 225–232. Amer. Elsevier, New York.
Snart, R. S., Siepard, R. F., and Agarwal, M. K. (1972). *Hormones* **3**; 36.
Svedmayr, N., Andersson, R., Bergh, N. P., and Malmberg, R. (1970). *Scand. J. Resp. Dis.* **51**, 171.
Szporny, L., Hajos, G. T., Szeberenyi, S., and Fekete, G. (1968). *Advan. Exp. Med. Biol.*, **2**, 196–202.
Talamo, R. C. (1971). *J. Allergy. Clin. Immunol.* **48**, 248.
Tassman, G. C. (1965). *J. Dent. Med.* **20**, 51.
Travis, J., and Coan, M. H. (1972). *In* "Pulmonary Emphysema and Proteolysis (C. Mittman, ed.), pp. 341–348. Academic Press, New York.

Tsomides, J., and Goldberg, R. I. (1969). *Clin. Med.* **76**, 40.

Verly, W. G., Deschamps, Y., Pushpathadam, J., and Desrosiers, M. (1971). *Can. J. Biochem.* **49**, 1376.

Voorhess, J. J., and Duell, E. A. (1971). *Arch. Dermatol.* **104**, 352.

Weiss, P., and Kavanau, J. L. (1957). *J. Gen. Physiol.* **41**, 1.

Whitehouse, M. W. (1969). *Pure Appl. Chem.* **19**, 35.

Windsor, T. (1972). *J. Clin. Pharmacol,* **12**, 325.

Winter, C. A., Risley, E. A., and Nuss, G. W. (1964). *Fed. Proc., Fed. Amer. Soc. Exp. Biol.* **23**, 284.

Wolfsen, A. R., McIntyre, H. B., and Odell, W. D. (1972). *J. Clin. Endocrinol. Metab.* **34**, 684.

Yalow, R. S., and Berson, S. A. (1971). *Biochem. Biophys. Res. Commun.* **44**, 439.

Yamashiro, D., and Li, C. H. (1973). *J. Amer. Chem. Soc.* **95**, 4.

Author Index

Numbers in italics refer to the pages on which the complete references are listed.

Subject Index

A

Abbott-29590, 189-190

2-Acetamido-1-N-(β-L-aspartyl)-2-deoxy-β-glucopyranosylamine, 202

5-Acetyl-4-hydroxythiophenes, 151-152

Acetylsalicylic acid, *see* Aspirin

ACTH
  assays for, 366
  biological effects of, 366-368
  clinical use, 368-369
  composition, 364-365
  corticosteroid therapy and levels of,
    283-285
  half-life, 367

ACTH analogs, 260-261

Acute gout, *see* Gout, acute

N-Acylsulfonamides, 54, 175-176

Adjuvant arthritis
  gold compounds in, 214-215, 235-239
  steroids in, 250

Adrenal function, *see* Corticosteroids

Adrenocorticotropic hormones, *see* ACTH

Alclofenac, 97

Allergic rhinitis, 279

Allergy
  ACTH treatment, 369
  steroid treatment, 287-288

Allochrysine, 213, *see also* Gold compounds

Allocolchicine, 311

Allopurinol, 13-14, 342-353
  effect on pyrimidine biosynthesis, 351-352
  mechanism of action, 13, 343-346
  use in gout, 13, 342-343

Amethopterin, *see* Methotrexate

Anilinobenzoic acids, 53, *see also* N-Aryl-anthranilic acids

Anilinophenylacetic acids, 71-72

Anilinophenylcinnamic acids, 73

Anilinophenylpropionic acids, 73

Anilinothiophenecarboxylic acids, 67-68

Ankylosing spondylitis, 14

Anti-human-lymphocyte globulin (ALG),
  for renal transplantation, 21

Antiinflammatory agents, *see also* specific
  classes and agents
  biological spectrum of, 182-183
  interaction potential, 30
  new classes, 180-184
  nonacidic, nonsteroidal, 184-203

Antimitotic agents
  chalones, 376-380
  colchicine, 325

α_1-Antitrypsin (AT), 374-375

Apazone, *see* Azapropazone

Arachidonic acids, 34

Arylalkanoic acids, 91-127
  absolute configuration, 36, 38, 120
  receptor site for, 119-121
  structure-activity relationships, summary,
    119-121
  toxicity, 121

N-Arylanthranilic acids, 46-64
  heterocyclic isosteres, 64-70
  homologs of, 71-73
  structure-activity relationships, 47-54
    carboxylic acid function, 53-54
    replacement of nitrogen with other
      groups, 51-53

411

A 4
B 5
C 6
D 7
E 8
F 9
G 0
H 1
I 2
J 3